Smart Healthcare: Challenges, Directions and Future Predictions

Smart Healthcare: Challenges, Directions and Future Predictions

Editor: Lakia Stevens

hayle medical

New York

Hayle Medical,
750 Third Avenue, 9th Floor,
New York, NY 10017, USA

Visit us on the World Wide Web at:
www.haylemedical.com

ISBN 978-1-64647-566-7 (Hardback)

Cataloging-in-Publication Data

Smart healthcare : challenges, directions and future predictions / edited by Lakia Stevens.
p. cm.
Includes bibliographical references and index.
ISBN 978-1-64647-566-7
1. Medical informatics. 2. Medical technology. 3. Medical care--Technological innovations.
4. Medical care--Information services. 5. Artificial intelligence--Medical applications.
6. Information storage and retrieval systems--Medicine. 7. Information stor I. Stevens, Lakia.
R858 .S63 2023
610.285--dc23

Contents

Preface

The main aim of this book is to educate learners and enhance their research focus by presenting diverse topics covering this vast field. This is an advanced book which compiles significant studies by distinguished experts in the area of analysis. This book addresses successive solutions to the challenges arising in the area of application, along with it; the book provides scope for future developments.

Smart healthcare makes use of the new generation of information technologies to change the conventional medical system in a comprehensive manner, and make the healthcare more personalized, convenient and efficient. It is responsible for accessing information, connecting institutions, materials and people, which are linked in healthcare systems. It is also engaged in managing and responding to the requirements of the medical ecosystem in a smart manner. There are various applications of smart healthcare, including prevention and risk monitoring of diseases, drug research, assistance in the treatment and diagnosis of diseases, providing virtual assistants and playing an important role in developing smart hospitals. Some of the current challenges in smart healthcare include a lack of programmatic documents and macro guidance that results in non-achievement of the desired goals and eventually leads to the wastage of resources. This book aims to understand the challenges, directions and future predictions of smart healthcare. Researchers and students in this field will be assisted by it.

It was a great honour to edit this book, though there were challenges, as it involved a lot of communication and networking between me and the editorial team. However, the end result was this all-inclusive book covering diverse themes in the field.

Finally, it is important to acknowledge the efforts of the contributors for their excellent chapters, through which a wide variety of issues have been addressed. I would also like to thank my colleagues for their valuable feedback during the making of this book.

Editor

1

Feature Selection and Classification of Ulcerated Lesions Using Statistical Analysis for WCE Images

Shipra Suman [1,*], Fawnizu Azmadi Hussin [1], Aamir Saeed Malik [1], Shiaw Hooi Ho [2], Ida Hilmi [2], Alex Hwong-Ruey Leow [2] and Khean-Lee Goh [2]

1 Center for Intelligent Signal & Imaging Research, Universiti Teknologi PETRONAS, Seri Iskandar 32610, Malaysia; fawnizu@utp.edu.my (F.A.H.); aamir_saeed@utp.edu.my (A.S.M.)

2 Department of Medicine, University of Malaya Medical Center, Kuala Lumpur 50603, Malaysia; shooiho@yahoo.com (S.H.H.); i_hilmi@um.edu.my (I.H.); alexleow@gmail.com (A.H.-R.L.); klgoh56@gmail.com (K.-L.G.)

* Correspondence: suman.shipra@ieee.org

Abstract: Wireless capsule endoscopy (WCE) is a technology developed to inspect the whole gastrointestinal tract (especially the small bowel area that is unreachable using the traditional endoscopy procedure) for various abnormalities in a non-invasive manner. However, visualization of a massive number of images is a very time-consuming and tedious task for physicians (prone to human error). Thus, an automatic scheme for lesion detection in WCE videos is a potential solution to alleviate this problem. In this work, a novel statistical approach was chosen for differentiating ulcer and non-ulcer pixels using various color spaces (or more specifically using relevant color bands). The chosen feature vector was used to compute the performance metrics using SVM with grid search method for maximum efficiency. The experimental results and analysis showed that the proposed algorithm was robust in detecting ulcers. The performance in terms of accuracy, sensitivity, and specificity are 97.89%, 96.22%, and 95.09%, respectively, which is promising.

Keywords: wireless capsule endoscopy; feature selection; color space selection; statistical analysis; support vector machine; grid search; overlapping area; classification

---

1. Introduction

Gastrointestinal tract (GIT) diseases, such as ulcer, bleeding, Crohn's disease, cancer or chronic diarrhea are common nowadays. Bleeding and ulcer are some common lesions which affect the small and large bowel. In the United States, approximately 1.6 million Americans currently are currently suffering from inflammatory bowel disease (IBD), representing an increase of about 200,000 since 2011.There are approximately 70,000 new cases of IBD diagnosed each year, and there may be as many as 80,000 children who are suffering from Crohn's disease (CD) or ulcerative colitis (UC) currently. Additionally, as illustrated reported in the first paper of this issue [1], the incidence number of occurrences of IBD is increasing worldwide [2]. The growth of IBD cases in newly-industrialized countries has paralleled its growth on par with that of the Western world 30 to 40 years ago. Genetic and environmental studies performed in these countries may provide new clues to the pathogenesis of IBD. However, it adds another layer of complexity since risk factors and gene-environment interactions may vary by continents and ethnicities [3]. Traditional endoscopy has been adopted for many years in order to diagnose abnormalities of GIT, whereby a physician controls a flexible endoscope to examine the lower and upper parts of GIT. This technique is limited to inspecting bowel of average length 7–8 m. It imposes high level of discomfort on the patient as well.

Wireless capsule endoscopy (WCE) [4,5] is a recent technology introduced by Given Imaging Ltd. (Yokne'am Illit, Israel) to visualize the entire GIT painlessly. It offers an efficient and comfortable way for visualizing the complete GIT. It has eight skin antennas mounted to the abdomen wall. While moving through the complete GIT, the capsule captures numerous images at approximately 2–4 frames per second (fps), and transfers them wirelessly to the data logger (DL) or recorder unit. This DL is hooked up to the patient waist and the videos/images are stored. Once the examination is complete (i.e., the WCE exits patient's body after 8 h), the images can be downloaded to a dedicated computer from DL and inspected by clinical experts through specific software. This procedure produces more than 60,000 images per examination and experts spend about 4–5 h to inspect the whole video footage very carefully. In some mild cases, clinicians have to go through each frame manually, leading to visual fatigue. This tedious and time-consuming process is the main drawback of WCE. Various image processing techniques for automatic disease detection (based on size, shape, and depth, including performance matrices) have been developed. Automatic lesion detection, on the other hand, is more efficient for chronic cases.

In this particular work, we have extracted color features for various color spaces. We have analyzed each band in order to separate the ulcer and non-ulcer pixels. Furthermore, it was combined with cross-correlation measure in order to add similarity between two images or matrices. Classification task was performed using support vector machine with and without grid search method in order to quantify the result. The main contribution of this work is the implementation of a novel computer-aided diagnostic method which is used to discriminate ulcer pixels from non-ulcerated ones with high performance in terms of sensitivity, specificity, and accuracy.

This paper is organized in the following manner: Section 2 describes the research background and the related works. Section 3 demonstrates the methodology, and Section 4 describes experimental setup, results, and discussions. Section 5 concludes the current work.

2. Background and Literature

Researchers have ventured into the technology of using automated computer-aided design (CAD) tools, such as WCE for ulcer screening. Precious clinical information in some important lesion areas can be displayed on an image [6–9]. Deeba [6] has used Retinex theory and the salient region detection method for various pathologies, such as stenosis, chylous cysts, lymphangiectasis, polypoid, bleeding, angioectasia, and ulcers. They have used a color enhancement method to improve the diagnostic yield of the CAD system. A significant improvement in detection performance using the Retinex-based color enhancement method has been achieved. An unsupervised method [10] has been used to localize the region-of-interest in order to detect angioectasia. The utility of IHb index for angioectasia detection has been pioneered to detect other abnormalities.

Yuan [8] has used a saliency detection method based on multi-level super pixel representation in order to outline the ulcer candidates. They have evaluated the corresponding saliency in accordance with the texture and the color feature of each level in the super pixel region. The images have been categorized by using saliency max-pooling with locality-constrained linear coding (LLC).

Iakovidis [9] has presented a method to detect various abnormalities in GIT by considering color as a discriminative feature. This method has been tested on a WCE model. Here, the single image (instead of the complete WCE video footage) has been analyzed. The author [11] has reviewed some current CAD methods employed in enhanced video capsule endoscopy. Various hardware and software problems have been highlighted in a review article [12] for detecting lesions in the small bowel.

Peptic ulcers are usually found in the duodenum (duodenal ulcer) and in the stomach (gastric ulcer). They can be found in small and large bowel areas of the GIT as well. They may cause severe gastrointestinal perforation or gastrointestinal bleeding [13]. Usually, it appears as a white spot in WCE images. In severe cases, these ulcers are accompanied by bleeding and other abnormalities. Ulcer lesions and normal tissue can be differentiated by using color and texture features (see Figure 1).

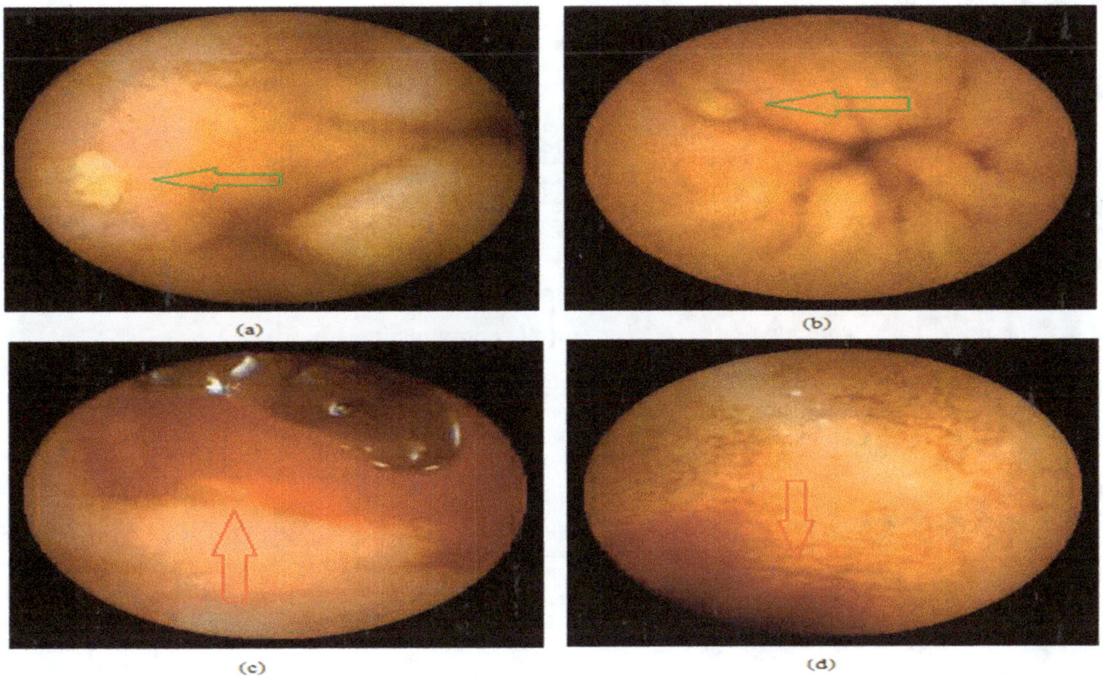

Figure 1. WCE images with bleeding and ulcer. (**a**,**b**) Ulcer image; and (**c**,**d**) bleeding images.

Feature selection [14] as practiced in machine learning is beneficial for supporting the WCE findings [15–17]. In general, feature extraction involves creating many new features mixed with the current ones. Due to the fact that the characterization of complete data variance is not possible after dimensional reduction, a highly-discriminative selecting feature [10] is undoubtedly necessary.

In order to classify the area of interest for capsule endoscopic images, first-order-histogram-based features extracted from various color spaces are very important. Relevant information can be extracted using various color spaces in order to describe the pattern of assured class. In case of bleeding detection, different color spaces [18] such as RGB (Red, Green, Blue), CMYK (Cyan, Magenta, yellow and Key [Black]), YIQ (Luma, chrominance information), CIE Lab, and HSI have been extensively investigated.

Yeh [13] used an improved CH algorithm (chosen name for the color coherence vector, CCV) to extract the color feature. The grey level co-occurrence matrix (GLCM) has been used to extract texture information. In our previous work [19], RGB and Lab color spaces have been chosen for statistical analyses of ulcer and non-ulcerated pixels. This paper extends the work of [19] by incorporating various color bands for statistical analysis.

Figueiredo et al. [20] has proposed a geometry-based automatic colorectal polyp detection method that has motivated the current work. The authors [21] have proposed a new computer-assisted bleeding detector for differentiating between bleeding and non-bleeding regions. The utilized second component from the CIE Lab color space with enhancement and segmentation techniques involves anisotropic diffusion.

3. Methodology

While analyzing the features, it is necessary to perform a few prior steps which are related to image processing. This section shows the complete flow of work. The proposed work focuses on reducing the analysis time while processing huge number of images. RGB color space is the most popular color scheme in visual system [22]; however, it has a few major disadvantages for natural images where high correlation between components can be observed [23]. Figure 2 depicts the flow of methodology for feature classification and extraction.

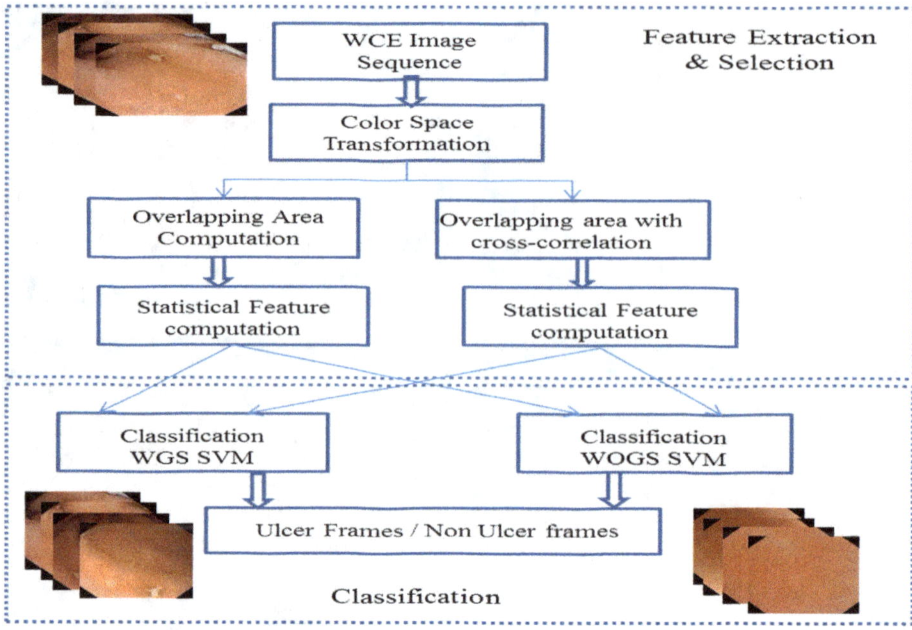

Figure 2. Methodology of proposed feature selection and classification.

3.1. *Image Processing and Enhancement*

The video generated after WCE examination is usually saved in a raw format and it cannot be processed directly by any programming platform. Endocapsule software (MAJ-2039) (EC 10, Olympus, Seri Iskandar, Perak, Malaysia, 2014) was used to import raw video in Audio Video Interleave (AVI) format. Subsequently, MATLAB was used to extract all images from the entire video footage in tagged image file format (TIFF) format. We have chosen the TIFF format to represent the WCE color image because it has greatest strength to support the full range of image size, color depth, and resolution. It also supports various compression techniques, where lossless compression allows this format to maintain image resolution without loss of any detail related to image [24]. Image enhancement is essential before applying any techniques in image processing. It is a technique that is able to eliminate non-essential information from an image [25]. In this particular work, we have used wavelet de-noising [26] with three levels of decomposition. Additionally, the db2 wavelet with soft thresholding method was applied to eliminate redundant noise.

3.2. *Feature Extraction and Feature Selection*

In this section, we have generated various normalized color spaces for feature analysis. RGB, HSV, YCbCr, CIE Lab, YUV, XYZ, and CMYK color spaces have been chosen for feature extraction and feature selection. By using these secen color spaces, we have analyzed 22 separate color bands individually. These bands contain various information of lesion and it is essential to identify the best band for the classification step.

We have used two methods to identify the best suitable band by separating foreground (non-ulcerated) and ulcer pixels. These methods involve statistical analysis of foreground and ulcer pixels in each band. We have implemented the first method (or Method 1) named as the overlapping area (OA) to measure the overlapping area between ulcer and foreground pixels. The normal distribution curve for foreground and ulcer pixels is analyzed from each pixel set. Here, we are able to highlight the index of separation for each band which shows overlapping area between foreground and ulcer pixels. Of course, lesser overlapping area signifies better separation in a particular band. The second method (or Method 2) uses overlapping area with cross-correlation (OACCorr) value in each band. Cross-correlation [27] is a standard measure for determining similarity between two images or matrices. It is more accurate and computationally more efficient. Additionally, it depends on the calculation of covariance between two bands.

The method of fast normalized cross-correlation is fast, independent, and accurate (in terms of pixel contrast and brightness values) in computing image similarity. This technique involves the estimation of correlation between all bands in the data cube of band i. Equation (1) was used to estimate the correlation values of other bands in j data cube:

$$NCC_{i,j} = \frac{\Sigma_{xy}\left[\left(D_i(x,y) - \overline{D_i}\right) \times \left(D_j(x,y) - \overline{D_j}\right)\right]}{\sqrt{\Sigma_{xy}\left(D_i(x,y) - \overline{D_i}\right)^2} \times \sqrt{\Sigma_{xy}\left(D_j(x,y) - \overline{D_j}\right)^2}} \quad (1)$$

where $NCC_{i,j}$ is the normalized cross-correlation between band i and j, $D_i(x,y)$. is the intensity of pixel, (x, y) are the pixel indices within one band, and $\overline{D_i}$ is the mean of pixel intensity values of band i.

Table 1 shows the OA and OACCorr values for 22 color bands used in extracting the color features. We have used seven color spaces in the following order: RGB, HSV, YCbCr, CIE Lab, YUV, XYZ, and CMYK. The first color space is RGB with rgbR, rgbG, and rgbB color bands with allotted band numbers of 1, 2 and 3, respectively. The second color space is HSV with hsvH, hsvS, and hsvV color bands. Their allotted band numbers are 4, 5 and 6, respectively. The third color space is YCbCr with ycbcrY, ycbcrCB, and ycbcrCR color bands. Their allotted band numbers are 7, 8 and 9, respectively. The fourth color space is CIE Lab with CIE LabL, CIE LabA, and CIE LabB color bands. Their allotted band numbers are 10, 11 and 12, respectively. The fifth color space is YUV with yvuY, yvuU, and yuvV color bands of allotted band numbers 13, 14 and 15, respectively. The sixth color space is XYZ with xyzX, xyzY, and xyzZ color bands of allotted band numbers 16, 17 and 18, respectively. Finally, the seventh color space is CMYK with four bands, i.e., cmykC, cmykM, cmykY, and cmykK. Their allotted band numbers are 19, 20, 21 and 22, respectively. These entire bands are used as feature vector for further classification.

From Table 1 (columns 2 and 3), the overlapping areas of the respective band number and band name obtained using Method 1 are displayed in an incremental manner. For Method 2 (see columns 4 and 5 in Table 1), the overlapping areas added with standard measure of degree of similarity between two images are displayed in an incremental manner as well. For example, if the serial number 1 for feature extraction is analyzed using Method 1, it shows a chromium component (ycbcrCR) of YCbCr with band number 9 that has a lesser overlapping area between ulcer and foreground pixels. If the result of Method 2 is analyzed, the same band (ycbcrCR) is selected as well.

Table 1. Comparison of overlapping area with overlapping area and cross-correlation method.

Serial No.	OA		OACCorr	
	Band No.	**Band Name**	**Band No.**	**Band Name**
1	9	ycbcrCR	9	ycbcrCR
2	11	CIE LabA	21	cmykY
3	4	hsvH	11	CIE LabA
4	17	yuvU	4	hsvH
5	21	cmykY	3	rgbB
6	3	rgbB	17	yuvU
7	15	xyzZ	5	hsvS
8	5	hsvS	15	xyzZ
9	20	cmykM	8	ycbcrCB
10	16	yuvY	20	cmykM
11	8	ycbcrCB	16	yuvY
12	12	CIE LabB	12	CIE LabB

Table 1. *Cont.*

Serial No.	OA		OACCorr	
	Band No.	**Band Name**	**Band No.**	**Band Name**
13	19	cmykC	19	cmykC
14	22	cmykK	22	cmykK
15	1	rgbR	1	rgbR
16	6	hsvV	6	hsvV
17	13	xyzX	13	xyzX
18	2	rgbG	2	rgbG
19	7	ycbcrY	7	ycbcrY
20	14	xyzY	14	xyzY
21	18	yuvV	18	yuvV
22	10	CIE LabL	10	CIE LabL

3.3. Machine Learning

SVMs are accurate as they contain appropriate kernels that work well even if the data is not linearly separable in the base future space. By using the kernel functions of SVM [28], one can perform a non-linear classification more accurately by mapping its input to high-dimensional feature spaces [29]. There are various hyperplanes that separate the classes; however, it is important to select the best one which has the largest distance to the nearest data point of two classes. Grid search [30] is the conventional method of performing the optimization of hyper parameter utilizing parameter sweep or grid search through a manually specified subset of the hyper parameter of a learning algorithm. This algorithm must be guided by some performance metric, normally measured by evaluation on a held-out validation set or by cross-validation of the training dataset. For this work, we are using an SVM classifier with an RBF kernel having at least two parameters (regularization constant C and kernel hyper parameter γ) that need to be tuned to achieve high performance on the testing data. The mathematical descriptor is shown below for a binary classification problem: $\{(x_1, y_1), (x_2, y_2), \ldots, (x_k, y_k)\}$, where $x_i \in R_n$ represents the n-dimensional feature vectors, and $y_i \in \{1, -1\}$ is the corresponding class label. The SVM requires the solution of the following optimizing problem:

$$\min\left(\frac{1}{2}\omega^T\omega + C\sum_{i=1}^{k}\varepsilon_i\right)$$
$$\text{Subjected to } y_i\left(\omega^T\varphi(x_i)+b\right) \geq 1-\varepsilon_i,\ \varepsilon_i \geq 0,\ i = 1, \ldots, k \quad (2)$$

Here, ε_i is the slack variable for misclassified examples, and C is the penalty parameter of error term. In addition, $K(x_i, x_j) = \varphi(x_i)^T\varphi(x_j)$ is the kernel function. Basically, there are four kernel functions used for pattern recognition and classification: linear kernel, polynomial kernel, radial basis function (RBF), and sigmoid kernel. We have adopted the RBF [28] kernel in this paper:

$$K(x_i, x_j) = \exp\left(-\gamma \parallel x_i - x_j \parallel^2\right),\ \gamma > 0 \quad (3)$$

Here, γ is the parameter which must be carefully selected in the experiment. The optimum values for parameter C and $\log_2 \gamma$ were selected from the range: $(-8, 7, 6, \ldots, 6, 7, 8)$. The grid method [29] was adopted as the searching procedure (a 0.8 step was used). Each γ and C value pair was used in the training data with ten-fold cross-validation in order to evaluate the model performance. Once the optimal values of γ and C were found, they were adopted to train a new SVM model.

4. Experimental Results and Discussions

This work was assisted by the expertise from the endoscopy unit in University of Malaya Medical Centre (UMMC), Kuala Lumpur, Malaysia for medical/clinical advises. The UTP team, on the other hand, was responsible in providing the engineering solutions. We accumulated 30 videos of various abnormalities. Moreover, the experts provided us the ground truth for these videos with labelled ulcerated lesions. This dataset serves as the reference data set for our subsequent analysis. The WCE pill used for generating the dataset was Endocapsule developed by Olympus. The resolution of the dataset provided was 288 × 288. The processor used for this work was Intel (R) Core(TM) i7-2600 CPU @3.20 GHz (Dell Optiplex 990, Seri Iskandar, Malaysia) with 8 GB memory. The chosen programming platform was MATLAB R2017a (Matlab 9.2, MathWorks, Malaysia, 2017).

4.1. Dataset Selection

Our dataset consisted of 48,000 WCE images. These images (16,000 of them) were divided into three groups. In each group, we used 8000 images to create our training set (5000 images were ulcer samples and 3000 images were normal samples) and 8000 images in testing set (5000 images were ulcer samples and 3000 images were normal samples). These images were accumulated from 30 patients and manually-labelled by gastroenterologists.

4.2. Results of Statistical Analysis

The results are presented in Table 1.

From Table 1, it is apparent that the overlapping area method (Method 1) can better reveal the ulcer information with the following bands (arranged in the descending performance): ycbcrCR, cmykY, CIE LabA, hsvH, rgbB, yuvU, and CIE LabL. Similarly, by using overlapping area with cross-correlation (Method 2), bands such as ycbcrCr, cmykY, rgbB, and hsvS contains more information for ulcer lesion. In Figure 3, we have extracted the feature vector for each band using Method 1 and Method 2. By choosing 50% of overlapping area and cross-correlation, it gives us six color bands such as ycbcrCR, cmykY, CIE LabA, hsvH, rgbB, and yuvU (i.e., the first six output rows of Table 1) using Method 1 and four color bands such as ycbcrCr, cmykY, rgbB and hsvS (i.e., the first four rows in Table 1) using Method 2. We found that the performance classifiers such as sensitivity, specificity, and accuracy are similar when more than 50% of overlapping area and cross-correlation are chosen. Otherwise, the performance is degraded and we might not be able to extract sufficient features.

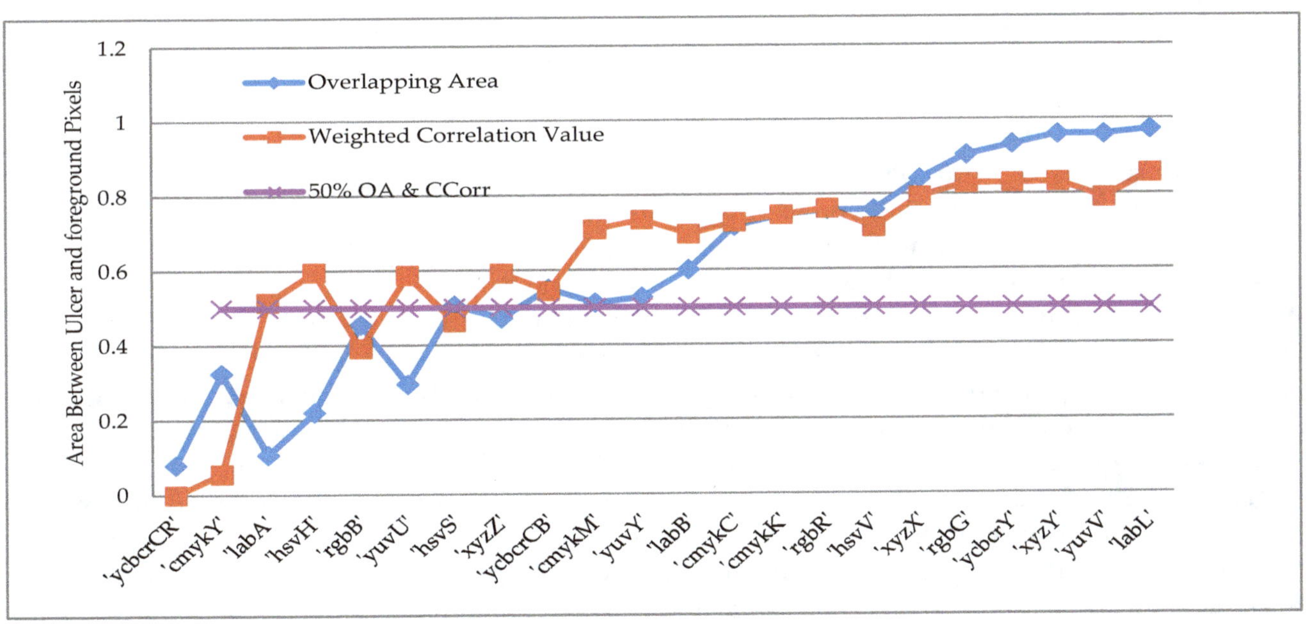

Figure 3. Comparison of overlapping area and Weighted correlation value.

The x-axis in Figure 3 shows the color bands for Method 2 (i.e., similar to column 5 in Table 1). A total of 50% of overlapping area (six feature vectors) and cross-correlation (four feature vectors) is taken as feature vector for Method 1 and Method 2. For Method 1 (OA), data on blue line containing ycbcrCR, cmykY, CIE LabA, hsvH, rgbB, and yuvU are chosen as feature vector as they have less overlapping area between ulcer and foreground pixels. For Method 2 (OACCorr), data on red line containing ycbcrCR, cmykC, rgbB, and hsvS are chosen as feature vector the overlapping areas added with standard measure of degree of similarity between two images are displayed in an incremental manner. The selected feature vectors were further fed into the classifier in order to analyze the algorithm performance in terms of sensitivity, specificity, and accuracy.

These bands provide the best result in terms of separating the ulcerated and non-ulcerated pixels. To enhance the result of classification, we fed the selected band to the SVM classifier. In this classifier, we used radial basis function (RBF) as kernel for the SVM. The result of classification for performance matrices is shown in Table 2.

Table 2. Sensitivity, specificity, and accuracy using SVM classifier.

Methods		Color Bands					
		Cr, Y, A, H, B, U		*Cr, Y, A, H, B*		*Cr, Y, A, H*	
Method 1	SVM (OA)	Sen 90.32	Spe 90.55	Sen 91.98	Spe 91.56	Sen 91.58	Spe 91.23
		Cr, Y, B, S		*Cr, Y, B*		*Cr, Y*	
Method 2	SVM (OACCorr)	Sen 92.58	Spe 91.84	Sen 93.76	Spe 92.91	Sen 93.08	Spe 91.36

4.3. Performance Metrics

Performance metrics such as accuracy (Acc), sensitivity (Sen), and specificity (Spe) were computed to evaluate the effectiveness of the proposed method. For the experimentation on GIT image data set, the positive sample represents lesion images and the negative sample represents normal images. The equations for sensitivity and specificity can be expressed as:

$$\text{Accuracy (Acc)} = \text{TP} + \text{TN}/(\text{TP} + \text{TN} + \text{FP} + \text{FN}) \tag{4}$$

$$\text{Sensitivity (Sen)} = \text{TP}/(\text{TP} + \text{FN}) \tag{5}$$

$$\text{Specificity (Spe)} = \text{TN}/(\text{FP} + \text{TN}) \tag{6}$$

where TP represents the number of true positives, TN represents the number of true negatives, FP represents the incorrect positive image samples identified and FN represents the incorrect negative image samples identified. From the clinical experts, sensitivity defines the probability of a positive analysis and specificity is the probability of a negative analysis.

In Table 2, SVM (OA) is depicted as Support vector machine for overlapping area. It is computed for seven bands, six bands, and five bands and the results are shown in Table 2. Similarly, SVM (OACCorr) is a support vector machine for overlapping area with cross-correlation value and it is computed for four bands, three bands, and two bands. Here, *Cr, Y, A, H* and *B* give better results for Method 1 (OA). On the other hand, *Cr, Y* and *B* give the best result with Method 2 (OACCorr). Specifically, Method 2 is more promising than Method 1. The above results shows that combining various color bands can provide more meaningful results.

Figure 4 shows the analyses of SVM (OACCorr) by using grid search method (WGS) and without grid search method (WOGS). The accuracies of 3 datasets have been compared. From the results taken from *Cr, Y, B* color bands, the extracted feature is more obvious using grid search method. For this method, the average accuracy, sensitivity, and specificity are 97.89%, 96.22% and 95.09%, respectively.

Additionally, we have compared our results of classification with others as presented in Table 3. It is important to note the dataset provided by other authors might be extracted from different capsule. Therefore, for comparison purpose, the dataset employed in the current work has been used for all methods, including those reported by other researchers (Table 3 shows the dataset used by other authors). The authors in [31] combined the merits of both Contourlet transform and Log Gabor filter in HSV color space; however, their dataset was very small. Author from [13] utilized RGB and HSV color space and classification was performed using MLP neural network. By using color coherence vector (CCV), a promising result was attained. As reported in [32], color wavelet covariance feature was used on various color spaces, and Texton boost was applied to classify normal and abnormal tissues. It is interesting to note that the proposed method shows higher sensitivity and higher specificity even for a very large dataset.

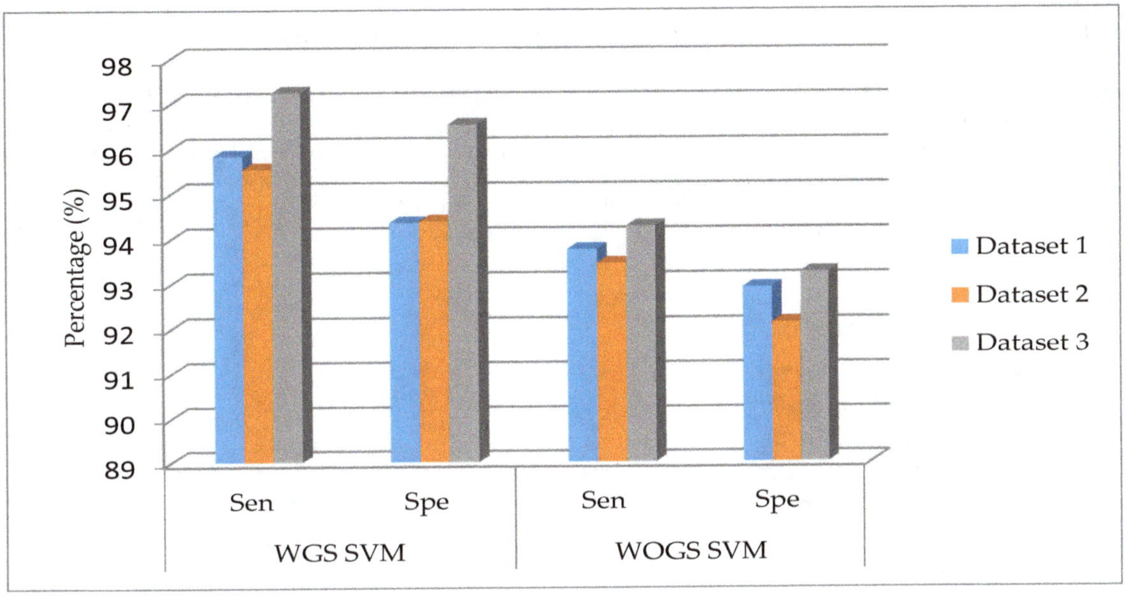

Figure 4. Performance of the proposed method.

Table 3. Comparison of performance with other author work.

Author	Color Space/Bands	Classifier	Dataset	Acc (%)	Sen (%)	Spe (%)
[31]	HSV	SVM	137 images	94.83	91.89	97.16
[13]	RGB, HSV, CCV	MLP	448 images	86.93	89.03	85.56
[32]	Various color space	Joint boost	100 images	NA	91.67	84.73
Proposed	*Cr, Y, B*	WGS SVM (OACCorr)	48,000 images	97.89	96.22	95.09

5. Conclusions

This paper has outlined a new method for detecting ulcer in an entire GIT. This method utilizes the divide-and-conquers technique to extract ulcer frame from a complete video footage. Statistical analysis has been performed to achieve higher separation between ulcer and non-ulcerated pixels. This technique has sub-parts for computing feature vectors in order to reveal highly-relevant information for ulcer and non-ulcer pixel discrimination which includes image enhancement, transformation of various color space, statistic feature computation, and classification. Statistical analysis has been performed to achieve higher separation between ulcer and non-ulcerated pixels by using this technique. The pixels have been classified using seven color spaces. Instead of using any single color space, it is more important to extract band information using various color spaces in order to achieve more accurate results. In this proposed method, Cr, Y, and B bands have been selected from YCbCr, CMYK, and RGB color spaces, respectively. Additionally, overlapping area with correlation using grid search method has increased the performance in separating the ulcerated pixels from normal pixels. Grid method has been adopted as the searching procedure (0.8 step was used). Each γ and C value pair has been used in the training data with ten-fold cross-validation in order to evaluate the model performance. A large dataset has been used to create training and testing dataset in order to obtain meaningful result. In this work, the sensitivity and the specificity of ulcer classification using the grid search method in SVM are 96.22% and 95.09%, respectively, which are substantially higher than those of classification without grid search method (93.76% and 92.91%, respectively). The main contribution of this work is the implementation of a novel computer aided diagnostic method which can be used to discriminate ulcer pixel from non-ulcerated pixel. The method exhibits promising performance in terms of sensitivity, specificity, and accuracy. The current work has paved the way to providing a reliable computer-aided WCE diagnosis system.

Acknowledgments: This research work is supported by the Centre for Intelligent Signal and Imaging Research (CISIR) and the Graduate Assistantship (GA) scheme, Universiti Teknologi PETRONAS, Perak, Malaysia.

Author Contributions: Shipra Suman finished the draft of this paper. Fawnizu Azmadi Hussin contributed in the design of the experimental work. Aamir Saeed malik contributed in feature extraction and feature selection algorithm for better discrimination between ulcer and foreground pixel. Shiaw Hooi Ho and Ida Hilmi contributed in the labelling of Ulcer dataset used in the experiment. Alex Hwong-Ruey Leow and Khean-Lee Goh have contribution towards disease specification and other challenges found throughout the writing and other reviewing procedure. All authors reviewed and approved the contents of this paper.

Abbreviations

AVI	Audio Video Interleaved
CAD	Computer Aided Design
CCV	Color Coherence Vector
DL	Data Logger
GIT	Gastrointestinal Tract
GLCM	Grey Level Co-Occurrence Matrix
LLC	Locality-constrained Linear Coding
OA	Overlapping Area
OACCorr	Overlapping area with Cross-correlation
RBF	Radial Basis Function
SVM	Support Vector Machine
WCE	Wireless Capsule Endoscopy
WGS	With Grid Search
WOGS	Without Grid Search

References

1. Kaplan, G.G.; Ng, S.C. Understanding and preventing the global increase of inflammatory bowel disease. *Gastroenterology* **2017**, *152*, 313–321. [CrossRef] [PubMed]
2. Kaplan, G.G.; Jess, T. The changing landscape of inflammatory bowel disease: East meets West. *Gastroenterology* **2016**, *150*, 24–26. [CrossRef] [PubMed]
3. Colombel, J.-F.; Mahadevan, U. Inflammatory Bowel Disease 2017: Innovations and Changing Paradigms. *Gastroenterology* **2017**, *152*, 309–312. [CrossRef] [PubMed]
4. Iddan, G.; Meron, G.; Glukhovsky, A.; Swain, P. Wireless capsule endoscopy. *Nature* **2000**, *405*, 417. [CrossRef] [PubMed]
5. Ghoshal, U.C. Capsule Endoscopy: A New Era of Gastrointestinal Endoscopy. In *Endoscopy of GI Tract*; InTech: Rijeka, Crotia, 2013.
6. Deeba, F.; Mohammed, S.K.; Bui, F.M.; Wahid, K.A. Unsupervised Abnormality Detection Using Saliency and Retinex Based Color Enhancement. In Proceedings of the 2016 IEEE 38th Annual International Conference of the Engineering in Medicine and Biology Society (EMBC), Orlando, FL, USA, 16–20 August 2016; pp. 3871–3874.
7. Deeba, F.; Mohammed, S.K.; Bui, F.M.; Wahid, K.A. A Saliency-Based Unsupervised Method for Angioectasia Detection in Capsule Endoscopic Images. *CMBES Proc.* **2016**, *39*, 1–11.

8. Yuan, Y.; Wang, J.; Li, B.; Meng, M.Q.-H. Saliency based ulcer detection for wireless capsule endoscopy diagnosis. *IEEE Trans. Med. Imaging* **2015**, *34*, 2046–2057. [CrossRef] [PubMed]
9. Iakovidis, D.K.; Koulaouzidis, A. Automatic lesion detection in capsule endoscopy based on color saliency: Closer to an essential adjunct for reviewing software. *Gastrointest. Endosc.* **2014**, *80*, 877–883. [CrossRef] [PubMed]
10. Charisis, V.S.; Katsimerou, C.; Hadjileontiadis, L.J.; Liatsos, C.N.; Sergiadis, G.D. Computer-Aided Capsule Endoscopy Images Evaluation Based on Color Rotation and Texture Features: An Educational Tool to Physicians. In Proceedings of the 2013 IEEE 26th International Symposium on Computer-Based Medical Systems (CBMS), Porto, Portugal, 20–22 June 2013; pp. 203–208.
11. Iakovidis, D.K.; Koulaouzidis, A. Software for enhanced video capsule endoscopy: Challenges for essential progress. *Nat. Rev. Gastroenterol. Hepatol.* **2015**, *12*, 172–186. [CrossRef] [PubMed]
12. Koulaouzidis, A.; Iakovidis, D.K.; Karargyris, A.; Plevris, J.N. Optimizing lesion detection in small-bowel capsule endoscopy: From present problems to future solutions. *Exp. Rev. Gastroenterol. Hepatol.* **2015**, *9*, 217–235. [CrossRef] [PubMed]
13. Yeh, J.-Y.; Wu, T.-H.; Tsai, W.-J. Bleeding and ulcer detection using wireless capsule endoscopy images. *J. Softw. Eng. Appl.* **2014**, *7*, 422. [CrossRef]
14. Mohammed, S.K.; Deeba, F.; Bui, F.M.; Wahid, K.A. Feature Selection Using Modified Ant Colony Optimization for Wireless Capsule Endoscopy. In Proceedings of the IEEE Annual Ubiquitous Computing, Electronics & Mobile Communication Conference (UEMCON), New York, NY, USA, 20–22 October 2016; pp. 1–4.
15. Suman, S.; Hussin, F.A.B.; Walter, N.; Malik, A.S.; Ho, S.H.; Goh, K.L. Detection and Classification of Bleeding Using Statistical Color Features for Wireless Capsule Endoscopy Images. In Proceedings of the International Conference on Signal and Information Processing (IConSIP), Vishnupuri, India, 6–8 October 2016; pp. 1–5.
16. Suman, S.; Hussin, F.A.; Walter, N.; Malik, A.S.; Hilmi, I. Automatic Detection and Removal of Bubble Frames from Wireless Capsule Endoscopy Video Sequences. In Proceedings of the 2016 6th International Conference on Intelligent and Advanced Systems (ICIAS), Kuala Lumpur, Malaysia, 15–17 August 2016; pp. 1–5.
17. Suman, S.; Hussin, F.A.; Nicolas, W.; Malik, A.S. Ulcer Detection and Classification of Wireless Capsule Endoscopy Images Using RGB Masking. *Adv. Sci. Lett.* **2016**, *22*, 2764–2768. [CrossRef]
18. Ibraheem, N.A.; Hasan, M.M.; Khan, R.Z.; Mishra, P.K. Understanding color models: A review. *ARPN J. Sci. Technol.* **2012**, *2*, 265–275.
19. Suman, S.; Walter, N.; Hussin, F.A.; Malik, A.S.; Ho, S.H.; Goh, K.L.; Hilmi, I. Optimum colour space selection for ulcerated regions using statistical analysis and classification of ulcerated frames from wce video footage. In *Neural Information Processing, Part I, Proceedings of the 22nd International Conference, ICONIP 2015, Istanbul, Turkey, 9–12 November 2015*; Arik, S., Huang, T., Lai, W.K., Liu, Q., Eds.; Springer: Cham, Switzerland, 2015; pp. 373–381.
20. Figueiredo, P.N.; Figueiredo, I.N.; Prasath, S.; Tsai, R. Automatic polyp detection in pillcam colon 2 capsule images and videos: Preliminary feasibility report. *Diagn. Ther. Endosc.* **2011**, *2011*. [CrossRef] [PubMed]
21. Figueiredo, I.N.; Kumar, S.; Leal, C.; Figueiredo, P.N. Computer-assisted bleeding detection in wireless capsule endoscopy images. *Comput. Methods Biomech. Biomed. Eng.* **2013**, *1*, 198–210. [CrossRef]
22. Colantoni, P. Color Space Transformations. Available online: http://faculty.kfupm.edu.sa/ics/lahouari/Teaching/colorspacetransform-1.0.pdf (accessed on 8 June 2017).
23. Pascale, D. A review of rgb color spaces ... from xyy to r′g′b′. *Babel Color* **2003**, *18*, 136–152.
24. Wiggins, R.H.; Davidson, H.C.; Harnsberger, H.R.; Lauman, J.R.; Goede, P.A. Image file formats: Past, present, and future. *Radiographics* **2001**, *21*, 789–798. [CrossRef] [PubMed]
25. Suman, S.; Hussin, F.A.; Malik, A.S.; Walter, N.; Goh, K.L.; Hilmi, I.; Ho, S.h. Image Enhancement Using Geometric Mean Filter and Gamma Correction for WCE Images. In Proceedings of the 21st International Conference on Neural Information Processing, Kuching, Malaysia, 3–6 November 2014; pp. 276–283.
26. Saevarsson, B.B.; Sveinsson, J.R.; Benediktsson, J.A. Combined Curvelet and Wavelet Denoising. In Proceedings of the 7th Nordic Signal Processing Symposium, NORSIG 2006, Rejkjavik, Iceland, 7–9 June 2006; pp. 318–321.
27. Ahmed, A.; Sharkawy, M.E.; Ramly, S.E. Analysis of Inter-band Spectral Cross-Correlation Structure of Hyperspectral Data. In Proceedings of the WSEAS International Conference Recent Advances in Computer Engineering Series, Istanbul, Turkey, 21–23 August 2012.

28. Chang, C.-C.; Lin, C.-J. LIBSVM: A library for support vector machines. *ACM Trans. Intell. Syst. Technol. (TIST)* **2011**, *2*, 27. [CrossRef]
29. Hsu, C.-W.; Chang, C.-C.; Lin, C.-J. *A Practical Guide to Support Vector Classification*; National Taiwan University: Taipei City, Taiwan, 2003.
30. Bengio, Y. Practical recommendations for gradient-based training of deep architectures. In *Neural Networks: Tricks of the Trade*; Springer: Berlin/Heidelberg, Germany, 2012; pp. 437–478.
31. Koshy, N.E.; Gopi, V.P. A New Method for Ulcer Detection in Endoscopic Images. In Proceedings of the 2015 2nd International Conference on Electronics and Communication Systems (ICECS), Coimbatore, India, 26–27 Febuary 2015; pp. 1725–1729.
32. Liu, X.; Gu, J.; Xie, Y.; Xiong, J.; Qin, W. A New Approach to Detecting Ulcer and Bleeding in Wireless Capsule Endoscopy Images. In Proceedings of the 2012 IEEE-EMBS International Conference on Biomedical and Health Informatics (BHI), Hong Kong, China, 5–7 January 2012; pp. 737–740.

2

In Vivo Optogenetic Modulation with Simultaneous Neural Detection Using Microelectrode Array Integrated with Optical Fiber

Penghui Fan [1,2], Yilin Song [1,2], Shengwei Xu [1,2], Yuchuan Dai [1,2], Yiding Wang [1,2], Botao Lu [1,2], Jingyu Xie [1,2], Hao Wang [1,2] and Xinxia Cai [1,2,*]

1 Aerospace Information Research Institute Chinese Academy of Sciences, Beijing 100190, China; fan_ph@163.com (P.F.); ylsong@mail.ie.ac.cn (Y.S.); swxu@mail.ie.ac.cn (S.X.); hongri1991@126.com (Y.D.); wangyiding18@mails.ucas.ac.cn (Y.W.); lslbt96@163.com (B.L.); xiejingyu16@mails.ucas.ac.cn (J.X.); wanghao161@mails.ucas.ac.cn (H.W.)

2 University of the Chinese Academy of Sciences, Beijing 100049, China

* Correspondence: xxcai@mail.ie.ac.cn

Abstract: The detection of neuroelectrophysiology while performing optogenetic modulation can provide more reliable and useful information for neural research. In this study, an optical fiber and a microelectrode array were integrated through hot-melt adhesive bonding, which combined optogenetics and electrophysiological detection technology to achieve neuromodulation and neuronal activity recording. We carried out the experiments on the activation and electrophysiological detection of infected neurons at the depth range of 900–1250 μm in the brain which covers hippocampal CA1 and a part of the upper cortical area, analyzed a possible local inhibition circuit by combining opotogenetic modulation and electrophysiological characteristics and explored the effects of different optical patterns and light powers on the neuromodulation. It was found that optogenetics, combined with neural recording technology, could provide more information and ideas for neural circuit recognition. In this study, the optical stimulation with low frequency and large duty cycle induces more intense neuronal activity and larger light power induced more action potentials of neurons within a certain power range (1.032 mW–1.584 mW). The present study provided an efficient method for the detection and modulation of neurons in vivo and an effective tool to study neural circuit in the brain.

Keywords: optogenetics; micro-electrode array; in situ detection; electrophysiology; neural circuit recognition

---

1. Introduction

Optogenetic technology has been widely used in the research of behavior, diseases and other aspects of neural mechanism since it was put forward in 2005 [1], and not only on the central nervous system; it also had effects on the peripheral nervous system [2,3]. Optogenetic technology can modulate the activities of target neuron cells with high spatial-temporal resolution by combining photonics and genetic techniques and has been one of the most important neuroscience research tools [4–6]. The core of optogenetics is light-sensitive protein, also called opsins, which are mainly found in micro-organisms. The opsin gene is introduced into the subject's brain through viral vectors, and is eventually expressed in targeted cells after transcription [7,8]. The light-sensitive protein expressed in the cell membrane acts as an ion channel or pump controlled by light in a specific wavelength range. Channelrhodopsin-2 (ChR2) is one of the most commonly used opsin tools, which promotes cell depolarization when exposed to blue light.

When optogenetic technology was used to modulate neural activity, a large amount of neuronal activity needed to be recorded, mined and utilized to help us better understand the neurophysiology of the nervous system. Optogenetics combined neuronal recording can also help to identify neuronal subtypes and circuit [9]. Therefore, a tool that can simultaneously transmit light to targeted cells and detect electrophysiological information is particularly important. Microelectrode array (MEA), based on the Micro-Electro-Mechanical System (MEMS) method, is considered to be an ideal platform to detect the neural activity of a single neuron, which also has the potential of electrochemical detection. At present, the integrated device combining optical interface and MEA, also called optrode, which can be classified according to integrated optical fiber, waveguide and micro light emitting diode (μ-LED), has attracted attention [10,11]. The optrode integrating optical fiber is a kind of mature and effective optogenetic tool [12,13]. HyungDal Park formed the V-groove on the MEA by KOH wet etching process to assist the alignment of the optical fiber and electrode [14]. Wang and colleagues bonded a cannula to the open hole on the backside of the MEA to guide the fiber [15]. This method can be successfully applied to the field of optogenetics, but requires considerable time and effort to develop. The optrode based on waveguide is completed by directly depositing the waveguide material (usually SU-8) on the MEA through the MEMS technology. Since the optical waveguide only act as optical transmission medium, it is difficult to couple the light source and the optical waveguide, which usually generates a large light loss and increases cost [16–18]. The μ-LED itself is a low-power light source, and can directly stimulate tissues with minimal light loss, so it is often integrated on MEA [19,20]. Furthermore, the manufacturing technology is usually forming the μ-LED structure on silicon probe through metalorganic vapor phase epitaxy (MOVPE) or directly bonding the commercial μ-LED to the MEA. However, this method is complicated and even cause tissue damage due to overheating of the light source [21,22].

Considering the cost and operability, we produced an optrode that combines optical fiber and MEA through hot-melt adhesive. We used a homemade MEA that has been connected to Printed Circuit Board (PCB) which increased the operable space and provided a larger and harder contact area for fiber bonding. The device had the characteristics of low cost, easy operation and reusability for acute in vivo experiment. Here, we verified the performance of the integrated device, analyzed a possible circuit based on the performance of neurons under the optogenetic control and explored the effect of optical patterns and light powers on neuronal activity. This study provided an efficient tool for optogenetic neuromodulation and simultaneous in vivo electrophysiological detection.

2. Materials and Methods

2.1. Fabrication and Preparation of MEA Integrated with Optical Fiber

The Silicon-based MEA was fabricated based on MEMS technology as previously reported [23], which consisted of four 6 mm shanks. Each shank was 100 μm in width, 30 μm in thickness and 80 μm spacing. There were four electrode sites (16 μm in diameter) on the tip of every shank forming a 4 × 4 array. The fabrication process is shown as Figure 1a: (1) the SiO_2 layer was deposited on the silicon-on-insulator (SOI, 30 μm Si/2 μm SiO_2/450 μm Si) substrate to insulate the microelectrode from the substrate; (2) then, the Pt/Ti conductive layer pattern (including recording sites, bonding pads and conductive lines) was formed by photolithography, sputtering and lift-off process; (3) the SiO_2/Si_3N_4 insulating layer was deposited via plasma enhanced chemical vapor deposition (PECVD) and the recording sites and bonding pads were exposed by the second photolithography and CHF_3 reactive ion etching (RIE); (4) the shape of the MEA was established by the third photolithography and inductively coupled plasma deep reactive ion etching (ICP DRIE); (5) the backside silicon was wet etched and the silicon probes were released by self-stop etching in KOH solution. Then, the pads of individual probe were connected to the printed circuit board (PCB) through wire bonding and embedded in silicone rubber (Nanda 705#, Liyang Kangda Chemical Co. Ltd., Liyang, China) to isolate electrical connection. Finally, the assembled MEA was electroplated with platinum nanoparticles to improve recording performance.

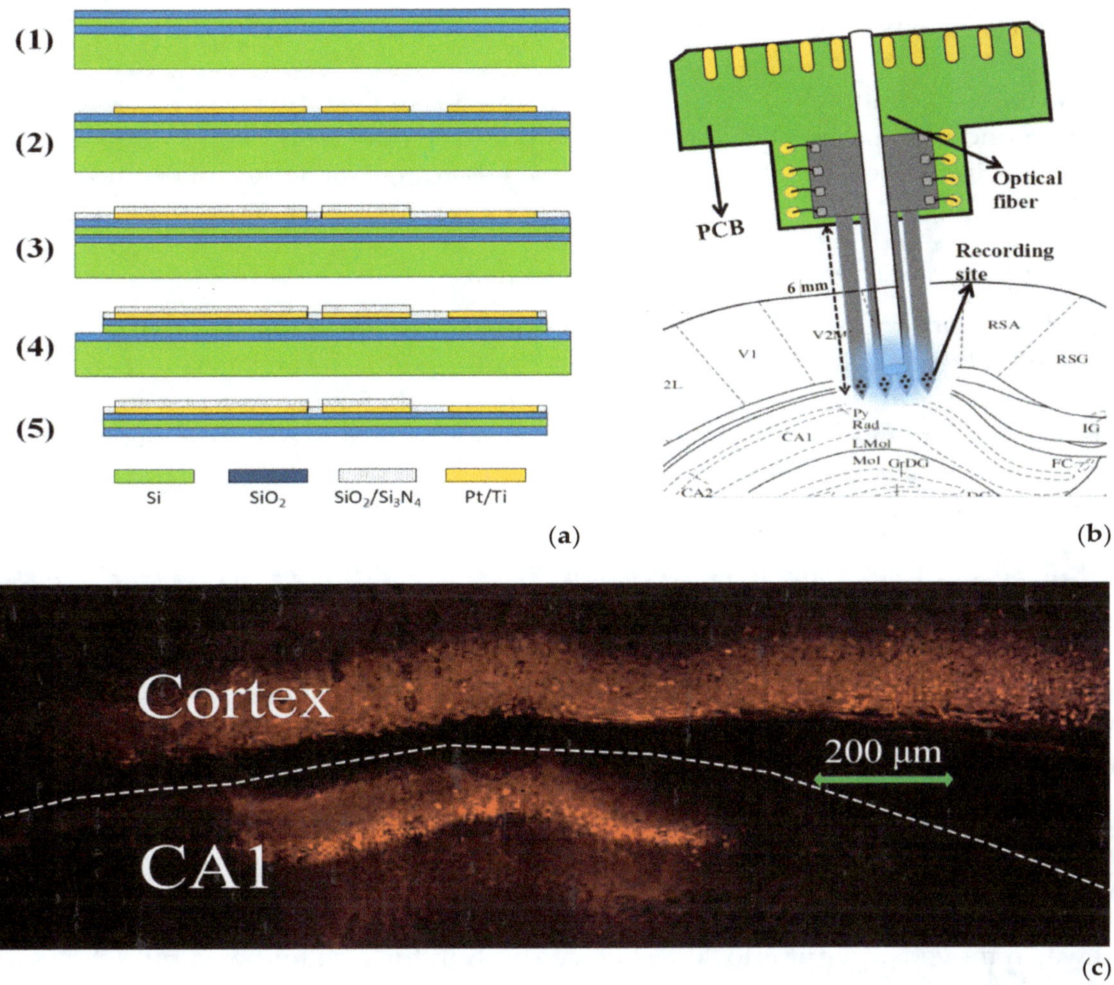

Figure 1. (**a**) Microelectrode array (MEA) manufacturing process: (1) Deposition of a layer of SiO_2 on silicon-on-insulator (SOI). (2) Photolithography, sputtering and lift-off to form conductive layer. (3) Deposition of the insulating layer and exposure of recording sites and bonding pads. (4) Formation of the shape of the MEA. (5) Release of the MEA from the substrate. (**b**) Schematic diagram of the integrated device inserted into hippocampal CA1 of brain. (**c**) The fluorescence image of brain area infected by rAAV.

In order to integrate with the optical interface, a 20 mm optical fiber (200 μm in diameter, NA = 0.39, CFMLC12L20, Thorlabs, USA) was closely attached to the PCB of the assembled MEA. Then the fiber was adjusted to be as parallel as possible with probes, and the fiber tip was about 200 μm above the recording sites. Finally, hot-melt adhesive was used to bond the optical fiber and MEA to ensure mechanical stability (Figure 1b). This method was simple in operation, short in time and low in light loss. The fiber and MEA could even be separated under heating, which undoubtedly improved their utilization rates. At the same time, the integrated device could be reused for acute experiments.

2.2. ChR2 Transduction and Optrode Implantation

The experimental procedures were conducted with the permission of Beijing Association on Laboratory Animal Care. The C57 mouse (7-week-old, 25 g) was anesthetized by the isoflurane anesthesia apparatus (RWD520, RWD Life Science, Shenzhen, China) and fixed in the stereotaxic frame (51, 600, Stenting, Wood Dale, IL, USA). The craniotomy was centered at AP = −2.3 mm and ML = 1.5 mm for targeting the mouse hippocampus. Then 0.5 μL adeno-associated viruses (rAAV-hSyn-hChR2(H134R) -mCherry-WPRE-hGH PolyA, BrainVTA, Wuhan, China) were injected into the mouse brain at a depth of 1 mm (Corresponding to the pyramidal cell layer of hippocampal CA1). After the injection, the scalp was sutured, and penicillin was applied to the wound to prevent infection. Then the mouse was placed on a soft cotton pad and returned to the rearing cage after being fully awake.

After 4 weeks, the integrated device was implanted into the target brain area at the same site for virus injection under anesthesia using a micropositioner (model 2662, David KOPF instrument, USA) for testing. The depth of electrophysiological signal recording is mainly concentrated from 800 μm to 1250 μm. The schematic diagram of device implantation is shown in Figure 1b.

2.3. Electrophysiological Recording and Optical Stimulation

For real-time electrophysiological recordings, the MEA was connected to the recordings system (USB-ME16-FAI-System, MultiChannel Systems, Reutlingen, Germany) via a 16-channel headstage. The electrophysiological signals were sampled at the rate of 25 kHz. A high pass filter (200 Hz) was used to obtain action potentials (spikes), and a low pass filter (200 Hz) was applied to obtain local field potentials (LFPs). During recording, the background noise was about ±13 μV, and the action potentials trigger threshold was set to −40 μV to ensure that the signal-to-noise ratio of the signal was greater than 3.

For optical stimulation, the light was applied by fiber-coupled LED (M450F, 450 nm, Throlabs, Newton, NJ, USA), and the optical fiber on the optrode was coupled to the light source through a ceramic mating sleeve. We used the Labview program to drive the LED light source, and change the output power of the LED by setting the driving voltage. The maximum driving voltage was 5000 mV, which corresponded to the maximum output power of the LED. The schematic diagram of the experiment is shown in Figure S1a.

2.4. Histology

Following completion of test, the mouse was injected with 10% chloral hydrate into deep anesthesia and perfused through the heart with 0.9% NaCl and 4% paraformaldehyde in sequence. After perfusion, the brain was removed and put into 20% sucrose solution for 24 h followed by 30% sucrose solution for 48 h for postfication. Then 40 μm thick sections were prepared with a freezing microtome and mounted on glass slides, and sections were viewed and photographed under the confocal fluorescence microscopy. The fluorescence image is shown as Figure 1c, due to the spread of the virus, the infection area covers the hippocampal CA1 and part of the cortex above CA1. The estimated spread of ChR2 was 400 μm in the vertical plane.

2.5. Statistics

We used a mouse in this article to verify the device performance and made repeated experiments to ensure the accuracy of the conclusion. There is enough blank time between different experiments to eliminate the interference between them. Therefore, all tests were administrated independently. Spike data were sent to Offline Sorter for sorting and clustering analyses. Spike waveforms were purified and extracted by principal component analysis (PCA). Then sorted spike data and LFP data were further analyzed by NeuroExplorer as the following:

(1) Spike firing rate analysis was defined as the mean number of spikes per second each bin. Here we took the average of multiple recording channels.
(2) Interspike interval (ISI) analysis was defined as the number of spikes each bin of the discharge interval (from 0–100 ms).
(3) Auto-correlation analysis was defined as the number of neuron firing time differences (from −50 to 50 ms) in each time window.

(4) LFP power was defined as the integral of the mean squared LFP. Here we took the average of multiple recording channels.

Statistical analyses and graphs were administrated by Origin Software and all results were expressed as mean ± SD unless otherwise specified.

3. Results

3.1. Optical Stimulation Enhances Neuronal Activity

We conducted in vivo experiments with the integrated devices, first tested the response of neurons under optical stimulation and proved the performance of the MEA. In the region where the neurons successfully expressed ChR2, optical stimulation induced more neuronal activity. As shown in Figure 2a, the background noise of the electrode hardly changed before and during the illumination period. However, the spike firing rate significantly increased during the illumination period (Figure 2b). The LFP power also increased in the during-light period (Figure 2c). We also tested in non-viral transfection areas (as shown in Figure S2). It could be seen that the background noise had almost no change before and during the illumination, and the optical stimulation did not induce more spikes and increase lager LFP power, which proved that the application of light alone did not enhance neuronal activity. This indicated that the device successfully modulated the neuronal activity and measured the electrophysiology information, and these two experiments together illustrated the authenticity of optical stimulation-induced neuronal activity in the virus-infected area.

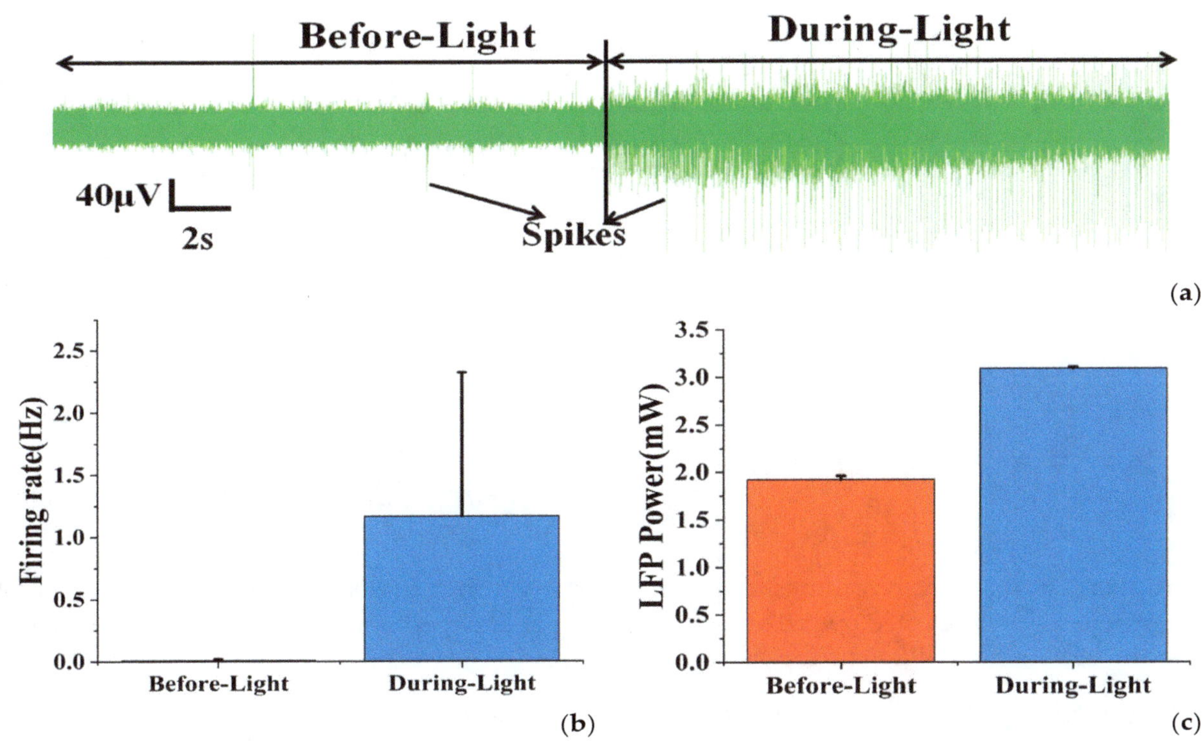

Figure 2. (**a**) The real-time recordings of electrophysiological signals before and during light illumination in viral transfection areas; (**b**) the average spike firing rate of neurons before and during optical stimulation; (**c**) the mean LFP power (0–30 Hz) of neurons before and during optical stimulation. Error bars indicate standard deviation of 3 channels.

The experiment verified that at least in the range of brain depth 900–1250 μm, optical stimulation enhanced neuronal activity, indicating the excellent performance of the device in modulation and detection. As shown in Figure 3a, spikes significantly increased during optical stimulation at different test depths. Figure 3b shows the spike waveform extracted from the recording channels, and the results indicated that the spike waveforms measured at different depths were different. Due to the different optical stimulation pattern and opsin expression level at different test depths, the neuronal activity during illumination is not the same, but their neuronal activity was all significantly enhanced compared to before light illumination.

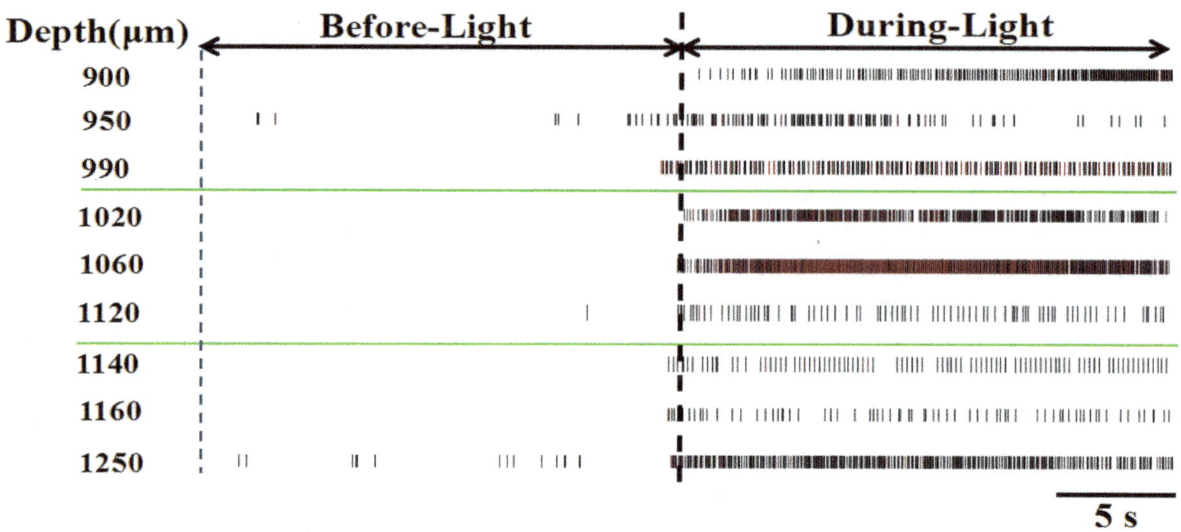

(a)

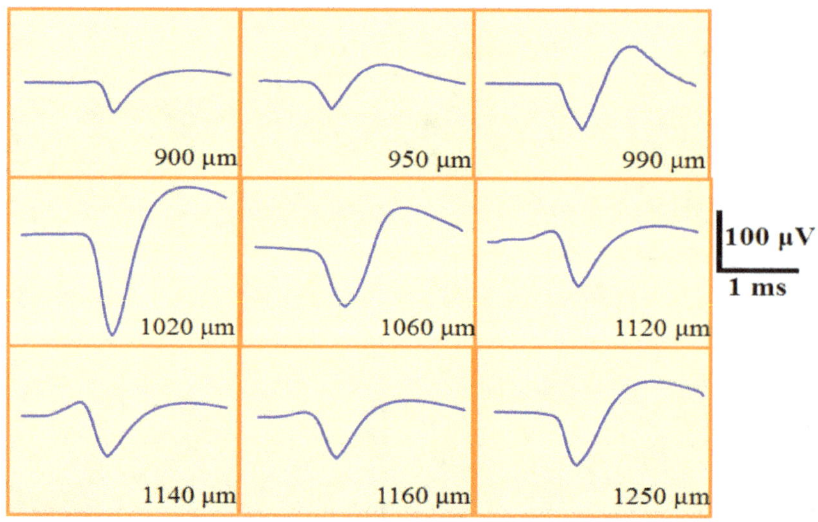

(b)

Figure 3. (**a**) The real-time recordings of spikes before and during blue light illumination at different depths (here we only selected one channel for each group of experiments as a display); (**b**) the spike waveform of neurons at different depths.

3.2. *Optical Stimulation Activates a Possible Local Inhibitory Circuit*

During the experiment, we attempted to analyze and study a local circuit combining optogenetics and electrophysiological recording. As shown in Figure 4a, the data was first recorded for 3 min without light, and then illumination (30 s light-on, 30 s light-off) lasting 6 min. Four neuron units were obtained (unit-a and unit-b were separated from the same recording channel) by principal component analysis and clustering from three recording channels. It can be seen from the figure that the spikes generated by unit-b,c,d increased significantly during optical stimulation. The spike firing rate of unit-b,c,d during optical stimulation was much greater than before optical stimulation (Figure 4b), which indicated that the neurons expressing ChR2 were successfully activated.

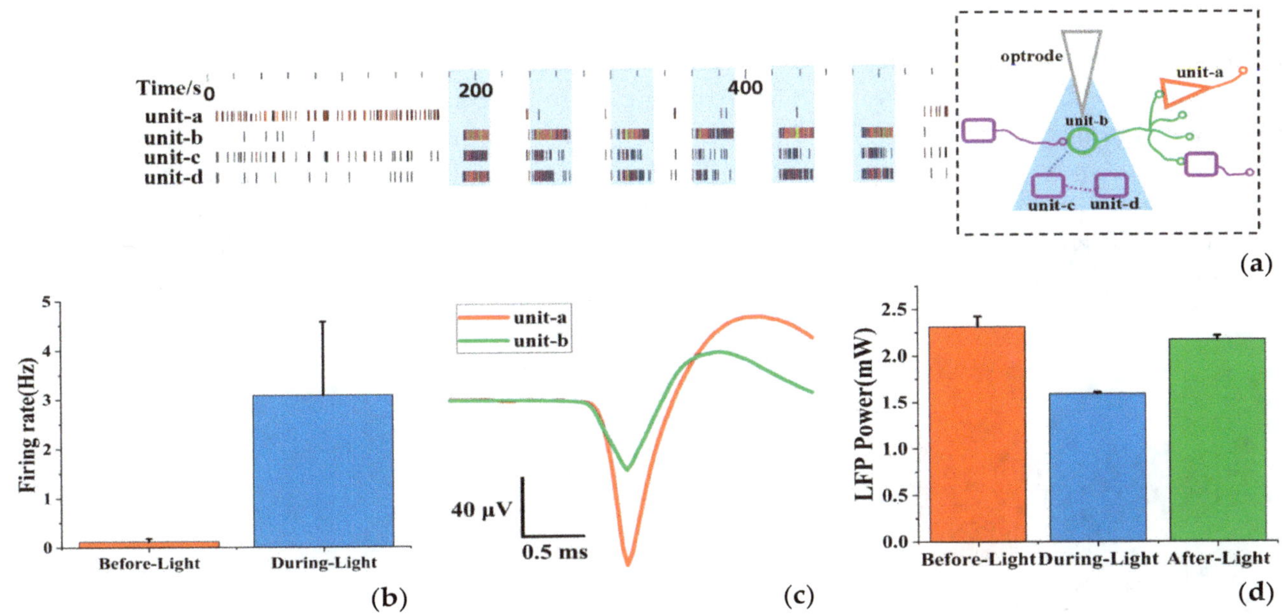

Figure 4. (**a**) The real-time recordings of spikes of 4 units separated from three recording channels (the shaded area is the period of during-light, 30sm) and inferred local circuit (the green circle represents the interneuron, the red triangle represents pyramidal neuron, the purple rectangles represent unknown type of neurons and dotted lines between neurons indicate uncertain connections); (**b**) the average spike firing rate of neurons before and during optical stimulation; (**c**) spike waveform of unit-a and unit-b; (**d**) the mean LFP power (0–8 Hz) of neurons before, during and after optical stimulation. Error bars indicate standard deviation of 3 channels and N = 6 (N is the number of experiments).

It was also found that the neuronal activity did not increase for unit-a, and even weakened during optical stimulation. In order to explore the reasons, we did a further analysis. Figure S3 shows the auto-correlograms and ISI histograms of unit-a (Figure S3a,c) and unit-b (Figure S3b,d). The ISI histogram of unit-a (yellow) showed a short and sharp peak, and its auto-correlation analysis showed a decreasing trend, indicating that it had obvious cluster-like spike characteristics. For the unit-b (green) auto-correlation analysis, several equally spaced peaks appeared, indicating that it has periodic spike characteristics under optical stimulation. In terms of spike waveform, the amplitude of unit-a was almost twice that of unit-b (Figure 4c). Combined with their respective auto-correlation analysis, we speculated that unit-a may be a putative pyramidal neuron, while unit-b may be a putative interneuron [24]. Furthermore, we speculated that they were in a local circuit (dotted box in the Figure 4a), and the direction of synaptic transmission was from interneuron to pyramidal neuron, i.e., unit-b was the upstream neuron. The types of unit-c and unit-d were unclassified and their connection with others was not clear. When optical stimulation activated unit-b interneurons, its neuronal activity increased and its inhibitory effect on unit-a also enhanced. Therefore, spikes of unit-a were reduced during light. The LFP power (0–8 Hz) during illumination was lower than before and after illumination (Figure 4d), which also seems to prove our speculation. Figure S3e showed the LFP power (0–30 Hz) before, during and after optical stimulation, which had the same trend as 0–8 Hz. Figure S3f showed the power of LFP in different frequency bands. It was found that LFP was mainly concentrated in 0–8 Hz, so the subsequent LFP analysis was mainly concentrated at 0–8 Hz.

3.3. *Effects of Different Optical Stimulation Patterns on Optogenetic Neuromodulation*

The spikes of the three channels in different optical stimulation patterns were recorded (see Figure S4a). According to the statistical average spike firing rate during optical stimulation, it was found that under the same duration, the spikes induced by s1 optical stimulation pattern were more than s2 optical stimulation pattern, the spikes induced by s2 optical stimulation pattern were more than s3 optical stimulation pattern (as shown in Figure 5a), the spike firing rate of the three channels had the same trend (Figure S4b). On the whole, within a certain range, the lower the light frequency and the greater the duty cycle, the stronger the neuronal activity were caused. At the same time, we calculated the LFP power (0–8 Hz) under different optical stimulation patterns. The power under s1 was greater than that of s2 and s3, but there was no significant difference between s2 and s3 (Figure 5b). This may be due to the fact that LFP depended on thousands of neurons in a wide range, and there may be inhibition or excitation circuits in this area, which had complex effects on neuronal activity. In short, we believed that different optical stimulation patterns had an effect on the intensity of induced neuronal activity.

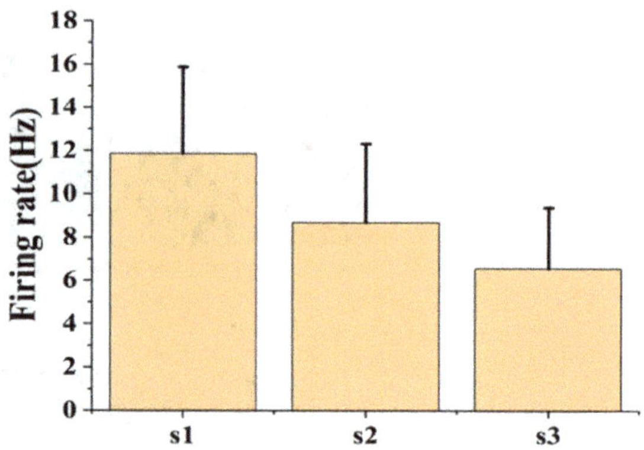

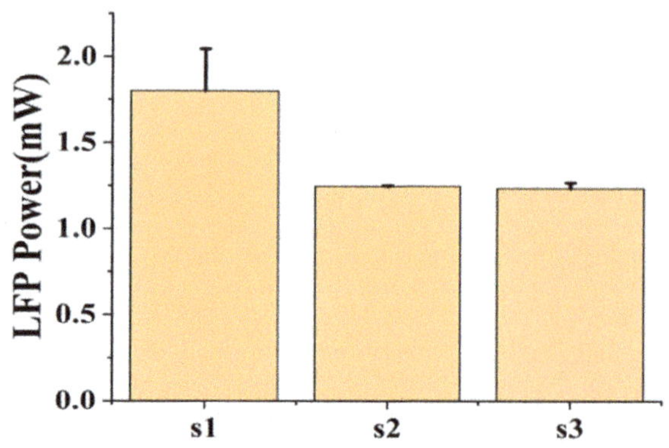

Figure 5. (**a**) The average spike firing rate of neurons under different optical stimulation patterns (s1: 10 Hz, duty ratio = 50%, 2 min; s2: 10 Hz, duty ratio = 25%, 2 min; s3: 16.6 Hz, duty ratio = 25%, 2 min); (**b**) The mean LFP power (0–8 Hz) of neurons under different optical stimulation patterns. Error bars indicate standard deviation of 3 channels.

3.4. Effects of Different Light Powers on Optogenetic Neuromodulation

The output power of LED light source (P_s) and the tip of optrode (P_t) under different driving voltages is shown in Figure S5a (unless otherwise specified, the output power refers to the output power of the optrode tip P_t). We could see the maximum tip output power was 1.7 mW. We also simulated the power density at a certain distance from the fiber tip of the integrated device [13,25,26], see supplementary materials and Figure S5b for detailed process. Since the distance between the optical fiber tip and the recording site was 200 μm, the neurons were exposed to less than 10 mW/mm^2 and the light would not cause great damage to the recorded neurons from the perspective of power density.

Then, the effect of different light power on neural activity was explored. We used 5000 mV, 4000 mV, 3000 mV, 2000 mV and 2500 mV to drive the laser one by one. The time of each stage was 2 min (after 40 s of illumination, the light was closed for 20 s, and the cycle was twice). According to the statistics of spike firing rate under different light power (Figure 6a), it was found that when the driving voltage of 2500 mV (corresponding to 1.032 mW output power) or above was used, the optical stimulation produced the effect of enhancing the activities of neurons; when the driving voltage of 2000 mV was used for optogenetic control, there was almost no obvious modulation effect. This showed that optogenetics required the light intensity to reach a certain threshold (1.032 mW in this study). At the same time, it was found that within a certain power range (1.032 mW–1.584 mW), the firing rate increased as the light power increased. When the driving voltage exceeds 4000 mV (corresponding to 1.584 mW), the firing rate decreased instead. On the one hand, it might be related to the switching property of photoreceptor itself, on the other hand, it might be due to the heat generated by light, resulting in the increase of neurons' temperature, which might have a inhibition effect on the activity of neurons. There was also no obvious relationship between LFP power and light power (Figure 6b).

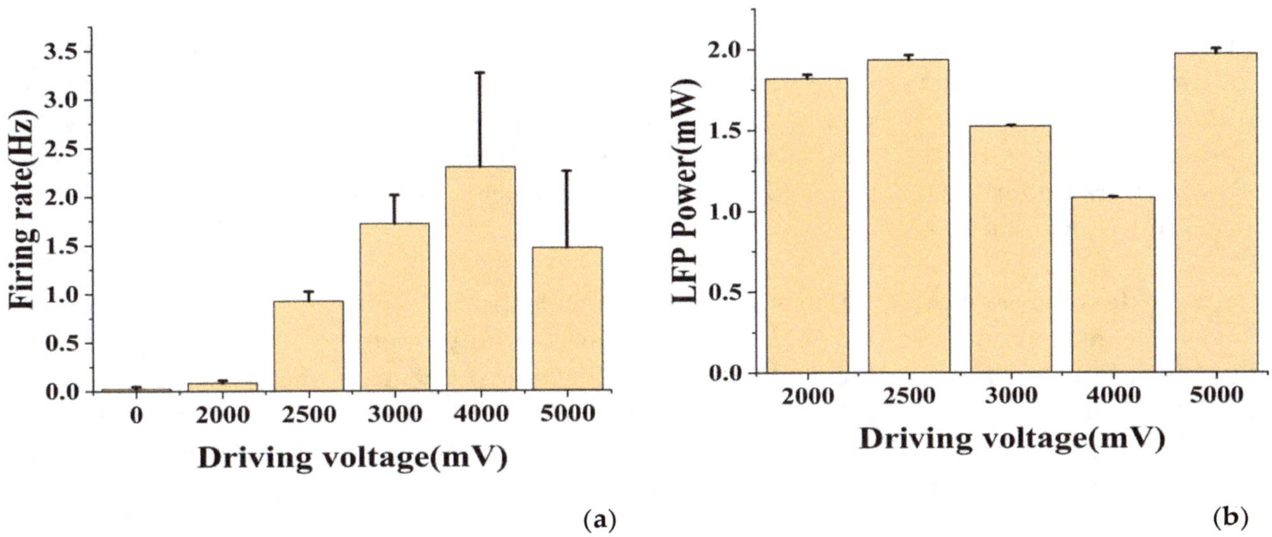

Figure 6. (**a**) The average spike firing rate of neurons under different driving voltages; (**b**) The mean LFP power (0–8 Hz) of neurons under different driving voltages. Error bars indicate standard deviation of 3 channels and N = 2 (N is the number of experiments).

4. Conclusions

In this paper, we employed a physical bonding method to integrate an optical fiber onto an MEA. This allowed us to characterize the activity of neural circuits in vivo, using optogenetic light delivery, and hence quantifying neural firing patterns. The changes of neuronal activity in a large range (depth from 900 to 1250 μm in the brain) under optogenetic control were detected and the infected neurons were successfully activated by optical stimulation, which proved the excellent performance of the integrated device. Furthermore, a possible circuit is analyzed by optogenetic modulation and electrophysiological detection, which provided a new method for circuit research. At the same time, we also studied the effect of different optical stimulation patterns and different light powers on the neuromodulation. We found that the optical stimulation patterns with lower frequency and larger duty cycle induced more intense neuronal activity. The light power needed to reach a certain response threshold (1.032 mW in this study), and greater optical power induced more intense neuronal activity within a certain power range.

In our work, the optical fibers are only used to transmit light. However, as far as we know, some new sensors based on optical fiber have great application potential in neuroscience research and attract many people's attention. For example, researchers integrate high-resolution twist/torsion optical fiber sensors to monitor eventual movements of the patients utilizing the electromagnetic interference independency (EMI) of optical fibers [27]. Furthermore, some optical fiber-based sensors also are studied for MRI (Magnetic Resonance Imaging) interventions [28]. The optical fiber force sensors can help to provide force sensing in the MRI interventions, which increases the safety or accuracy of interventions. If the optical fiber on our integrated device is combined with photo sensor and customized circuit, it will have the potential to become an optical fiber force sensor. However, there are many other issues to consider in order to make it MRI-compatible. First of all, small fiber diameter and small footprint should be used to meet the requirement of sensor miniaturization. Secondly, we should choose the materials carefully. Polymer optical fiber can be considered for better flexibility and compatibility and the electrode can be based on polyimide, which matches brain tissue well in magnetic susceptibility. Finally, due to the potential of the electric current inducing imaging artifacts, some measures should be taken to prevent the interference of electrophysiology detection on MRI. In summary, our devices have the potential to be compatible with MRI. At the same time, we can also add in vivo electrochemical analysis function of neurotransmitters to the MEA. Many events in the nervous system are accompanied by the release of neurotransmitters, so the detection of neurotransmitters is particularly important. Electrochemical analysis need to modify multilayer polymers and enzymes at the electrode sites and the measurement is carried out in the three electrodes system, which are compatible with our devices [29]. Furthermore, it is also possible to measure the concentration of different neurotransmitters on an MEA by using different polymers or enzymes. These ideas will make it possible to simultaneously detect electrophysiological signals and neurotransmitters under the neuromodulation of optogenetics, which will undoubtedly promote the development of neuroscience.

With the development of materials science, flexible electrodes have great advantages in the field of biosensors due to their close contact with brain tissue, many microelectrodes or optical devices based on flexible substrates have been studied [30,31]. The μ-LED array based on flexible substrate can accurately stimulate the brain at multiple points. Mccall and colleagues have made cellular-scale microscale, inorganic light-emitting diodes (μ-ILED, 6.45 μm thick, 50 × 50 μm^2), and the μ-ILED is transferred to Polyethylene terephthalate (PET, polyester film) substrate for long-term implantation [32]. The thickness of organic light-emitting diodes (OLED) can even be less than 1 μm, which is more suitable for implantation in the brain [33]. Therefore, we can combine flexible electrode and optical interface to explore long-term optogenetic modulation and multi-mode sensor integration in the future [34,35]. In a word, the method proposed in this paper was an effective and feasible way of optogenetic neuromodulation and simultaneous neural detection, which can be applied to the study of neuroscience mechanism.

Author Contributions: P.F., Y.S. and X.C. conceived and designed the experiments; P.F., Y.D. and Y.W. performed the experiments; P.F., S.X., B.L., J.X. and H.W. analyzed the data; P.F., Y.S. and X.C. wrote the paper. All authors have read and agreed to the published version of the manuscript.

References

1. Boyden, E.S.; Zhang, F.; Bamberg, E.; Nagel, G.; Deisseroth, K. Millisecond-timescale, genetically targeted optical control of neural activity. *Nat. Neurosci.* **2005**, *8*, 1263–1268. [CrossRef] [PubMed]
2. Hibberd, T.J.; Feng, J.; Luo, J.; Yang, P.; Samineni, V.K.; Gereau, R.W.t.; Kelley, N.; Hu, H.; Spencer, N.J. Optogenetic induction of colonic motility in mice. *Gastroenterology* **2018**, *155*, 514–528 e516. [CrossRef] [PubMed]
3. Spencer, N.J.; Hu, H. Enteric nervous system: Sensory transduction, neural circuits and gastrointestinal motility. *Nat. Rev. Gastroenterol. Hepatol.* **2020**, *17*, 338–351. [CrossRef]
4. Aston-Jones, G.; Deisseroth, K. Recent advances in optogenetics and pharmacogenetics. *Brain. Res.* **2013**, *1511*, 1–5. [CrossRef] [PubMed]
5. Chow, B.Y.; Boyden, E.S. Optogenetics and Translational Medicine. *Sci. Transl. Med.* **2013**, *5*, 177ps5. [CrossRef]
6. Yizhar, O.; Fenno, L.E.; Davidson, T.J.; Mogri, M.; Deisseroth, K. Optogenetics in neural systems. *Neuron* **2011**, *71*, 9–34. [CrossRef]
7. Zhang, F.; Vierock, J.; Yizhar, O.; Fenno, L.E.; Tsunoda, S.; Kianianmomeni, A.; Prigge, M.; Berndt, A.; Cushman, J.; Polle, J.; et al. The Microbial opsin family of optogenetic tools. *Cell* **2011**, *147*, 1446–1457. [CrossRef]
8. Bernstein, J.G.; Boyden, E.S. Optogenetic tools for analyzing the neural circuits of behavior. *Trends. Cogn. Sci.* **2011**, *15*, 592–600. [CrossRef]
9. Buzsaki, G.; Stark, E.; Berenyi, A.; Khodagholy, D.; Kipke, D.R.; Yoon, E.; Wise, K.D. Tools for probing local circuits: High-density silicon probes combined with optogenetics. *Neuron* **2015**, *86*, 92–105. [CrossRef]
10. Goncalves, S.B.; Ribeiro, J.F.; Silva, A.F.; Costa, R.M.; Correia, J.H. Design and manufacturing challenges of optogenetic neural interfaces: A review. *J. Neural Eng.* **2017**, *14*, 041001. [CrossRef]

11. Zhao, H. Recent progress of development of optogenetic implantable neural probes. *Int. J. Mol. Sci.* **2017**, *18*, 1751. [CrossRef]
12. Royer, S.; Zemelman, B.V.; Barbic, M.; Losonczy, A.; Buzsaki, G.; Magee, J.C. Multi-array silicon probes with integrated optical fibers: Light-assisted perturbation and recording of local neural circuits in the behaving animal. *Eur. J. Neurosci.* **2010**, *31*, 2279–2291. [CrossRef] [PubMed]
13. Stark, E.; Koos, T.; Buzsaki, G. Diode probes for spatiotemporal optical control of multiple neurons in freely moving animals. *J. Neurophysiol.* **2012**, *108*, 349–363. [CrossRef] [PubMed]
14. Park, H.; Shin, H.-J.; Cho, I.-J.; Yoon, E.-S.; Suh, J.-K.F.; Im, M.; Yoon, E.; Kim, Y.-J.; Kim, J.; IEEE. The First Neural Probe Integrated with Light Source (Blue Laser Diode) for Optical Stimulation and Electrical Recording. In Proceedings of the 2011 Annual International Conference of the IEEE Engineering in Medicine and Biology Society, Boston, MA, USA, 30 August–3 September 2011; pp. 2961–2964.
15. Wang, J.; Wagner, F.; Borton, D.A.; Zhang, J.; Ozden, I.; Burwell, R.D.; Nurmikko, A.V.; van Wagenen, R.; Diester, I.; Deisseroth, K. Integrated device for combined optical neuromodulation and electrical recording for chronic in vivo applications. *J. Neural Eng.* **2012**, *9*, 016001. [CrossRef] [PubMed]
16. Schwaerzle, M.; Seidl, K.; Schwarz, U.T.; Paul, O.; Ruther, P. Ultracompact optrode with integrated laser diode chips and su-8 waveguides for optogenetic applications. In Proceedings of the 26th IEEE International Conference on Micro Electro Mechanical Systems, Taipei, China, 20–24 January 2013; pp. 1029–1032.
17. Son, Y.; Lee, H.J.; Kim, J.; Shin, H.; Choi, N.; Lee, C.J.; Yoon, E.S.; Yoon, E.; Wise, K.D.; Kim, T.G.; et al. In vivo optical modulation of neural signals using monolithically integrated two-dimensional neural probe arrays. *Sci. Rep.* **2015**, *5*, 15466. [CrossRef]
18. Huang, W.C.; Chi, H.S.; Lee, Y.C.; Lo, Y.C.; Liu, T.C.; Chiang, M.Y.; Chen, H.Y.; Li, S.J.; Chen, Y.Y.; Chen, S.Y. Gene-embedded nanostructural biotic-abiotic optoelectrode arrays applied for synchronous brain optogenetics and neural signal recording. *ACS Appl. Mater. Interfaces* **2019**, *11*, 11270–11282. [CrossRef]
19. Cao, H.; Gu, L.; Mohanty, S.K.; Chiao, J.C. An integrated mu LED optrode for optogenetic stimulation and electrical recording. *IEEE Trans. Biomed. Eng.* **2013**, *60*, 225–229. [CrossRef]
20. Wu, F.; Stark, E.; Ku, P.C.; Wise, K.D.; Buzsaki, G.; Yoon, E. Monolithically integrated muLEDs on silicon neural probes for high-resolution optogenetic studies in behaving animals. *Neuron* **2015**, *88*, 1136–1148. [CrossRef]
21. Scharf, R.; Tsunematsu, T.; McAlinden, N.; Dawson, M.D.; Sakata, S.; Mathieson, K. Depth-specific optogenetic control in vivo with a scalable, high-density muLED neural probe. *Sci. Rep.* **2016**, *6*, 28381. [CrossRef]
22. Reddy, J.W.; Kimukin, I.; Stewart, L.T.; Ahmed, Z.; Barth, A.L.; Towe, E.; Chamanzar, M. High density, double-sided, flexible optoelectronic neural probes with Embedded muLEDs. *Front. Neurosci.* **2019**, *13*, 745. [CrossRef]
23. Fan, X.; Song, Y.; Ma, Y.; Zhang, S.; Xiao, G.; Yang, L.; Xu, H.; Zhang, D.; Cai, X. In situ real-time monitoring of glutamate and electrophysiology from cortex to hippocampus in mice based on a microelectrode array. *Sensors* **2016**, *17*, 61. [CrossRef] [PubMed]
24. Kuang, H.; Tsien, J.Z. Large-scale neural ensembles in mice: Methods for recording and data analysis. In *Electrophysiological Recording Techniques*; Vertes, R.P., Stackman, R.W., Eds.; Humana Press: Totowa, NJ, USA, 2011; Volume 54, p. 103126.
25. Aravanis, A.M.; Wang, L.-P.; Zhang, F.; Meltzer, L.A.; Mogri, M.Z.; Schneider, M.B.; Deisseroth, K. An optical neural interface:in vivocontrol of rodent motor cortex with integrated fiberoptic and optogenetic technology. *J. Neural Eng.* **2007**, *4*, S143–S156. [CrossRef] [PubMed]
26. Binding, J.; Ben Arous, J.; Leger, J.F.; Gigan, S.; Boccara, C.; Bourdieu, L. Brain refractive index measured in vivo with high-NA defocus-corrected full-field OCT and consequences for two-photon microscopy. *Opt. Express.* **2011**, *19*, 4833–4847. [CrossRef] [PubMed]
27. Zhang, X.; Chen, J.; González-Vila, Á.; Liu, F.; Liu, Y.; Li, K.; Guo, T. Twist sensor based on surface plasmon resonance excitation using two spectral combs in one tilted fiber Bragg grating. *J. Opt. Soc. Am. B* **2019**, *36*, 1176–1182. [CrossRef]
28. Su, H.; Iordachita, I.I.; Tokuda, J.; Hata, N.; Liu, X.; Seifabadi, R.; Xu, S.; Wood, B.; Fischer, G.S. Fiber optic force sensors for mri-guided interventions and rehabilitation: A Review. *IEEE Sens. J.* **2017**, *17*, 1952–1963. [CrossRef]

29. Xiao, G.; Xu, S.; Song, Y.; Zhang, Y.; Li, Z.; Gao, F.; Xie, J.; Sha, L.; Xu, Q.; Shen, Y.; et al. In situ detection of neurotransmitters and epileptiform electrophysiology activity in awake mice brains using a nanocomposites modified microelectrode array. *Sens. Actuators B Chem.* **2019**, *288*, 601–610. [CrossRef]
30. Noh, K.N.; Park, S.I.; Qazi, R.; Zou, Z.; Mickle, A.D.; Grajales-Reyes, J.G.; Jang, K.I.; Gereau, R.W.t.; Xiao, J.; Rogers, J.A.; et al. Miniaturized, battery-free optofluidic systems with potential for wireless pharmacology and optogenetics. *Small* **2018**, *14*, 1702479. [CrossRef]
31. Park, S.I.; Shin, G.; McCall, J.G.; Al-Hasani, R.; Norris, A.; Xia, L.; Brenner, D.S.; Noh, K.N.; Bang, S.Y.; Bhatti, D.L.; et al. Stretchable multichannel antennas in soft wireless optoelectronic implants for optogenetics. *Proc. Natl. Acad. Sci. USA* **2016**, *113*, E8169–E8177. [CrossRef]
32. Kim, T.I.; McCall, J.G.; Jung, Y.H.; Huang, X.; Siuda, E.R.; Li, Y.; Song, J.; Song, Y.M.; Pao, H.A.; Kim, R.H.; et al. Injectable, cellular-scale optoelectronics with applications for wireless optogenetics. *Science* **2013**, *340*, 211–216. [CrossRef]
33. Matarese, B.F.E.; Feyen, P.L.C.; de Mello, J.C.; Benfenati, F. Sub-millisecond Control of Neuronal Firing by Organic Light-Emitting Diodes. *Front. Bioeng. Biotechnol.* **2019**, *7*, 278. [CrossRef]
34. McCall, J.G.; Kim, T.I.; Shin, G.; Huang, X.; Jung, Y.H.; Al-Hasani, R.; Omenetto, F.G.; Bruchas, M.R.; Rogers, J.A. Fabrication and application of flexible, multimodal light-emitting devices for wireless optogenetics. *Nat. Protoc.* **2013**, *8*, 2413–2428. [CrossRef] [PubMed]
35. Schwaerzle, M.; Pothof, F.; Paul, O.; Ruther, P. High-Resolution Neural Depth Probe with Integrated 460 Nm Light Emitting Diode For Optogenetic Applications. In Proceedings of the 18th International Conference on Solid-State Sensors, Actuators and Microsystems, Anchorage, AK, USA, 21–25 January 2015; pp. 1774–1777.

3

Assessment of Gold Bio-Functionalization for Wide-Interface Biosensing Platforms

Lucia Sarcina [1], Luisa Torsi [1,2,3], Rosaria Anna Picca [1,2], Kyriaki Manoli [1,2,*] and Eleonora Macchia [3]

1 Dipartimento di Chimica, Università degli Studi di Bari Aldo Moro, 70125 Bari, Italy; lucia.sarcina@uniba.it (L.S.); luisa.torsi@uniba.it (L.T.); rosaria.picca@uniba.it (R.A.P.)
2 CSGI (Centre for Colloid and Surface Science), Department of Chemistry, 70125 Bari, Italy
3 The Faculty of Science and Engineering, Åbo Akademi University, FI-20500 Turku, Finland; eleonora.macchia@abo.fi
* Correspondence: kyriaki.manoli@uniba.it

Abstract: The continuous improvement of the technical potential of bioelectronic devices for biosensing applications will provide clinicians with a reliable tool for biomarker quantification down to the single molecule. Eventually, physicians will be able to identify the very moment at which the illness state begins, with a terrific impact on the quality of life along with a reduction of health care expenses. However, in clinical practice, to gather enough information to formulate a diagnosis, multiple biomarkers are normally quantified from the same biological sample simultaneously. Therefore, it is critically important to translate lab-based bioelectronic devices based on electrolyte gated thin-film transistor technology into a cost-effective portable multiplexing array prototype. In this perspective, the assessment of cost-effective manufacturability represents a crucial step, with specific regard to the optimization of the bio-functionalization protocol of the transistor gate module. Hence, we have assessed, using surface plasmon resonance technique, a sustainable and reliable cost-effective process to successfully bio-functionalize a gold surface, suitable as gate electrode for wide-field bioelectronic sensors. The bio-functionalization process herein investigated allows to reduce the biorecognition element concentration to one-tenth, drastically impacting the manufacturing costs while retaining high analytical performance.

Keywords: surface plasmon resonance; biosensors; bio-functionalization optimization; cost-effective biosensors; lab-on-a-chip

---

1. Introduction

Single-molecule detection is a crucial task to accomplish [1,2], which could in fact allows to gather digital tracking of a biomarker from its physiologic to its pathogenic level. Such an analytical tool will enable to define the onset from a healthy to diseased patient. Early diagnostics in progressive diseases would, hence, become possible well before any symptom appears. Single-molecule biomarker detection would further allow marker quantification non-invasively, in readily available biofluids such as saliva, sweat, or even tears where they can be present at much lower concentrations. Along the same line, it would make possible ultrasensitive liquid biopsy, i.e., the assay of peripheral biofluids such as plasma, serum, or even saliva, a feasible medical procedure replacing the invasive inspection of diseased tissues. Among the single-molecule detection methods proposed so far, only a few are exploitable for real clinical sensing. This approach, addressed as wide-field sensing [2], involves the assay of a biomarker at the attomolar (aM, 10^{-18} M) or even zeptomolar (zM, 10^{-21} M) limit-of-detection with a large-area interface that is functionalized with a huge number of biorecognition elements (10^{11}–10^{12} cm^{-2}). Large-area organic-bioelectronic devices endowed with an electronic-interface capable to detect recognition element/biomarker complexes intrinsic properties, such as the electrostatic or dielectric ones, are emerging as a powerful tool capable of selective, label-free, and fast biomarker detection at the physical limit in real biofluids. Bioelectronic thin-film transistors (TFTs) [3–5], gated via an ionically-conducting and electronically-insulating electrolyte [6–8], are generating a lot of interest as they can potentially be produced by scalable large-area low-cost approaches. Such sensors [9,10] are capable of high selectivity via the bio-functionalization of the organic semiconductors (OSCs) [10] or the gate metal surface [11]. Electrolyte-gated TFTs (EG-TFTs) have been successfully engaged, lately, as wide-field bioelectronic sensors exhibiting limits of detection at zM - aM level also in real bio-fluids [12,13]. In the Single-Molecule with a large-Transistor (SiMoT) platform, based on an EG-TFT device [12], the gate is bio-functionalized [14] with 10^{12} cm^{-2} recognition elements covalently attached to a 0.5 cm^2 gold gate. The SiMoT platform has been demonstrated to successfully perform label-free detection at the physical limit of immunoglobulin-M [13], C-reactive protein in saliva [15], and HIV-p24 [16,17], as well as genomic biomarkers [18]. However, in clinical practice, to gather enough information to formulate a diagnosis, multiple biomarkers are normally quantified from the same biological sample. Therefore, it is necessary to develop a technology capable to perform multiplexing [19] and thus realized with an array of 96 or more transducing elements, so that the standard solutions, the negative-controls, and the sample can be assayed, with all the replicates for each biomarker, at the same time. All this calls for translating the lab-based SiMoT device into a cost-effective portable multiplexing array prototype that integrates, with a modular approach, novel materials, and standard components/interfaces. In this perspective, the assessment of cost-effective manufacturability represents a crucial step, with specific regard to the optimization of the bio-functionalization protocol of the gate modules. Therefore, in this study, we have developed, with the aid of surface plasmon resonance (SPR) technique, a novel and reliable cost-effective process to successfully bio-functionalize a gold surface suitable as gate electrode in a SiMoT-based platform. An uncommon approach has been chosen in the SPR settings by using a method that can be easily translated to bioelectronic device surface modifications. In particular, the bio-functionalization process herein proposed allows to reduce to one-tenth the concentration of the biorecognition elements. This can drastically reduce the manufacturing costs without sacrificing the sensing performance in terms of sensitivity. In general, for a biomolecular reaction to occur, the two reagents need to be confined in an adequately small volume for a sufficiently long time. The recognition element can be attached on a surface that serves as detecting interface. Regardless, the interaction cross-section of the two reagents has to be reasonably high. In this respect, a volume of 1 μm^3 (1 femtoliter - fL) has been proven sufficiently small for a single enzyme to interact with its substrate (present in excess concentration though) on the minute time-scale [20,21]. Indeed, a solution comprising $n = 1 \pm 1$ ($\sqrt{n}$ = Poisson error) molecules in each 1fL sub-volumes has a concentration of $\sim 1 \times 10^{-9}$ mol $\times$ l^{-1} (nM). Smaller volumes (attoliter, aL, or zeptoliter, zL), each occupied by a single molecule, entails even larger concentrations. Since the number of molecules in a volume V = 100 μL of a solution of molar concentration [c] is $n = [c]{\cdot}V{\cdot}N_A$ (N_A = Avogadro's number), 1 nM equals $\sim 10^{11}$ molecules or, equivalently, $\sim 10^{11}$ 1 fL sub-volumes. As two molecules need to be confined in a volume of 1 fL or smaller to rapidly interact, at least one of them is to be present at a concentration of 1 nM. Every 1 fL (or lower) statistically contains one reagent, so wherever the other single reagent is, there is always one fL sub-volume comprising both reagents. A single-molecule interaction can, therefore, occur when the recognition-elements are present at nM concentration (or higher) along with a single biomarker or the opposite way around. In clinical assays, the former is to be preferred. Therefore, the aim of the study herein presented is to determine which is the minimum biorecognition element concentration requested to achieve a sufficiently high surface coverage. Interestingly, it has been demonstrated that it is possible to reduce to one tenth the biorecognition elements concentration without impacting on the analytical performances, thus optimizing the biofunctionalization protocol of the SiMBiT platform as well as of other bioelectronic devices [22–24]. This study paves the way toward a multiplexing single molecule technology that will open to a massive use of high-throughput array-based assay not only in clinical laboratory analysis but also in point-of-care and low resources settings.

2. Materials and Methods

2.1. Materials

3-mercaptopropionic acid (3-MPA), 11-mercaptoundecanoic acid (11-MUA), 1-ethyl-3-(3-dimethylaminopropyl)-carbodiimide (EDC), N-hydroxysulfosuccinimide sodium salt (NHSS), ethanolamine hydrochloride (EA), and 66 kDa molecular weight bovine serum albumin (BSA) were purchased from Sigma–Aldrich and used with no further purification. HPLC-grade water, ethanol grade puriss. p.a. assay, ≥99.8%, ammonium hydroxide solution (NH_4OH) 28.0–30.0%, hydrogen peroxide (H_2O_2) 30% (w/w) in H_2O were purchased from Sigma–Aldrich and used with no further purification. Anti-human immunoglobulin M (anti-IgM) produced in goat polyclonal antibodies was purchased from Sigma–Aldrich and used with no further purification. Human IgM (~950 kDa) affinity ligand, purchased from Sigma–Aldrich, was isolated from pooled normal human serum and used with no further purification. Phosphate buffered saline (PBS pH 7.4, Sigma-Aldrich- Merck KGaA, Darmstadt, Germany) solution was prepared according to previous works [12]. 2-(N-morpholino)ethane-sulfonic acid (MES) buffer (Sigma-Aldrich- Merck KGaA, Darmstadt, Germany) 0.1 M was adjusted with sodium hydroxide solution (NaOH 1 M) at pH 4.8–4.9.

2.2. Preparation of Mixed Self-Assembled Monolayers

The sensor slides (SPR Navi-200), comprising a 50 nm gold on glass, were cleaned in a freshly prepared "basic piranha" $NH_4OH/H_2O_2/H_2O$ solution (1:1:5 v/v) at c.a. 80–90 °C for 10 min. The slides were rinsed with HPLC water, dried with N_2, and then treated for 10 min in ozone cleaner. For the assembly of the chemical SAM (chem-SAM) on the gold surface, the slides were immediately immersed in a 10 mM thiol solution of 11-MUA: 3-MPA (1:10 molar ratio) in degassed ethanol. The slides were kept in contact with the mixed thiol solution for 18 h at 22 °C under a nitrogen atmosphere in the dark. Afterward, the samples were rinsed with ethanol and mounted in the SPR apparatus, drying the glass back-surface of the chip with N_2.

2.3. Surface Plasmon Resonance Real-Time Functionalization

A BioNavis Multi-parameter Surface plasmon resonance (MP-SPR) Navi^{TM} instrument, in the Kretschmann configuration, was used. The SPR instrument, equipped with two laser sources (670 and 785 nm wavelengths) was used to study the gold surface bio-functionalization in situ, by using the 670 nm source for both sampling areas. A wide angular range (50–78 °C) was measured, with real angular resolution of 0.001 °C. The variation of the plasmon peak angular response was monitored over time. All the experiments were performed at 22 °C in a one-channel cell in which the solutions were manually injected and kept in static conditions. This configuration allows the exposure of a gold area of c.a. 0.42 cm^2 to be functionalized. The strong gold-sulfur interaction results in the exposure of the carboxylic groups of thiols anchored to the sensor surface. For the immobilization of the biorecognition element, the COOH activation can be performed by the well-known EDC/NHSS chemistry [25,26]. Two sensor slides modified with the chem-SAM were tested by using two different concentrations for the functionalizing antibody. In the first protocol, addressed as protocol A, the modified slide was exposed first to HPLC water to acquire a stable SPR response as baseline. Then, 1 mL of an EDC (200 mM) and NHSS (50 mM) aqueous solution was injected through the cell (internal volume 100 μL, plus 100 μL capillary tubing) and left in contact for 2 h. The surface was subsequently rinsed first with H_2O and then PBS to inject 500 μL of a 100 μg/mL anti-IgM solution in PBS. The antibody was left in contact until a complete bio-conjugation was achieved, i.e., a plateau response was observed in the sensogram (SPR angle vs time). Then, the sensor slide was rinsed thoroughly with PBS to remove unbound antibodies. This preconcentration step was followed by the injection of 1 M ethanolamine

PBS solution (EA) for 45 min. The bio-functionalization was completed with the injection of 0.1 mg/mL bovine serum albumin (BSA) solution in PBS, to gain a more compact SAM, less prone to the nonspecific adsorption [27]. The modified sensor surface was then exposed to an IgM solution in PBS (50 nM) for testing the antibody binding efficacy. Protocol A has been described in detail elsewhere [14]. In the second protocol, addressed as protocol B and adapted from Reference [28] (Figure 2c), the baseline was set by injecting, instead of water, MES buffer through the chem-SAM modified surface. The solution of EDC/NHSS, prepared also in MES, was then injected and left in the SPR cell for 15 min. After the surface was washed with MES, PBS was injected to acquire a new baseline. At this stage, the activated chem-SAM gold surface was exposed to 500 μL of 10 μg/mL anti-IgM solution, and the conjugation was monitored in the sensogram, until a plateau was observed. The succeeding steps involving EA and BSA were performed as in protocol A. Finally, the IgM solution in PBS was injected through the functionalized sensor surface, recording the immunoglobulin binding response.

3. Results and Discussion

The amount of anti-IgM capturing proteins immobilized on the gate with the two bio-functionalization protocols A and B was estimated by measuring the SPR shift $\Delta\theta$ occurring when the anti-IgM capturing proteins are conjugated to the activated chem-SAM. The final capturing SAM segregated on the SPR slide is schematically depicted in Figure 1. It is well known that SPR technique ensures the direct correlation of plasmon peak shift with the thickness and optical properties of the medium that contacts the metal surface [29]. The activated carboxylic groups of SAM thiols on the modified gold surface can stably bind antibody primary amines. Thus, when antibodies approach the sensor slide, a new layer can be created at the surface and an increase of the detected angle in the sensogram is observed [30]. The efficacy of each step in the functionalization process can be verified by the SPR real-time monitoring for both the investigated protocols.

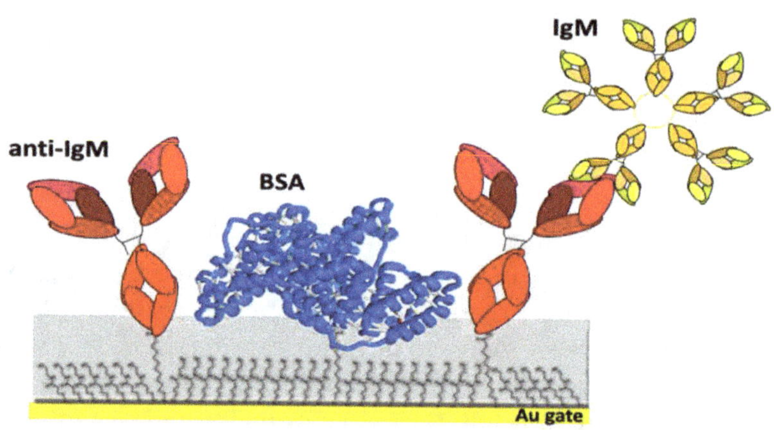

Figure 1. Capturing SAM, comprising both a chem-SAM of activated-and-blocked 3-mercaptopropionic acid (3-MPA) and 11-mercaptoundecanoic acid (11-MUA) and a bio-SAM of capturing antibodies.

The experimental trend for the immobilization of anti-IgM loaded at different concentrations is shown in Figure 2. In protocol A, shown in Figure 2a,b, a saturating trend for the preconcentration of anti-IgM is observed and completed soon after 60 min from the exposure to the solution. The high provision of ligand to the surface entails the typical fast increase of SPR angle within the first minutes of incubation [31]. Then, a slower rate of binding occurs until all the available sites on the surface are covered and an equilibrium state is reached. The injection of the PBS buffer (crossed arrow) removes excess of anti-IgM not anchored to the chem-SAM. A successful binding can be confirmed, as no significant decrease of the signal is registered after the PBS injection. The receptor conjugation is completed by injecting the EA solution, after which the unreacted carboxylic groups are deactivated and the electrostatically bound antibodies are washed over [32].

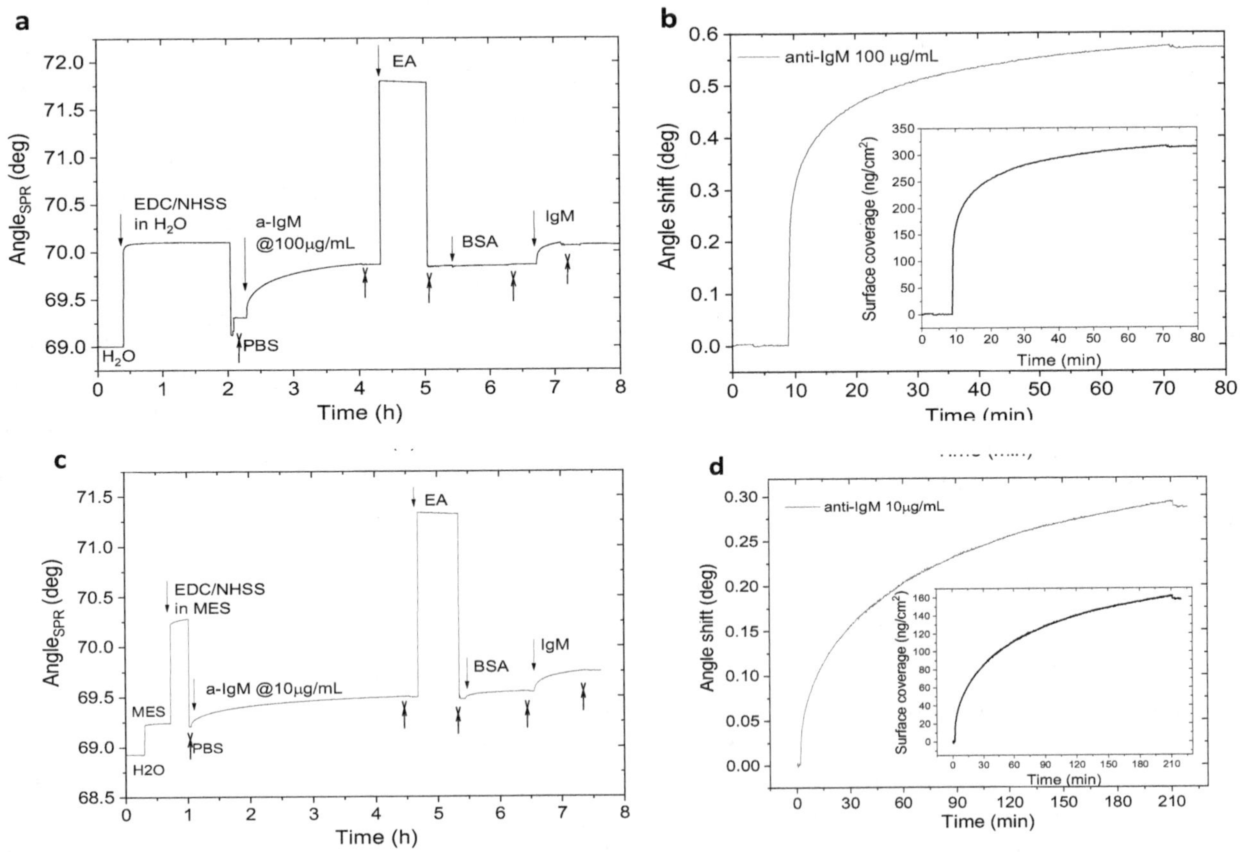

Figure 2. SPR real-time functionalization in which top-down arrows refer to injected solutions and reverse crossed-arrows to phosphate buffered saline (PBS) rinsing steps. (**a**) Sensogram for the immobilization of anti-IgM on the gold surface pre-modified with mixed SAM. (**b**) Zoom of the angular response (angle shift vs time) for anti-IgM exposure at 100 μg/mL and inset showing the corresponding surface coverage (ng/cm^2). (**c**) Sensogram for anti-IgM immobilization performed with reduced antibody concentration and (**d**) zoom in the 10 μg/mL anti-IgM preconcentration step with surface coverage (ng/cm^2) in the inset.

The SPR signal after the rinsing of EA will be related to the amount of effectively bound receptors as reported in Table 1. This angular shift does not differ significantly from the one recorded in the preconcentration. Moreover, the final step involving BSA does not produce significant changes in the angular response, thus a partial insertion of this blocking agent in the well-packed biolayer can be assumed [12,27].

Table 1. Surface plasmon resonance (SPR) response as angle shift ($\Delta\theta$) recorded for the anchored anti-human immunoglobulin M (IgM) and IgM exposure in nM range for both protocols. Calculated surface coverage expressed in ng/cm^2 and number of immobilized molecules for cm^2 surface area.

		SPR $\Delta\theta$ *(°)*	***SC* Γ (ng/cm^2)**	***SC (particles/cm^2)***
Protocol A	*Anti-IgM* # *100 μg/mL*	0.53	294	1.2×10^{12}
	IgM ##	0.23	127	8.0×10^{10}
Protocol B	*Anti-IgM* # *10 μg/mL*	0.27	146	5.9×10^{11}
	IgM ##	0.21	116	7.3×10^{10}

*SC: Surface coverage; # anti IgM MW 150 kDa; ## IgM MW 950 kDa.

The sensogram recorded for immobilization protocol B is reported in Figure 2c, with a zoom on the injection of anti-IgM 10 μg/mL in Figure 2d. Independently of the used solvent, the optimization of the procedure can be settled first with a decrease in the reaction time of EDC/NHSS solution, without substantial consequences on the activation efficacy. Indeed, the EDC action is completed within 20 min, so that an extended reaction will only result in a longer functionalization time with no enhancement in the subsequent binding rate of the receptor [33]. Moreover, the control over the pH obtained by means of MES buffer for the activating solution (pH ~5) leads to a more efficient reaction [34]. In a two-step reaction, to gain best results, the first activation step (i.e., EDC/NHSS) should be performed in a MES buffer at pH 5–6, then the pH should be raised to 7.2–7.5 with a phosphate buffer for a more effective reaction with the amine-containing groups of the antibody (anti-IgM) [35]. The pH plays an important role during the immobilization since the ligand is uncharged or positively charged in the preconcentration process to promote an electrostatic attraction between the amino group of the antibody and the negatively charged SAM surface. A pH 0.5–1 units below the isoelectric point of the ligand (typically ~ 8) is needed while preserving the negative charge on the sensor surface keeping the pH above 4 [36–38]. Optimal reaction conditions have been chosen in the present work according to the results already reported for other receptors [28].

As soon as the activation solution is washed away by the buffer, the ligand solution in PBS is injected into the SPR cell.

The main observed difference, related to the usage of a more diluted solution, relies on the time required to reach the steady state. Indeed, the first 30 min give a slower increase of the signal (Figure 2d) if compared to protocol A (Figure 2b). In static conditions, the molecule replenishment to the surface will be mostly related to their concentration in the bulk, since there is no flow that opposes the depletion of ligands near the surface [39,40]. Hence, for reaching the equilibrium state at a lower concentration, the time needed for the incubation of anti-IgM is at least 3.5 h. Once a plateau in the antibody binding signal is reached, the buffer is slotted over the cell. After rinsing, the signal does not drop-down thus the binding can be considered effective and the functionalization can be completed through the injection of EA and BSA afterward. A slight increase of the SPR angle is observed after BSA step for the second protocol (c.a. 0.07 °C shift from anti-IgM level). For this different behavior, major adsorption of BSA on the SAM can be assumed considering that the amount of the anti-IgM immobilized is half of that obtained in the first protocol. This means that the anchored receptors are more spaced and BSA can stabilize them by prominent steric hindrance, producing an appreciable signal onto the sensor surface.

The assessment of sensor surface modification is fundamental when developing a biolayer-based device since the properties of the biorecognition element regarding its orientation, surface density, and activity toward the binding analyte can dramatically influence the assay analytical performances [41,42]. In SPR direct assays, the typical explored analyte concentration returns limit of detections in the 1–10 nM range [43,44], with further improvement only by using nanostructures or sandwich assays [45]. Hence, for testing the response of the functionalized surface at saturating concentrations, in this study, the sensor slides for both protocols were exposed to a standard solution of IgM at nominal concentration of 50 nM (10^{-9} M), recording the corresponding SPR angle variation. The response obtained as angle shift and the equivalent surface density is compared in Table 1. This evaluation is done according to the literature [46], which states the relation between surface coverage (Γ, in ng/cm^2) and the plasmon resonance shift by means of the Feijter's equation: $\Gamma = (n_a - n_b)d_a \cdot (dn/dC)^{-1}$ [47]. Here, the coverage is related to the difference in refractive index between the antibody layer (n_a) and the bulk solution (n_b), the average thickness (d_a) of bounded species, and the refractive index increment (*dn*/*d*C). The difference in average refractive index corresponds to $(n_a - n_b) = \Delta\theta \cdot k$, where $\Delta\theta$ is the measured angular shift and k is the wavelength dependent sensitivity coefficient. For thin layer beyond the evanescent field depth (less than 200 nm) at a source wavelength of 670 nm, the equation can be simplified: the product ($k \cdot d_a$) is approximated to 1.0×10^{-7} cm/deg and *dn/dc* to 0.182 cm^3/g. Thus, the equation becomes $\Gamma = \Delta\theta \cdot 550$ (ng/cm^2) [12,14]. The conversion into a surface coverage expressed in number of molecules per cm^2 can be performed by considering the molecular weight of the species under investigation. At a fixed analyte concentration, by comparing the total bound IgM obtained with the two protocols, an analogous result is achieved (Table 1). Knowing the average response at this saturating analyte concentration for the same sensing platform used in protocol A [13,14], the reduction to one-tenth of biorecognition elements concentration still produces comparable analytical performances, as can be stated considering the response obtained with protocol B. Although the number of anti-IgM available on the surface is slightly lower (5.9×10^{11} particles/cm^2) with this latter protocol, the available binding sites are indeed enough to measure the same response of protocol A. By fitting the exponential growth relative to the analyte binding, a plateau was obtained correspondent to: $\Delta\theta = (0.238 \pm 0.005)$ °C for the exposure in the anti-IgM (100 μg/mL) modified SAM of protocol A, and $\Delta\theta = (0.227 \pm 0.002)$ °C for the anti-IgM (10 μg/mL) modified SAM of protocol B. Although the response is comparable in both protocols, one should notice that the 90% of the signal can be reached for protocol A soon after 16 min, meanwhile, 43 min are necessary for protocol B. This highlights the importance of selecting the correct time of analyte exposure within the assay for getting results not affected by time-dependent signals. Interestingly, protocol B leads to an improvement in the functionalization process, drastically reducing the concentration of capturing antibodies in the preconcentration solution, without affecting the assay readout. Moreover, the observed angular shifts for the antibody immobilization is consistent with values already reported in literature [48–50]. The main goal in a biosensing platform based on a wide-field approach is that of having a high density of receptor on the sensor surface, for the investigation of extremely low analyte concentrations [2]. These working conditions are hardly tied with low consumption of costly reagents, especially if compared with other miniaturized sensing techniques [42]. As SPR has been largely employed as surface-sensitive technique, many standardized protocols are reported in literature [51–53]. The usage of a SAM modified surface allows a controlled antibody binding, and the consequent usage of EA and BSA is well-established [26,54]. However, they were mostly focused on the flow-system facility, which enables the consumption of low volume of reagents while continuous replenishment of molecules to the surface. However, the applicability of these protocols to other sensing methods, such as wide-interface bioelectronics, is not straightforward. The assessment of a robust protocol by means of the SPR apparatus in non-conventional ways is presented here. The authors suggest an improvement in the fabrication of the sensor bio-active surface already tested for an immunoassay application, in the SiMoT device described elsewhere [55,56]. The SPR experimental conditions (i.e., solution volume loaded, the gold area exposed, and the manual injections) have been set to be feasible also for the SiMoT, as well as further bioelectronic platforms. After testing the proposed protocol for the bio-functionalization with a real-time technique like SPR, the modification of the gold electrode used in the electronic sensor can be optimized accordingly.

4. Conclusions

In conclusion, a modified bio-functionalization protocol of a gold surface is proposed and compared with the one previously adopted for gold gate electrodes in the ultrasensitive SiMoT biosensing platform. The two protocols are compared using SPR technique. The amount of anti-IgM capturing proteins immobilized on the mm^2 gate area with the two protocols was estimated by measuring the SPR angle shift $\Delta\theta$ when the anti-IgM capturing proteins are conjugated in real-time to the activated chem-SAM. It was shown that the amount of the capturing antibodies can be reduced at least ten times, up to 10 μg/mL, without affecting the assay analytical performance. The new protocol allows better control of the pH during the different steps of bio-functionalization and reduces the cost of the process, therefore, the cost of the SiMoT platform production. Indeed, this study sets the ground for the assessment of scalable manufacturability of biosensing platform based on EG-TFT devices such as multiplexing single-molecule technologies.

Author Contributions: Conceptualization, E.M., L.T. and K.M.; methodology, R.A.P, K.M. and E.M.; formal analysis, E.M., L.S.; investigation, E.M., L.S., R.A.P.; data curation, L.S., K.M. and E.M.; writing—original draft preparation, E.M. and L.S.; writing—review and editing, L.S., L.T., R.A.P. and K.M.; supervision, E.M. and K.M.; resources and funding acquisition, L.T. All authors have read and agreed to the published version of the manuscript.

Acknowledgments: The authors would like to thank Ronald Österbacka and Davide Blasi for useful discussions.

References

1. Jain, A.; Liu, R.; Ramani, B.; Arauz, E.; Ishitsuka, Y.; Ragunathan, K.; Park, J.; Chen, J.; Xiang, Y.K.; Ha, T. Probing cellular protein complexes using single-molecule pull-down. *Nature* **2011**, *473*, 484–488. [CrossRef]
2. Gooding, J.J.; Gaus, K. Single-molecule sensors: Challenges and opportunities for quantitative analysis. *Angew. Chem. Int. Ed.* **2016**, *55*, 11354–11366. [CrossRef]
3. Torsi, L.; Farinola, G.M.; Marinelli, F.; Tanese, M.C.; Omar, O.H.; Valli, L.; Babudri, F.; Palmisano, F.; Zambonin, P.G.; Naso, F. A sensitivity-enhanced field-effect chiral sensor. *Nat. Mater.* **2008**, *7*, 412–417. [CrossRef] [PubMed]
4. Gualandi, I.; Marzocchi, M.; Achilli, A.; Cavedale, D.; Bonfiglio, A.; Fraboni, B. Textile organic electrochemical transistors as a platform for wearable biosensors. *Sci. Rep.* **2016**, *6*, 33637. [CrossRef] [PubMed]
5. Piro, B.; Wang, D.; Benaoudia, D.; Tibaldi, A.; Anquetin, G.; Noël, V.; Reisberg, S.; Mattana, G.; Jackson, B. Versatile transduction scheme based on electrolyte-gated organic field-effect transistor used as immunoassay readout system. *Biosens. Bioelectron.* **2017**, *92*, 215–220. [CrossRef] [PubMed]
6. Berggren, M.; Richter-Dahlfors, A. Organic bioelectronics. *Adv. Mater.* **2007**, *19*, 3201–3213. [CrossRef]
7. Kergoat, L.; Herlogsson, L.; Braga, D.; Piro, B.; Pham, M.-C.; Crispin, X.; Berggren, M.; Horowitz, G. A water-gate organic field-effect transistor. *Adv. Mater.* **2010**, *22*, 2565–2569. [CrossRef] [PubMed]
8. Pettersson, F.; Remonen, T.; Adekanye, D.; Zhang, Y.; Wilén, C.-E.; Österbacka, R. Environmentally friendly transistors and circuits on paper. *Chem. Phys. Chem.* **2015**, *16*, 1286–1294. [CrossRef] [PubMed]
9. Mulla, M.Y.; Tuccori, E.; Magliulo, M.; Lattanzi, G.; Palazzo, G.; Persaud, K.; Torsi, L. Capacitance-modulated transistor detects odorant binding protein chiral interactions. *Nat. Commun.* **2015**, *6*, 6010. [CrossRef]
10. Manoli, K.; Magliulo, M.; Mulla, M.Y.; Singh, M.; Sabbatini, L.; Palazzo, G.; Torsi, L. Printable bioelectronics to investigate functional biological interfaces. *Angew. Chem. Int. Ed.* **2015**, *54*, 12562–12576. [CrossRef]
11. Palazzo, G.; De Tullio, D.; Magliulo, M.; Mallardi, A.; Intranuovo, F.; Mulla, M.Y.; Favia, P.; Vikholm-Lundin, I.; Torsi, L. Detection beyond Debye's length with an electrolyte-gated organic field-effect transistor. *Adv. Mater.* **2015**, *27*, 911–916. [CrossRef] [PubMed]
12. Macchia, E.; Manoli, K.; Holzer, B.; Di Franco, C.; Ghittorelli, M.; Torricelli, F.; Alberga, D.; Mangiatordi, G.F.; Palazzo, G.; Scamarcio, G.; et al. Single-molecule detection with a millimetre-sized transistor. *Nat. Commun.* **2018**, *9*, 3223. [CrossRef] [PubMed]
13. Macchia, E.; Tiwari, A.; Manoli, K.; Holzer, B.; Ditaranto, N.; Picca, R.A.; Cioffi, N.; Di Franco, C.; Scamarcio, G.; Palazzo, G.; et al. Label-Free and Selective Single-Molecule Bioelectronic Sensing with a Millimeter-Wide Self-Assembled Monolayer of Anti-Immunoglobulins. *Chem. Mater.* **2019**, *31*, 6476–6483. [CrossRef]
14. Holzer, B.; Manoli, K.; Ditaranto, N.; Macchia, E.; Tiwari, A.; Di Franco, C.; Scamarcio, G.; Palazzo, G.; Torsi, L. Characterization of covalently bound anti-human immunoglobulins on self-assembled monolayer modified gold electrodes. *Adv. Biosyst.* **2017**, *1*, 1700055. [CrossRef]
15. Macchia, E.; Manoli, K.; Holzer, B.; Di Franco, C.; Picca, R.A.; Cioffi, N.; Scamarcio, G.; Palazzo, G.; Torsi, L. Selective single-molecule analytical detection of C-reactive protein in saliva with an organic transistor. *Anal. Bioanal. Chem.* **2019**, *411*, 4899–4908. [CrossRef] [PubMed]
16. Sailapu, S.K.; Macchia, E.; Merino-Jimenez, I.; Esquivel, J.P.; Sarcina, L.; Scamarcio, G.; Minteer, S.D.; Torsi, L.; Sabaté, N. Standalone operation of an EGOFET for ultra-sensitive detection of HIV. *Biosens. Bioelectron.* **2020**, *156*, 112103. [CrossRef]
17. Macchia, E.; Sarcina, L.; Picca, R.A.; Manoli, K.; Di Franco, C.; Scamarcio, G.; Torsi, L. Ultra-low HIV-1 p24 detection limits with a bioelectronic sensor. *Anal. Bioanal. Chem.* **2020**, *412*, 811–818. [CrossRef]

18. Macchia, E.; Manoli, K.; Di Franco, C.; Picca, R.; Osterbacka, R.; Palazzo, G.; Torricelli, F.; Scamarcio, G.; Torsi, L. Organic field-effect transistor platform for label-free single-molecule detection of genomic biomarkers. *ACS Sens.* **2020**, *5*, 1822–1830. [CrossRef]
19. He, X.P.; Hu, X.L.; James, T.D.; Yoon, J.; Tian, H. Multiplexed photoluminescent sensors: Towards improved disease diagnostics. *Chem. Soc. Rev.* **2017**, *46*, 6687–6696. [CrossRef]
20. Iino, R.; Lam, L.; Tabata, K.V.; Rondelez, Y.; Noji, H. Single-molecule assay of biological reaction in femtoliter chamber array. *Jpn. J. Appl. Phys.* **2009**, *48*, 6–11. [CrossRef]
21. Engvall, E.; Jonsson, K.; Perlmann, P. Antiserum, immunoglobulin fraction, and specific antibodies Iodinated proteins. *Biochim. Biophys. Acta.* **1971**, *251*, 427–434. [CrossRef]
22. Casalini, S.; Leonardi, F.; Cramer, T.; Biscarini, F. Organic field-effect transistor for label-free dopamine sensing. *Org. Electron.* **2013**, *14*, 156–163. [CrossRef]
23. Berto, M.; Diacci, C.; Theuer, L.; Di Lauro, M.; Simon, D.T.; Berggren, M.; Biscarini, F.; Beni, V.; Bortolotti, C.A. Label free urea biosensor based on organic electrochemical transistors. *Flex. Print. Electron.* **2018**, *3*, 24001. [CrossRef]
24. Yang, S.Y.; DeFranco, J.A.; Sylvester, Y.A.; Gobert, T.J.; Macaya, D.J.; Owens, R.M.; Malliaras, G.G. Integration of a surface-directed microfluidic system with an organic electrochemical transistor array for multi-analyte biosensors. *Lab Chip* **2009**, *9*, 704–708. [CrossRef] [PubMed]
25. Patel, N.; Davies, M.C.; Hartshorne, M.; Heaton, R.J.; Roberts, C.J.; Tendler, S.J.B.; Williams, P.M. Immobilization of protein molecules onto homogeneous and mixed carboxylate-terminated self-assembled monolayers. *Langmuir* **1997**, *13*, 6485–6490. [CrossRef]
26. Lee, J.W.; Sim, S.J.; Cho, S.M.; Lee, J. Characterization of a self-assembled monolayer of thiol on a gold surface and the fabrication of a biosensor chip based on surface plasmon resonance for detecting anti-GAD antibody. *Biosens. Bioelectron.* **2005**, *20*, 1422–1427. [CrossRef] [PubMed]
27. Hideshima, S.; Sato, R.; Inoue, S.; Kuroiwa, S.; Osaka, T. Detection of tumor marker in blood serum using antibody-modified field effect transistor with optimized BSA blocking. *Sens. Actuators B Chem.* **2012**, *161*, 146–150. [CrossRef]
28. Blasi, D.; Sarcina, L.; Tricase, A.; Stefanachi, A.; Leonetti, F.; Alberga, D.; Mangiatordi, G.F.; Manoli, K.; Scamarcio, G.; Picca, R.A.; et al. Enhancing the sensitivity of biotinylated surfaces by tailoring the design of the mixed self-assembled monolayers synthesis. *ACS Omega* **2020**, in press. [CrossRef]
29. Homola, J. Present and future of surface plasmon resonance biosensors. *Anal. Bioanal. Chem.* **2003**, *377*, 528–539. [CrossRef]
30. Biacore Sensor Surface Handbook. Available online: https://timothyspringer.org/files/tas/files/biacore3000-sensorsurface.pdf. (accessed on 29 June 2020).
31. Miura, N.; Sasaki, M.; Gobi, K.V.; Kataoka, C. Highly sensitive and selective surface plasmon resonance sensor for detection of sub-ppb levels of benzo [a] pyrene by indirect competitive immunoreaction method. *Biosens. Bioelectron.* **2003**, *18*, 953–959. [CrossRef]
32. Disley, D.M.; Cullen, D.C.; You, H.X.; Lowe, C.R. Covalent coupling of immunoglobulin G to self-assembled monolayers as a method for immobilizing the interfacial-recognition layer of a surface plasmon resonance immunosensor. *Biosens. Bioelectron.* **1998**, *13*, 1213–1225. [CrossRef]
33. Liu, L.; Deng, D.; Xing, Y.; Li, S.; Yuan, B.; Chen, J.; Xia, N. Activity analysis of the carbodiimide-mediated amine coupling reaction on self-assembled monolayers by cyclic voltammetry. *Electrochim. Acta* **2013**, *89*, 616–622. [CrossRef]
34. Thermofisher INSTRUCTIONS NHS and Sulfo-NHS. Available online: https://www.thermofisher.com/document-connect/document-connect.html?url=https%3A%2F%2Fassets.thermofisher.com%2FTFS-Assets%2FLSG%2Fmanuals%2FMAN0011309_NHS_SulfoNHS_UG.pdf&title=VXNlciBHdWlkZTogIE5IUyBhbmQgU3VsZm8tTkhT (accessed on 29 June 2020).
35. Grabarek, Z.; Gergely, J. Zero-length crosslinking procedure with the use of active esters. *Anal. Biochem.* **1990**, *185*, 131–135. [CrossRef]
36. de Mol, N.J.; Fischer, M.J.E. Surface plasmon resonance: Methods and protocols. *Life Sci.* **2010**, *627*, 255. [CrossRef]
37. Tsai, T.C.; Liu, C.W.; Wu, Y.C.; Ondevilla, N.A.P.; Osawa, M.; Chang, H.C. In situ study of EDC/NHS immobilization on gold surface based on attenuated total reflection surface-enhanced infrared absorption spectroscopy (ATR-SEIRAS). *Colloids Surf. B Biointerfaces* **2019**, *175*, 300–305. [CrossRef]

38. Goyon, A.; Excoffier, M.; Janin-Bussat, M.-C.; Bobaly, B.; Fekete, S.; Guillarme, D.; Beck, A. Determination of isoelectric points and relative charge variants of 23 therapeutic monoclonal antibodies. *J. Chromatogr. B* **2017**, *1065–1066*, 119–128. [CrossRef]
39. Erk, T. Gedig surface chemistry in SPR technology. In *Handbook of Surface Plasmon Resonance*; Richard, B.M.S., Ed.; The Royal Society of Chemistry: Cambridge, UK, 2017; pp. 173–220. ISBN 978-1-78801-028-3.
40. Glaser, R.W. Antigen-antibody binding and mass transport by convection and diffusion to a surface: A two-dimensional computer model of binding and dissociation kinetics. *Anal. Biochem.* **1993**, *213*, 152–161. [CrossRef]
41. León-Janampa, N.; Zimic, M.; Shinkaruk, S.; Quispe-Marcatoma, J.; Gutarra, A.; Le Bourdon, G.; Gayot, M.; Changanaqui, K.; Gilman, R.H.; Fouquet, E.; et al. Synthesis, characterization and bio-functionalization of magnetic nanoparticles to improve the diagnosis of tuberculosis. *Nanotechnology* **2020**, *31*, 175101. [CrossRef]
42. Darain, F.; Gan, K.L.; Tjin, S.C. Antibody immobilization on to polystyrene substrate—On-chip immunoassay for horse IgG based on fluorescence. *Biomed. Microdevices* **2009**, *11*, 653–661. [CrossRef]
43. Mariani, S.; Minunni, M. Surface plasmon resonance applications in clinical analysis. *Anal. Bioanal. Chem.* **2014**, *406*, 2303–2323. [CrossRef]
44. Puiu, M.; Bala, C. SPR and SPR imaging: Recent trends in developing nanodevices for detection and real-time monitoringof biomolecular events. *Sensors* **2016**, *16*, 870. [CrossRef]
45. Jiang, T.; Minunni, M.; Wilson, P.; Zhang, J.; Turner, A.P.F.; Mascini, M. Detection of TP53 mutation using a portable surface plasmon resonance DNA-based biosensor. *Biosens. Bioelectron.* **2005**, *20*, 1939–1945. [CrossRef]
46. Dubacheva, G.V.; Araya-Callis, C.; Geert Volbeda, A.; Fairhead, M.; Codée, J.; Howarth, M.; Richter, R.P. Controlling multivalent binding through surface chemistry: Model study on Streptavidin. *J. Am. Chem. Soc.* **2017**, *139*, 4157–4167. [CrossRef]
47. BioNavis MP-SPR Navi LayerSolver User Manual. Available online: http://www.bionavis.com/en/material-science/products/additional-options-and-consumables/software-mp-spr-navi/layersolver/ (accessed on 29 June 2020).
48. Baniukevic, J.; Kirlyte, J.; Ramanavicius, A.; Ramanaviciene, A. Comparison of oriented and random antibody immobilization techniques on the efficiency of immunosensor. *Procedia Eng.* **2012**, *47*, 837–840. [CrossRef]
49. Tsai, W.C.; Li, I.C. SPR-based immunosensor for determining staphylococcal enterotoxin A. *Sens. Actuators B Chem.* **2009**, *136*, 8–12. [CrossRef]
50. Frederix, F.; Bonroy, K.; Laureyn, W.; Reekmans, G.; Campitelli, A.; Dehaen, W.; Maes, G. Enhanced performance of an affinity biosensor interface based on mixed self-assembled monolayers of thiols on gold. *Langmuir* **2003**, *19*, 4351–4357. [CrossRef]
51. Kang, C.D.; Cao, C.; Lee, J.; Choi, I.S.; Kim, B.W.; Sim, S.J. Surface plasmon resonance-based inhibition assay for real-time detection of Cryptosporidium parvum oocyst. *Water Res.* **2008**, *42*, 1693–1699. [CrossRef] [PubMed]
52. Liang, H.; Miranto, H.; Granqvist, N.; Sadowski, J.W.; Viitala, T.; Wang, B.; Yliperttula, M. Surface plasmon resonance instrument as a refractometer for liquids and ultrathin films. *Sens. Actuators B Chem.* **2010**, *149*, 212–220. [CrossRef]
53. Mytych, D.T.; La, S.; Barger, T.; Ferbas, J.; Swanson, S.J. The development and validation of a sensitive, dual-flow cell, SPR-based biosensor immunoassay for the detection, semi-quantitation, and characterization of antibodies to darbepoetin alfa and epoetin alfa in human serum. *J. Pharm. Biomed. Anal.* **2009**, *49*, 415–426. [CrossRef]
54. Šípová, H.; Ševců, V.; Kuchař, M.; Ahmad, J.N.; Mikulecký, P.; Osička, R.; Malý, P.; Homola, J. Surface plasmon resonance biosensor based on engineered proteins for direct detection of interferon-gamma in diluted blood plasma. *Sens. Actuators B Chem.* **2012**, *174*, 306–311. [CrossRef]
55. Picca, R.A.; Manoli, K.; Macchia, E.; Sarcina, L.; Di Franco, C.; Cioffi, N.; Blasi, D.; Österbacka, R.; Torricelli, F.; Scamarcio, G.; et al. Ultimately sensitive organic bioelectronic transistor sensors by materials and device structures' design. *Adv. Funct. Mater.* **2019**, *30*, 1904513. [CrossRef]
56. Macchia, E.; Picca, R.A.; Manoli, K.; Di Franco, C.; Blasi, D.; Sarcina, L.; Ditaranto, N.; Cioffi, N.; Österbacka, R.; Scamarcio, G.; et al. About the amplification factors in organic bioelectronic sensors. *Mater. Horiz.* **2020**, *7*, 999–1013. [CrossRef]

4

A Plug and Play IoT Wi-Fi Smart Home System for Human Monitoring

Marco Bassoli, Valentina Bianchi * and Ilaria De Munari

Department of Engineering and Architecture, University of Parma, Parco Area delle Scienze, 181/A, 43124 Parma, Italy; marco.bassoli@studenti.unipr.it (M.B.); ilaria.demunari@unipr.it (I.D.M.)
* Correspondence: valentina.bianchi@unipr.it

Abstract: The trend toward technology ubiquity in human life is constantly increasing and the same tendency is clear in all technologies aimed at human monitoring. In this framework, several smart home system architectures have been presented in literature, realized by combining sensors, home servers, and online platforms. In this paper, a new system architecture suitable for human monitoring based on Wi-Fi connectivity is introduced. The proposed solution lowers costs and implementation burden by using the Internet connection that leans on standard home modem-routers, already present normally in the homes, and reducing the need for range extenders thanks to the long range of the Wi-Fi signal. Since the main drawback of the Wi-Fi implementation is the high energy drain, low power design strategies have been considered to provide each battery-powered sensor with a lifetime suitable for a consumer application. Moreover, in order to consider the higher consumption arising in the case of the Wi-Fi/Internet connectivity loss, dedicated operating cycles have been introduced obtaining an energy savings of up to 91%. Performance was evaluated: in order to validate the use of the system as a hardware platform for behavioral services, an activity profile of a user for two months in a real context has been extracted.

Keywords: smart homes; Internet of Things (IoT); Wi-Fi; human monitoring; behavioral analysis

---

1. Introduction

The concept of a Smart Home has evolved remarkably over the past few decades. Initially, the Smart Home coincided with Home Automation intended as technological solutions applied to the home environment to automatically manage some situations (e.g., open doors/curtains, control thermostat) and detect dangerous events (e.g., fire, flood), freeing the user from manual control [1]. Now, the evolution of ICT (Information and Communication Technologies) has allowed for the addition of many advanced features to smart homes over time, extending the possible applications. Among the advancements, the monitoring of human activity in the home environment has particular importance. Modern systems exploit human monitoring mainly to improve the energy management of the building [2–7]. However, data related to the users and how they live in their own home environment can find straightforward applications in health management, allowing for early detection of behavioral trends and anomalies possibly relevant to one's wellbeing [8–14].

To accomplish this task, some new devices have to be developed [15] aimed at considering the interaction of the user with the home environment (e.g., armchair sensors to monitor inactivity periods, toilet sensors, etc.). These devices must be able to send data over the Internet so that, once processed, they can be accessed by the various professionals involved, for example, medical doctors, caregivers, relatives, and the users themselves.

Applications based on such a system have been presented in past works. For example, an infrastructure based on a Passive InfraRed (PIR), bed and temperature sensors was reported in [16]. In this case, data transmission was based on the X10 wireless protocol, and a home server was exploited to process data and to send analyses and alerts to a third person (i.e., the clinician) through emails. Another monitoring system based on temperature, pressure, PIR sensors, and actuators was described in [17]. Sensors communicated with a local computer by means of a wireless ZigBee protocol. Data were processed to monitor the activities of elders, and the results determined which actions were taken. The system proposed in [18] leans on a mix of ZigBee and Power Line Communication (PLC) transmission protocols. The architecture was conceived with distinct ZigBee Wireless Sensor Networks (WSNs) in each room, which communicate with a central management station through a PLC. An infrastructure exploiting a custom wireless protocol, the so called Wellness protocol, was presented in [19]. The implementation was based on temperature, pressure sensors, PIR sensors, a manual alert button, and actuators. Another example of such a system was CARDEA (Computer-Aided, Rule-based Domestic Environment Assistant), developed at the University of Parma and specifically aimed at behavioral analysis. Originally based on the Ethernet protocol [20,21], the system's strength is flexibility. It is conceived to integrate different kinds of sensors and to support smart interfaces [22,23], in order to tailor the system's functions to the specific users' needs. By supporting a wireless protocol (i.e., IEEE 802.15.4/ZigBee) as well, further kinds of devices were introduced; the most remarkable is the wearable sensor MuSA (MUltiSensor Assistant) [24–27], designed for user motion analysis (e.g., fall monitoring) and for localization and identification purposes [28,29].

Most of the systems presented in the literature based their connectivity on wireless protocols, typically ZigBee [30–32], due to the low cost and power consumption. Coupling the low power required by a ZigBee transmission with recent developments in the field of energy harvesting, it is now possible to develop battery-less Internet of Things (IoT) nodes [33,34]. However, powering the ZigBee protocol tasks for prolonged periods of time (i.e., >10 s) with energy harvesters is not recommended [35]. Some advanced functions (e.g., localization or identification [36]), useful in smart home systems conceived for the continuous monitoring of the individual and for behavioral analysis, can be prevented. Moreover, the disadvantage of the ZigBee approach is mainly the necessity of a completely new and dedicated infrastructure in each home in which the system is going to be deployed, since, typically, a network compliant with these standards is not already present. Furthermore, a gateway device has to be considered as an interface between the home protocol and the Ethernet, in addition to a number of range extenders due to the low range featured by ZigBee [37].

In this paper, we present a new home monitoring system entirely based on Wi-Fi connectivity, in a fashion strictly compliant with the Internet of Thing (IoT) paradigm. Sensors connect to the Internet through a standard Wi-Fi home router, which is quite often already present in the homes. Some manufacturers are already producing chips for routers which are able to support Wi-Fi, Bluetooth, and ZigBee protocols in parallel (e.g., Qualcomm QCA4020 and QCA4024 [38]). These solutions could simplify the adoption of multiple protocols in the near future, but do not eliminate the need for building a complete infrastructure for the ZigBee sensors and in particular for deploying range extenders in the environment. On the contrary, Wi-Fi features a much wider range than ZigBee, so that no (or fewer) network extenders are needed, simplifying the overall approach, lowering the costs, and making the whole system more scalable. These characteristics open the market to the system making it particularly attractive to consumers. This, of course, comes at the expense of increasing power consumption, which may harm battery lifetime. Therefore, we carefully designed sensor platforms for low-power operation. An extensive account for the exploited design methodologies is given in [39], where it is shown that the obtained battery lifetimes are suitable for practical exploitation.

Based on such preliminary studies, we developed a complete set of specific sensor prototypes, providing expressive information relevant to behavioral inference. In [16,40–42] some examples on how the sensor data can be processed and elaborated to extract patterns in the behaviors of home occupants are given. The present work is an extension of a published conference paper [43] where a brief description of the sensors is given. Here, more details about the developed hardware are given, and the proposed system hardware infrastructure is validated. The sensors have been tested both in a laboratory and in a real home environment. Some measurements about the power consumption are presented.

Moreover, during the tests, the sensors' data were logged to carry out a possible activity profile of the users in order to test the system performance. It is worth stressing that the aim of this work is not to develop and demonstrate a new behavioral analysis method, but to present a new hardware architecture conceived to collect data usable by behavioral analysis models developed elsewhere [16,40–42]. These tests show the usability and convenience of data collected and demonstrate that it is possible to take advantage of the flexibility of the Wi-Fi platform while eliminating costs given by the need of additional hardware (i.e., home servers and routers, adopted in [13–16]).

The paper is organized in four sections. After an introduction, a detailed description of the Wi-Fi architecture is presented in Section 2. In Section 3, experimental results are discussed, then in Section 4, conclusions are drawn.

2. Materials and Methods: The Wi-Fi System

2.1. System Architecture

The general system architecture is sketched in Figure 1. It includes a set of sensing devices, a Wi-Fi router, and services installed on a cloud environment. We currently exploit the IBM Bluemix Watson IoT platform (IBM, Armonk, NY, USA). The system is open to third-party and new device addition. We plan to integrate both custom-designed and commercial Wi-Fi devices in a seamless fashion.

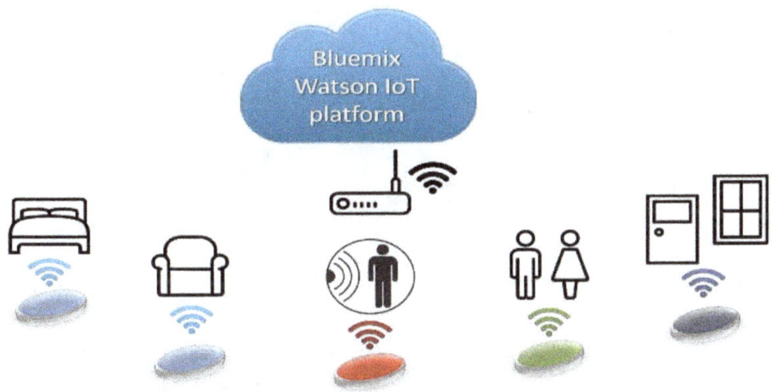

Figure 1. CARDEA (Computer-Aided, Rule-based Domestic Environment Assistant) Wi-Fi system architecture. IoT = Internet of Things.

Here, we discuss the custom design of a subset of sensors specifically aimed at behavioral analysis. Based on outcomes of previous European projects in which the ZigBee version was exploited [44], we defined the following device list:

- Armchair (or Bed) occupancy sensor, to monitor inactivity periods or sleep disorders;
- Passive InfraRed (PIR), to monitor the movements inside the house;
- Toilet sensor, to monitor the toilet accesses;
- Magnetic contact, to detect door and windows opening/closing. The same device can be used to monitor interaction with other meaningful objects (e.g., a cupboard door, to monitor feeding habits, or the medicine cabinet, for monitoring compliance with therapy prescriptions).

All sensors are directly and individually connected to the Internet through the Wi-Fi home router. The commissioning procedure is very simple and relies on the Wi-Fi Protected Setup (WPS) standard. No technical skill is required, so that consumers themselves could manage the installation procedure. Data are sent to the Watson IoT platform, inside the IBM Bluemix cloud services, via MQTT (Message Queue Telemetry Transport) protocol with a Quality of Service (QoS) equal to 2. This ensures the necessary reliability of the transmission process, since the protocol itself ensures that the message is received by the broker once and once only. The payload of the message is a string in a JSON (JavaScript Object Notation) format, reporting the sensor status. The device firmware, nevertheless, is suitable for connecting to other platforms as well (e.g., Amazon AWS (Amazon Web Services) (Amazon, Seattle, WA, USA), Microsoft Azure (Microsoft, Redmond, WA, USA), Thingspeak (MathWorks, Natick, MA, USA), etc.).

2.2. Sensors Prototypes

A Wi-Fi certified system-on-chip (SoC) (CC3200, Texas Instruments, Dallas, TX, USA [45]) was chosen as the core of all sensors. It integrates an 80 MHz clock MCU (MicroController Unit) with a 32-bit architecture and a network processor (compliant with the IEEE 802.11b/g/n network radio protocol).

For prototyping purposes, commercial development boards were exploited as the motherboard for all the devices. By connecting the same motherboard to different sensing devices, different sensors were built, sharing the architecture, thus reducing development costs. The sensors are shown in Figure 2.

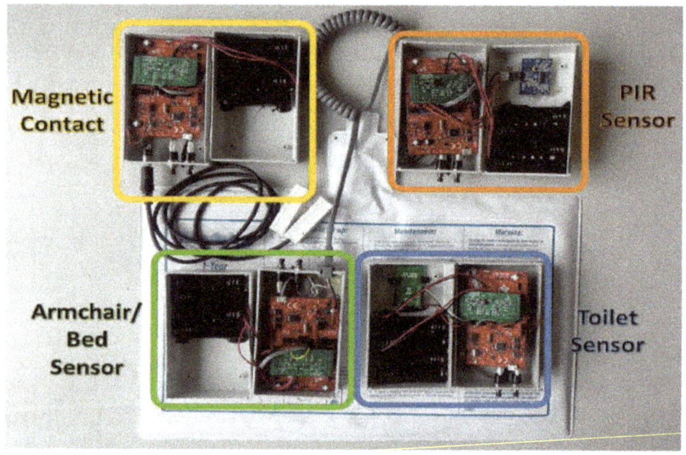

Figure 2. The sensors prototypes. PIR = Passive InfraRed.

All the devices can be powered from an AC (Alternating Current) outlet (through a standard USB port). This possibility eliminates the need to control and replace the batteries. However, the sensors' position is very important to efficiently monitor the users' activities. This position has to be independent of where the outlets have been set up in the house, but, at the same time, it is necessary to avoid wires in the room or to modify the existing home electrical system. For this reason, the devices are also conceived for battery-powered operation. In order to preserve battery lifetime, careful management of the energy budget was implemented. In particular, simple sensors do not need to fully exploit the Wi-Fi data transmission rate, since a limited quantity of data have to be exchanged over time. So, taking advantage of such an overabundant data rate, sleep phases are introduced in the operating cycle. The devices alternate active (data processing and transmission) and sleep intervals. Among available low power modes of the MCU, the Low-Power Deep Sleep (LPDS) and the HIBERNATE modes were exploited. In LPDS mode, the MCU stops its main clock while the radio module is active and maintains the connection with the network. The device is more reactive to external interrupts and features low wake up times. In HIBERNATE mode, the radio section is also turned off. Hence, HIBERNATE is the most effective in power saving, but, when awakening from hibernation, the device needs to re-connect to the network. Wake up times are in the order of tens of seconds, so hibernation is convenient when the sleep time is long enough. In our previous study [39], it was shown that the overall power performance of LPDS mode is better than HIBERNATE whenever a large enough frequency of messages (higher than 150 message/day) is to be managed. Considering the fact that all the sensors need to send a keep-alive message (every 15 minutes, in the application at hand), hibernation turns out to be practical whenever only a few tens of actual "events" per day are expected to occur. Among the sensors presented in this first implementation of the Wi-Fi system, this characteristic may fit with Armchair/Bed sensors, Toilet sensors and the several uses of the Magnetic contact. On the other hand, LPDS mode may be a better fit for higher frequency events, as happens for the PIR sensor. Based on such general assumptions, in the following specific implementation, details are given for each device.

- Armchair/Bed sensor: In [46], a characterization of three different chair sensor elements is presented: a strain gauge, a mechanical switch, and a vibration sensor. Highest detection accuracy is reported for the mechanical switch, but this kind of sensor is more difficult to integrate in an ordinary home chair/bed since it is not straightforward to cover the whole sitting area. For our application, the strain gauge seems the most indicated choice. Indeed, resistive pressure pads are being commercialized which can be placed under the bed mattress or over the chair seat. These pads have been selected as sensing elements. Resistance change is assessed through a simple voltage divider, which drives a binary threshold comparator. This, in turn, generates an interrupt to wake up the MCU. As mentioned, given the relatively low expected number of events, the HIBERNATE sleep mode is exploited during idle phases.
- Magnetic Contact: The sensing element is a reed switch, coupled to a magnet. When the two components are close to each other, the switch opens. This configuration is particularly convenient when drawers/doors are supposed to stay closed most of the time. Since the reed switch is open when they are closed, the sensor drains no current while in this state. Interrupts are generated to signal both transitions (close to open, open to close). In this case, selection of sleep mode depends on the actual device function. If, for instance, applied to the home main door, the HIBERNATE mode seems to be more effective again.
- Toilet sensor: The sensing element is a distance/proximity sensor. The sensor purpose is to allow for counting toilet visits (which may be relevant to many medical conditions), distinguishing them from generic bathroom presence (due to washing, for instance), which could be assessed though a PIR sensor. A short-enough, personalized reading range is therefore needed to cope with the actual placement of the sensor itself. The device has a reading range from 10 cm to 150 cm. The analog reading is fed to a comparator, which generates an interrupt signal to the system core. In our experiments, we found that calibrating the sensor threshold at 65 cm distance was effective in discriminating toilet actual usage from generic bathroom presence. The nature of this sensor should make it suitable to exploit the benefits of the HIBERNATE mode. However, due to the high current consumption of the sensing element during its on state, the system core needs to power it on only when a distance reading is needed, keeping it in the off state otherwise. In our tests, we found that a period of 3 seconds for power off followed by 0.5 s of power on gives the optimal system reactivity. Since the sensing element duty cycle is driven by the MCU, LPDS mode had to be adopted.
- PIR sensor: the sensing device is a standard passive-infrared motion sensor. It requires a supply voltage in the range of 3.3–5 V. In order to allow the system to be powered by AA batteries (as a common feature of all devices), a boost DC-DC regulator (direct current to direct current power converter that steps up voltage) has been added. The device already has embedded converters and provides a digital output signal, which is used to wake up the system core whenever a movement is detected. To avoid communication overload, PIR data are filtered on board; only status changes are transmitted, besides keep-alive messages. In the envisaged scenario, however, this results in a number of daily messages exceeding the above-mentioned threshold, which makes the adoption of hibernation not suitable and makes the adoption of LPDS mode preferable.

3. Results and Discussion

To evaluate the system, field tests were performed for two months.

For standby battery-lifetime evaluation, a full set of sensors was installed in a laboratory environment. The power consumption depended on the frequency of the occurring interactions with the sensor events. To determine a figure that allows for the comparison between sensors, only power consumption caused by the keep-alive events sent every 15 minutes were considered.

In order to estimate the battery lifetime in a working condition similar to the real one, another full set of sensors was installed in a real home environment inhabited by a family.

The sensors were deployed accordingly to their purpose:

- Armchair sensor: Sensor pad placed on a lunchroom chair.
- Magnetic contact: On the bedroom door.
- Toilet sensor: Inside the bathroom to sense toilet interactions.
- PIR sensor: Inside the bedroom.

The performance of the whole system was investigated, manually registering the user-sensor interactions and comparing them with the events reported by the sensors themselves.

Test details and results are given in the following subsections.

3.1. Power Consumption Analysis

In a previous work [39], preliminary laboratory tests about the sensors' power consumption were carried out. In this paper, we report an actual characterization of the system.

In the tests shown in [39], we assumed that the connection to the Wi-Fi network and to the Internet were reasonably stable. In real operation, this is not always true, and in order to consider possible disruptions that a consumer may experience, two main issues were evaluated:

- Sensor unable to connect to the Wi-Fi network: The system, after power on, is configured to search for the previously known network (through the WPS procedure) until connection succeeds; if the network connection is broken (e.g., because of a blackout), the device performs a reboot. The system always experiences an energy-expensive boot-loop until the network is restored;
- Sensor connected to the Wi-Fi network but without an active Internet access (e.g., because of Internet provider issues): This situation arises only after the previous condition is met. After power on, the device searches and connects to the known network; it tries to establish a connection with the online cloud. If the procedure fails (e.g., because the Internet connection is lost), a reboot is performed. The result is the same, with the system always in an energy-expensive boot-loop until the internet connection is restored.

To better understand the consequences of this behavior on the actual current consumption, each scenario was reproduced and current measurements were carried out using a digital oscilloscope with a bandwidth of 350 MHz, an ADC (Analog to Digital Converter) resolution of 12 bit, and a maximum sample rate of 1.25 GS/s. To measure the sensors current, a probe with a bandwidth of 50 MHz and a minimum sensitivity of 10 mA/div was exploited.

Results are shown in Figure 3. In Figure 3a, the device settles at an almost constant current absorption of 14.2 mA while waiting for the network connection, with an averaged 71.4 mA current while searching for a Wi-Fi connection. In Figure 3b, phases in which the system is not using the radio module (during reboot) with a 101 mA peak current absorption can be identified, as well as a 74.3 mA peak current when the Wi-Fi connection succeeded and tried to establish connection to the cloud.

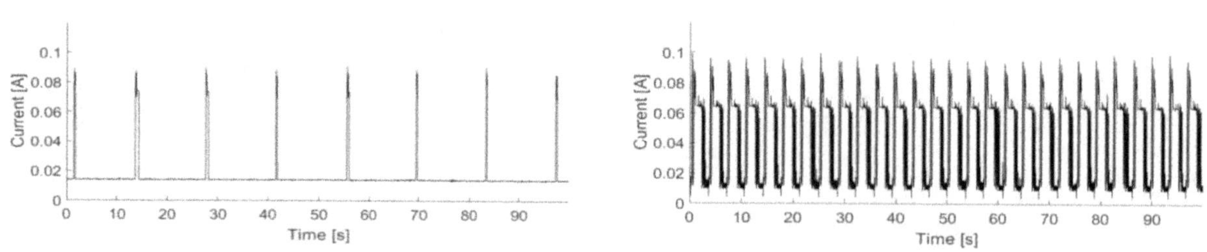

(a) (b)

Figure 3. Current absorption measurements: (**a**) scenario with missing Wi-Fi network connection; (**b**) scenario with sensor connected to Wi-Fi but without internet access.

By the analysis of those data, a total mean current of 17.3 mA can be extracted for the first scenario, and a total mean current of 34.5 mA for the second one. This behavior can significantly degrade sensors' energy performance. To overcome this problem, and hence to extend battery lifetime, the device is forced to follow a duty-cycled sequence of searching and sleeping phases, as shown in Figure 4.

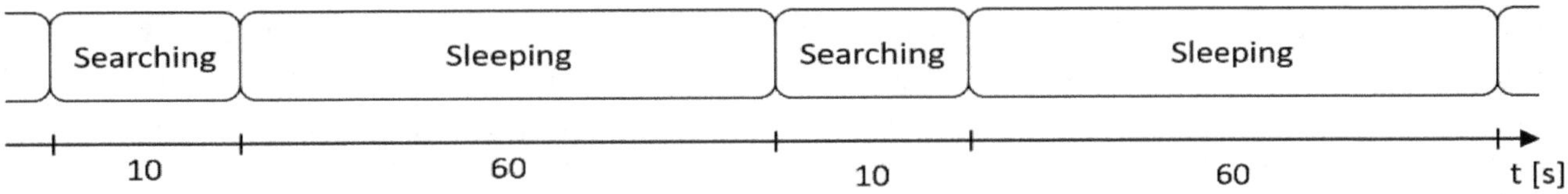

Figure 4. Working phases for both Wi-Fi and Internet absence scenarios.

The device is allowed to check for the presence of the Wi-Fi network or the Internet connectivity for a maximum period of 10 s. After this time, if the task fails, the system enters in a HIBERNATE sleep mode for 60 s to save energy and preserve battery charge. After the sleeping phase, a new search phase begins. This behavior has been tested and compared with the standard one for the same scenarios. The new current measurements are shown in Figure 5.

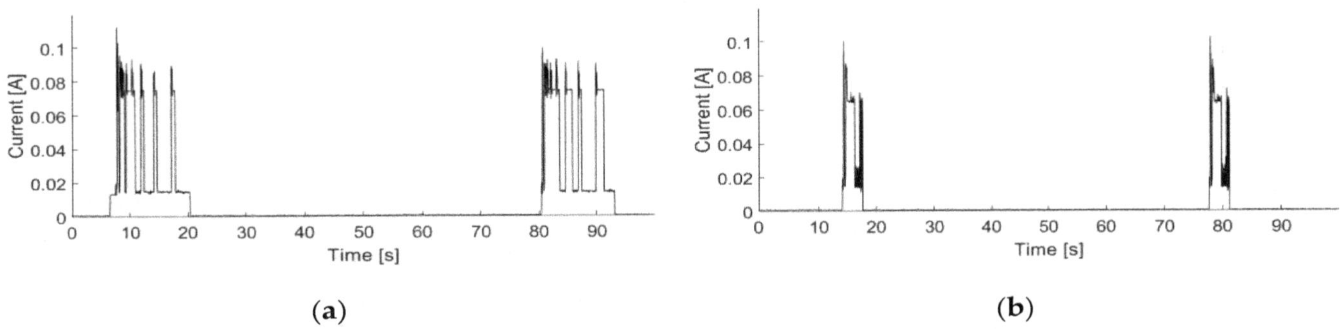

Figure 5. Current absorption measurements of sensors running with the introduced sleep periods: (**a**) scenario with missing Wi-Fi network connection; (**b**) scenario with sensor connected to Wi-Fi but without internet access.

After a larger initial current peak needed by the device to boot up, some current peaks are experienced during the Wi-Fi/Internet check phase and they reach the minimum in the sleep phase. In this case, the total mean currents over the period are 7.3 mA in the first scenario and 3.1 mA in the second one. Due to the unpredictability of these situations, the advantage in terms of battery lifetime is not quantifiable; however, with this method, the system is able to reduce the energy consumption by 42% in the case of Wi-Fi network absence and by 91% in the case of Internet connectivity absence. Hence, this behavior has been adopted for all sensors, and the actual battery lifetime during real operation has been evaluated.

As stated before, the sensors' energy performance was evaluated in both laboratory and home environments. All sensors were powered with parallel-series of four AA LR6 alkaline batteries. In the laboratory test, due to the different activity profile expected in a public environment, we tested only the stand-by power consumption. The only signals sent were periodic (15 min) keep-alive messages. In the real home environment, instead, the sensors were stressed during the day by three different members of a family.

After two months of testing, only the toilet sensor ran out of battery: For the other sensors, the laboratory set shows a residual charge of about 46%, while in the home environment this value is lower at 34%. It is worth considering that the battery lifetime in a real home environment strongly depends on the actual interaction with the sensors (e.g., the Magnetic contact can be stressed by more than one user, affecting the expected daily events and the sensor energetic performance). Moreover, as expected, the toilet sensor has a higher energy consumption because of the usage of LPDS mode and due to the higher power consumption of the sensible element. For this reason, the toilet battery lifetime was 30 days.

3.2. Behavioral Tests and Results

To evaluate the system accuracy, sensitivity, and specificity, one user manually took note of his interactions with the sensors for two months. These data were compared with the events generated by the sensors and automatically collected into the cloud platform. This analysis could effectively be done, in our scenario, only with the chair sensor, in fact, data for the Magnetic contact, Toilet and PIR sensors cannot be univocally assigned to a specific person, in an environment populated by more than one end-user. To resolve this situation a user identification mechanism should be considered [36,47].

In the case of the chair sensor, a total of 218 events were detected as follows: 99 True Positives (TP), 109 True Negatives (TN), 0 False Positives (FP), and 10 False Negatives (FN). Then, the accuracy, sensitivity, and specificity were carried out [48]:

$$Accuracy = \frac{TP + TN}{TP + TN + FP + FN} = 95\% \tag{1}$$

$$Sensitivity = \frac{TP}{TP + FN} = 91\% \tag{2}$$

$$Specificity = \frac{TN}{TN + FP} = 100\% \tag{3}$$

where TP, TN, FP, and FN are defined as reported in Table 1.

Table 1. Definition of True Positives (TP), True Negatives (TN), False Positives (FP), and False Negatives (FN).

Symbol	Position of the User	Where the User is Identified
TP	user seated on the chair	user detected as seated on the chair
TN	user not seated on the chair	user not detected as seated on the chair
FP	user not seated on the chair	user detected as seated on the chair
FN	user seated on the chair	user not detected as seated on the chair

The results presented show that our sensor is definitely capable of providing occupancy information in a real context. In [46], the reported averaged accuracy for a resistive strain gauge was 94%. This value is compatible with our results. We can conclude that the performance of our sensors are attributable to the resistive pressure pad. Nowadays, the pressure pad is the best choice due to its commercial availability and because it does not require specialized installation. Better performance could be obtained by replacing the sensing element, without affecting the system architecture.

Some elaborations on the data acquired from all the sensors has been performed to demonstrate the possibility of identifying patterns in the user's activity. For each sensor, two different cases have been considered:

- Daily activity: the distribution of the user-sensor interactions during a 24 h period was analyzed. In Figures 6a, 7a, 8a and 9a the probability of an event in a certain hour of the day is plotted. Values were obtained through the analysis of the activity per hour of every test day. The relative probability v_i was calculated with the equation

$$v_i = \frac{c_i}{N} \tag{4}$$

  where c_i is the number of events that occurred in the hour, \ and N is the total number of events observed during the test.
- Weekly activity: the interaction was assessed during a week, counting the events registered in different three-hour intervals in the same day of the week (Figures 6b–9b).

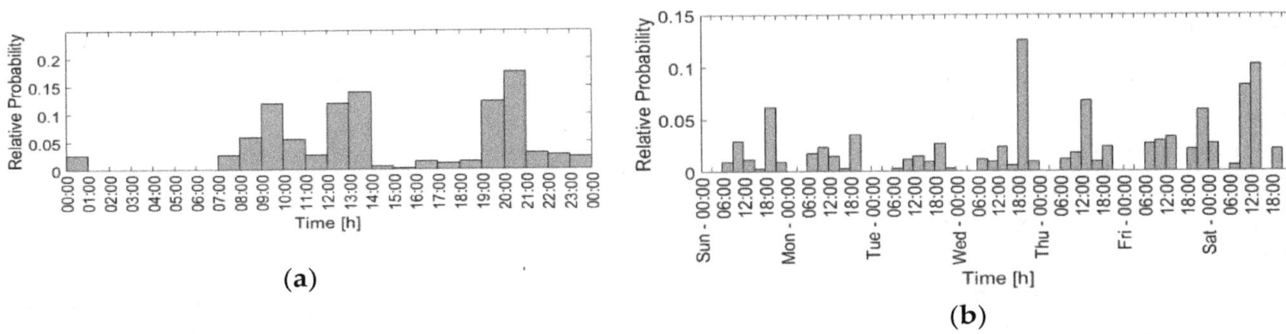

Figure 6. Armchair sensor activity during the day (**a**) and during the week (**b**).

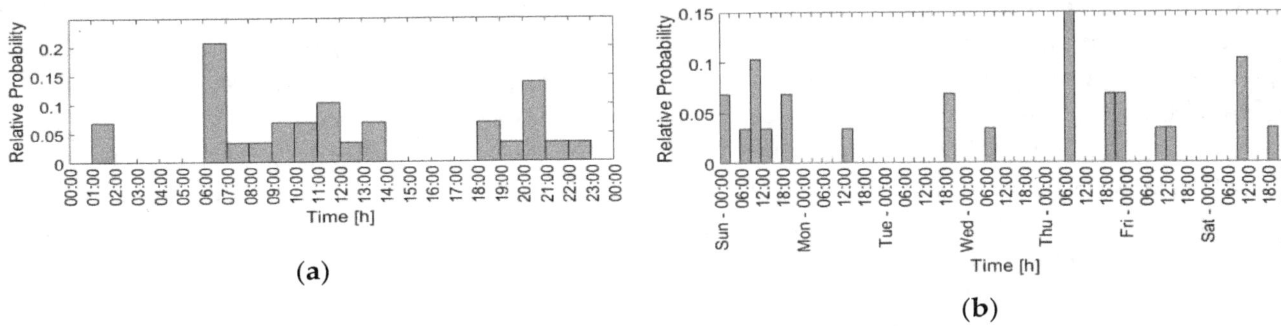

Figure 7. Magnetic contact (door sensor) activity during the day (**a**) and during the week (**b**).

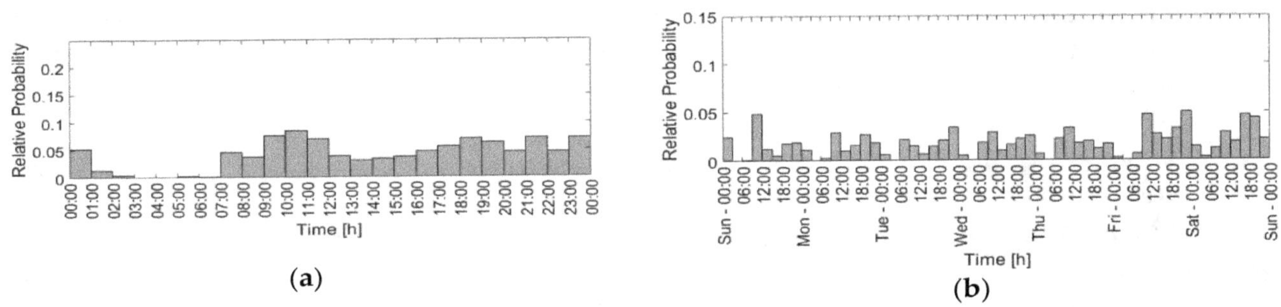

Figure 8. PIR sensor activity during the day (**a**) and during the week (**b**).

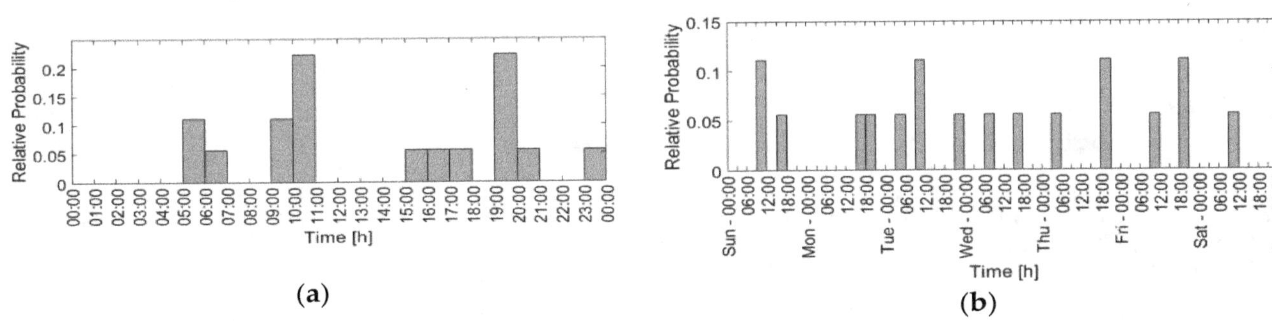

Figure 9. Toilet sensor activity during the day (**a**) and during the week (**b**).

Although the aim of this paper was not to present a complete behavioral analysis module, simple trend information might be extracted from the results, demonstrating data convenience. For instance, a high lunchroom chair interaction can be seen during meals; the door openings are concentrated during the weekend, when the user is usually not at work. This fact can be confirmed by the PIR weekly graphs, in which the activity distribution shows a higher presence starting from Friday. Looking at the Toilet sensor activity, a periodic usage can be seen around meal times and in the early morning after waking up. Moreover, as expected, no sensors recorded activities during nighttime, when the user is supposed to be sleep.

4. Conclusions

In this paper, a new Smart Home system architecture conceived for behavioral analysis and based on Wi-Fi connectivity has been presented. The aim is to present an alternative architecture compared to the more traditional ones based on protocols such as ZigBee. The ZigBee solutions are not typically already present in the home environment, and this causes some problems in the practical deployment, mainly due to the necessity of the set-up fo a new and complete network infrastructure for every system installation.

In the proposed architecture, the sensors are connected to the Internet through a standard Wi-Fi router, in an IoT compliant fashion, without the need to add a dedicated home gateway to ensure connectivity or the range extenders often needed when using other standard protocols. A complete set of new devices conceived to acquire data related to users' behaviors has been designed and developed.

Since the principal drawback of the Wi-Fi connectivity is the higher power consumption, low power design strategies have been considered and applied to demonstrate the possibility of using this architecture in the context of smart homes for behavioral monitoring. The whole system has been tested in a real environment to evaluate the feasibility of adopting it in a real situation.

For this study, two sets of sensors. composed of an Armchair sensor, a Magnetic contact, a Toilet sensor, and a PIR sensor, were run for two months. The first set was used to evaluate stand-by battery lifetime while the second one was placed in a real home environment, inhabited by a family, to evaluate real battery lifetime. After the two months of testing, only the Toilet sensor ran out of battery. For the other sensors, the laboratory set shows a residual charge of about 46%, while in the home environment this value was 34%. Furthermore, in some cases, the network could undergo connectivity issues; in these situations, dedicated operating cycles were introduced, instead of the standard ones, to reduce the impact on the battery lifetime. This lead to a reduction in the current absorption of 42% in the case of Wi-Fi network absence and of 91% in the case of a lack of Internet connectivity.

Moreover, in order to validate the possibility of using this system as a hardware platform for behavioral services, we have extracted, from the set of sensors installed in the home environment, a possible activity profile of an occupant. A user was assigned to take note of each interaction with the sensors for two months to test the system performance. The accuracy, sensitivity, and specificity were evaluated for the chair sensor (whose interaction, in our environment, can definitely be attributable to a single person) resulting in 95%, 91%, and 100%, respectively. These results show that our sensor is definitely capable of providing occupancy information in a real context.

In conclusion, exploiting Wi-Fi as an infrastructure for smart home systems conceived for human monitoring is a possible alternative to other systems based on protocols such as ZigBee, due to the low cost and ease of installation and use. The power consumption does not affect the usability, and the performance is not influenced by the system architecture.

Author Contributions: Conceptualization, V.B., I.D.M.; Methodology, V.B., I.D.M; Software, M.B.; Validation, V.B.; Formal Analysis, V.B., M.B.; Investigation, V.B., M.B.; Data Curation, V.B., M.B.; Writing-Original Draft Preparation, V.B., M.B.; Writing-Review and Editing, V.B., M.B., I.D.M.; Visualization, V.B., M.B, I.D.M.; Supervision, I.D.M; Project Administration, I.D.M.; Funding Acquisition, I.D.M.

Acknowledgments: The authors would like to acknowledge Federico Mendogni for the help with the experiments and prof. Paolo Ciampolini for his scientific guidance and advice.

References

1. Yerrapragada, C.; Fisher, P.S. Voice controlled smart house. In Proceedings of the IEEE 1993 International Conference on Consumer Electronics Digest of Technical, Rosemont, IL, USA, 8–10 June 1993. [CrossRef]
2. Shih, H.C. Automatic building monitoring and commissioning via human behavior recognition. In Proceedings of the 2016 IEEE 5th Global Conference on Consumer Electronics, Kyoto, Japan, 11–14 October 2016.

3. Hwang, I.K.; Lee, D.S.; Baek, J.W. Home network configuring scheme for all electric appliances using ZigBee-based integrated remote controller. *IEEE Trans. Consum. Electron.* **2009**, *55*, 1300–1307. [CrossRef]
4. Chen, C.-Y.; Liu, C.-Y.; Kuo, C.-C.; Yang, C.-F.; Chen, C.-Y.; Liu, C.-Y.; Kuo, C.-C.; Yang, C.-F. Web-Based Remote Control of a Building's Electrical Power, Green Power Generation and Environmental System Using a Distributive Microcontroller. *Micromachines* **2017**, *8*, 241. [CrossRef]
5. Lobaccaro, G.; Carlucci, S.; Löfström, E. A review of systems and technologies for smart homes and smart grids. *Energies* **2016**, *9*. [CrossRef]
6. Brusco, G.; Burgio, A.; Menniti, D.; Pinnarelli, A.; Sorrentino, N.; Scarcello, L.; Brusco, G.; Burgio, A.; Menniti, D.; Pinnarelli, A.; et al. An Energy Box in a Cloud-Based Architecture for Autonomous Demand Response of Prosumers and Prosumages. *Electronics* **2017**, *6*, 98. [CrossRef]
7. Froiz-Míguez, I.; Fernández-Caramés, T.; Fraga-Lamas, P.; Castedo, L.; Froiz-Míguez, I.; Fernández-Caramés, T.M.; Fraga-Lamas, P.; Castedo, L. Design, Implementation and Practical Evaluation of an IoT Home Automation System for Fog Computing Applications Based on MQTT and ZigBee-WiFi Sensor Nodes. *Sensors* **2018**, *18*, 2660. [CrossRef] [PubMed]
8. Ceccacci, S.; Generosi, A.; Giraldi, L.; Mengoni, M. An user-centered approach to design smart systems for people with dementia. In Proceedings of the 2017 IEEE 7th International Conference on Consumer Electronics-Berlin (ICCE-Berlin), Berlin, Germany, 3–6 September 2017.
9. Pal, D.; Funilkul, S.; Charoenkitkarn, N.; Kanthamanon, P. Internet-of-Things and Smart Homes for Elderly Healthcare: An End User Perspective. *IEEE Access* **2018**, *6*, 10483–10496. [CrossRef]
10. Vechet, S.; Hrbacek, J.; Krejsa, J. Environmental data analysis for learning behavioral patterns in smart homes. In Proceedings of the 2016 17th International Conference on Mechatronics-Mechatronika (ME), Prague, Czech Republic, 7–9 December 2016.
11. Thapliyal, H.; Nath, R.K.; Mohanty, S.P. Smart Home Environment for Mild Cognitive Impairment Population: Solutions to Improve Care and Quality of Life. *IEEE Consum. Electron. Mag.* **2018**, *7*, 68–76. [CrossRef]
12. Grossi, F.; Matrella, G.; De Munari, I.; Ciampolini, P. A flexible home automation system applied to elderly care. In Proceedings of the 2007 Digest of Technical Papers IEEE International Conference on Consumer Electronics, Las Vegas, NV, USA, 10–14 January 2007.
13. Saponara, S.; Donati, M.; Fanucci, L.; Celli, A.; Saponara, S.; Donati, M.; Fanucci, L.; Celli, A. An Embedded Sensing and Communication Platform, and a Healthcare Model for Remote Monitoring of Chronic Diseases. *Electronics* **2016**, *5*, 47. [CrossRef]
14. Sasakawa, D.; Honma, N.; Nakayama, T.; Iizuka, S.; Sasakawa, D.; Honma, N.; Nakayama, T.; Iizuka, S. Human Posture Identification Using a MIMO Array. *Electronics* **2018**, *7*, 37. [CrossRef]
15. Losardo, A.; Grossi, F.; Matrella, G.; De Munari, I.; Ciampolini, P. Exploiting AAL environment for behavioral analysis. *Assist. Technol. Res. Ser.* **2013**, *33*, 1121–1125. [CrossRef]
16. Skubic, M.; Guevara, R.D.; Rantz, M. Automated health alerts using in-home sensor data for embedded health assessment. *IEEE J. Transl. Eng. Heal. Med.* **2015**, *3*. [CrossRef] [PubMed]
17. Nag, A.; Mukhopadhyay, S.C. Occupancy Detection at Smart Home Using Real-Time Dynamic Thresholding of Flexiforce Sensor. *IEEE Sens. J.* **2015**, *15*, 4457–4463. [CrossRef]
18. Li, M.; Lin, H.-J. Design and Implementation of Smart Home Control Systems Based on Wireless Sensor Networks and Power Line Communications. *IEEE Trans. Ind. Electron.* **2015**, *62*, 4430–4442. [CrossRef]
19. Ghayvat, H.; Liu, J.; Mukhopadhyay, S.C.; Gui, X. Wellness Sensor Networks: A Proposal and Implementation for Smart Home for Assisted Living. *IEEE Sens. J.* **2015**, *15*, 7341–7348. [CrossRef]
20. Grossi, F.; Bianchi, V.; Matrella, G.; De Munari, I.; Ciampolini, P. Internet-Based Home Monitoring and Control. In *Assisted Technology: From Adapted Equipment to Inclusive Environment*; Assistive Technology Research Series; IOS Press: Amsterdam, The Netherlands, 2009; ISBN 9781607500421.
21. Losardo, A.; Bianchi, V.; Grossi, F.; Matrella, G.; De Munari, I.; Ciampolini, P. Web-Enabled Home Assistive Tools. In *Everyday Technology for Independence and Care*; Assistive Technology Research Series; IOS Press: Amsterdam, The Netherlands, 2011; Volume 29, pp. 448–455. [CrossRef]
22. Bianchi, V.; Grossi, F.; De Munari, I.; Ciampolini, P. *Multi-Modal Interaction in AAL Systems*; Assistive Technology Research Series; IOS Press: Amsterdam, The Netherlands, 2011; ISBN 9781607508137.

23. Mora, N.; Bianchi, V.; De Munari, I.; Ciampolini, P. Simple and efficient methods for steady state visual evoked potential detection in BCI embedded system. In Proceedings of the 2014 IEEE International Conference on Acoustics, Speech and Signal Processing (ICASSP), Florence, Italy, 4–9 May 2014.
24. Bianchi, V.; Grossi, F.; Matrella, G.; De Munari, I.; Ciampolini, P. A wireless sensor platform for assistive technology applications. In Proceedings of the 11th EUROMICRO Conference on Digital System Design Architectures, Methods and Tools, Parma, Italy, 3–5 September 2008.
25. Bianchi, V.; Guerra, C.; De Munari, I.; Ciampolini, P. A wearable sensor for AAL-based continuous monitoring. In *International Conference on Smart Homes and Health Telematics*; Springer: Cham, Switzerland, 2016; Volume 9677, pp. 383–394. [CrossRef]
26. Bianchi, V.; Grossi, F.; De Munari, I.; Ciampolini, P. MuSA: A multisensor wearable device for AAL. In Proceedings of the 2011 Federated Conference on Computer Science and Information Systems (FedCSIS), Szczecin, Poland, 18–21 September 2011; pp. 375–380.
27. Bianchi, V.; Grossi, F.; De Munari, I.; Ciampolini, P. Multi sensor assistant: A multisensor wearable device for ambient assisted living. *J. Med. Imaging Heal. Inform.* **2012**, *2*, 70–75. [CrossRef]
28. Montalto, F.; Guerra, C.; Bianchi, V.; De Munari, I.; Ciampolini, P. MuSA: Wearable multi sensor assistant for human activity recognition and indoor localization. *Biosyst. Biorobotics* **2015**, *11*, 81–92. [CrossRef]
29. Guerra, C.; Bianchi, V.; De Munari, I.; Ciampolini, P. CARDEAGate: Low-cost, ZigBee-based localization and identification for AAL purposes. In Proceedings of the 2015 IEEE International Instrumentation and Measurement Technology Conference (I2MTC) Proceedings, Pisa, Italy, 11–14 May 2015.
30. Gill, K.; Yang, S.H.; Yao, F.; Lu, X. A ZigBee-based home automation system. *IEEE Trans. Consum. Electron.* **2009**, *55*, 422–430. [CrossRef]
31. Hwang, K.; Choi, B.J.; Kang, S.H. Enhanced self-configuration scheme for a robust zigbee-based home automation. *IEEE Trans. Consum. Electron.* **2010**, *56*, 583–590. [CrossRef]
32. Zualkernan, I.A.; Al-Ali, A.R.; Jabbar, M.A.; Zabalawi, I.; Wasfy, A. InfoPods: Zigbee-based remote information monitoring devices for smart-homes. *IEEE Trans. Consum. Electron.* **2009**, *55*, 1221–1226. [CrossRef]
33. Cho, J.Y.; Kim, K.-B.; Jabbar, H.; Sin Woo, J.; Ahn, J.H.; Hwang, W.S.; Jeong, S.Y.; Cheong, H.; Yoo, H.H.; Sung, T.H. Design of optimized cantilever form of a piezoelectric energy harvesting system for a wireless remote switch. *Sens. Actuators A* **2018**, *280*, 340–349. [CrossRef]
34. Mallick, S.; Bin Habib, A.-Z.S.; Ahmed, A.S.; Alam, S.S. Performance appraisal of Wireless Energy Harvesting in IoT. In Proceedings of the 2017 3rd International Conference on Electrical Information and Communication Technology (EICT), Khulna, Bangladesh, 7–9 December 2017.
35. Amaro, J.P.; Cortesão, R.; Ferreira, F.J.T.E.; Landeck, J. Device and operation mechanism for non-beacon IEEE802.15.4/Zigbee nodes running on harvested energy. *Ad Hoc Networks* **2015**, *26*, 50–68. [CrossRef]
36. Bianchi, V.; Ciampolini, P.; De Munari, I. RSSI-Based Indoor Localization and Identification for ZigBee Wireless Sensor Networks in Smart Homes. *IEEE Trans. Instrum. Meas.* **2018**, 1–10. [CrossRef]
37. Al-Sarawi, S.; Anbar, M.; Alieyan, K.; Alzubaidi, M. Internet of Things (IoT) communication protocols: Review. In Proceedings of the 2017 8th International Conference on Information Technology (ICIT), Amman, Jordan, 17–18 May 2017.
38. QCA4020 | Qualcomm. Available online: https://www.qualcomm.com/products/qca4020 (accessed on 12 September 2018).
39. Bassoli, M.; Bianchi, V.; De Munari, I.; Ciampolini, P. An IoT approach for an AAL Wi-Fi-based monitoring system. *IEEE Trans. Instrum. Meas.* **2017**, *66*, 3200–3209. [CrossRef]
40. Moraru, S.; Perniu, L.; Kristaly, D.M.; Ungureanu, D.A.; Sandu, F.; Mo, A.A. Proceedings of the 2017 25th Mediterranean Conference on Control and Automation (MED), Valletta, Malta, 3–6 July 2017.
41. Kristaly, D.M.; Moraru, S.-A.; Stefan Petre, V.; Parvan, C.A.; Ungureanu, D.E.; Mosoi, A.A. A Solution for Mobile Computing in a Cloud Environment for Ambient Assisted Living. In Proceedings of the 2018 26th Mediterranean Conference on Control and Automation (MED), Zadar, Croatia, 19–22 June 2018.
42. Lago, P.; Roncancio, C.; Jiménez-Guarín, C. Learning and managing context enriched behavior patterns in smart homes. *Futur. Gener. Comput. Syst.* **2019**, *91*, 191–205. [CrossRef]
43. Bassoli, M.; Bianchi, V.; De Munari, I.; Ciampolini, P. An unobtrusive Wi-Fi system for human monitoring. In Proceedings of the IEEE International Conference on Consumer Electronics, Berlin, Germany, 3–6 September 2017.

44. Grossi, F.; Bianchi, V.; Matrella, G.; De Munari, I.; Ciampolini, P. Senior-friendly kitchen activity: The FOOD Project. *Gerontechnology* **2014**, *13*, 200. [CrossRef]
45. CC3200 SimpleLink Wi-Fi® and Internet-of-Things solution, a Single-Chip Wireless MCU | TI.com. Available online: http://www.ti.com/product/CC3200# (accessed on 12 September 2018).
46. Labeodan, T.; Aduda, K.; Zeiler, W.; Hoving, F. Experimental evaluation of the performance of chair sensors in an office space for occupancy detection and occupancy-driven control. *Energy Build.* **2016**, *111*, 195–206. [CrossRef]
47. Bianchi, V.; Guerra, C.; Bassoli, M.; De Munari, I.; Ciampolini, P. The HELICOPTER project: Wireless sensor network for multi-user behavioral monitoring. In Proceedings of the 2017 International Conference on Engineering, Technology and Innovation: Engineering, Technology and Innovation Management Beyond 2020: New Challenges, New Approaches, Funchal, Portugal, 27–29 June 2017.
48. Fawcett, T. An introduction to ROC analysis. *Pattern Recognit. Lett.* **2006**, *27*, 861–874. [CrossRef]

Towards a Predictive Analytics-Based Intelligent Malaria Outbreak Warning System

Babagana Modu [1,*], Nereida Polovina [2], Yang Lan [1], Savas Konur [1], A. Taufiq Asyhari [3] and Yonghong Peng [4]

1 School of Electrical Engineering and Computer Science, University of Bradford, Bradford BD7 1DP, UK; y.lan@bradford.ac.uk (Y.L.); s.konur@bradford.ac.uk (S.K.)
2 Manchester Metropolitan University Business School, Manchester Metropolitan University, Manchester M15 6BH, UK; n.polovina@mmu.ac.uk
3 Centre for Electronic Warfare, Information and Cyber, Cranfield University, Shrivenham SN6 8LA, UK; taufiq-a@ieee.org
4 Faculty of Computer Science, University of Sunderland, St Peters Campus, Sunderland SR6 0DD, UK; yonghong.peng@sunderland.ac.uk
* Correspondence: b.modu@bradford.ac.uk
† This paper is an extended version of our paper published in DIGITALISATION FOR A SUSTAINABLE SOCIETY Embodied, Embedded, Networked, Gothenburg, Sweden, 12–16 June 2017.

Abstract: Malaria, as one of the most serious infectious diseases causing public health problems in the world, affects about two-thirds of the world population, with estimated resultant deaths close to a million annually. The effects of this disease are much more profound in third world countries, which have very limited medical resources. When an intense outbreak occurs, most of these countries cannot cope with the high number of patients due to the lack of medicine, equipment and hospital facilities. The prevention or reduction of the risk factor of this disease is very challenging, especially in third world countries, due to poverty and economic insatiability. Technology can offer alternative solutions by providing early detection mechanisms that help to control the spread of the disease and allow the management of treatment facilities in advance to ensure a more timely health service, which can save thousands of lives. In this study, we have deployed an *intelligent malaria outbreak early warning system*, which is a mobile application that predicts malaria outbreak based on climatic factors using machine learning algorithms. The system will help hospitals, healthcare providers, and health organizations take precautions in time and utilize their resources in case of emergency. To our best knowledge, the system developed in this paper is the first publicly available application. Since confounding effects of climatic factors have a greater influence on the incidence of malaria, we have also conducted extensive research on exploring a new ecosystem model for the assessment of hidden ecological factors and identified three confounding factors that significantly influence the malaria incidence. Additionally, we deploy a smart healthcare application; this paper also makes a significant contribution by identifying hidden ecological factors of malaria.

Keywords: malaria; climatic factors; machine learning; prediction; mobile application; structural equation modelling; partial least squares model

---

1. Introduction

Malaria, as one of the most serious infectious diseases causing public health problems in the world, affects about two-thirds of the world population, with estimated resultant deaths close to a million annually [1]. Its prevalence can be significantly attributed to climate factors, usually worsened by human factors through poor sanitation, overwhelmed sewage and deforestation. These climatic factors were found to contribute to the incidence of malaria [2], which apparently imposes a greater challenge to human life today.

The effects of malaria are much more profound in third world countries due to very limited medical resources. When an intense outbreak occurs, most of these countries cannot cope with the high number of patients due to the lack of medicine, equipment and hospital facilities. The prevention or reduction of the risk factor of this disease is very challenging, especially in these countries, due to poverty, and economic insatiability. Technology can offer alternative solutions by providing early detection mechanisms that help to control the spread of the disease and allow the management of treatment facilities in advance to ensure a more timely health service, which can save thousands of lives. The availability of an early detection system will not only prevent or decrease the large spread of malaria by creating quarantine zones, but also help healthcare providers deliver the necessary medical care on time by managing resources and calling for international aid and support, if needed.

In this study, we aim to design and deploy an *intelligent malaria outbreak early warning system*, which is a mobile application, that predicts malaria outbreak based on climatic factors using machine learning algorithms. The system will help hospitals, healthcare providers, and health organizations take precautions in time and utilize their resources in case of emergency. To our best knowledge, the system developed in this paper is the first publicly available application.

As well as deploying a smart healthcare application, this paper also makes a significant contribution by identifying *hidden ecological factors* of malaria (e.g., temperature, humidity, wind, location, drought, floods, etc.). Since confounding effects of climatic factors have a greater influence on the incidence of malaria, we have also conducted extensive research on exploring a new ecosystem model for the assessment of hidden ecological factors and identified three confounding factors that significantly contribute to the outbreak of malaria.

In this paper, we use an efficient methodology, comprising four stages. In the first stage, we have collected data from some repositories. Unfortunately, most of this data was incomplete in terms of climate factors. We have completed the dataset with the climate variables using satellite-based meteorological data obtained from CFSR (Climate Forecast System Reanalysis).

In the second stage, we have identified hidden ecological factors of malaria. The fundamental concept behind this emanated from the fact that a causal relationship exists among the climatic factors [3]. Some recent studies [4,5] combined meteorological variables together with malaria incidence data and established time series models for predicting malaria incidence. Regression and correlation analysis modelling was applied and using meteorological variables the trend of malaria incidence was determined [6]. Also, one of the most recent studies presented in this direction [7] uses a hybrid approach for time-series modelling and lagged-regression analysis of climate data combined with reported malaria incidence cases. Their result showed that malaria incidence in the area studied has a significant association with relative humidity, whereas temperature and precipitation were found to have negligible effects. This finding might particularly reveal that malaria incidence can be strongly influenced by relative humidity alone. However, this methodology suffers weaknesses due to its inability to capture the pre-determined existing causal relationship among the climate factors.

In this study, we use the partial least squares path modelling (PLS-PM) [8] methodology to analyse the causal relationships among meteorological variables, e.g., minimum average temperature, maximum average temperature, relative humidity, wind speed, precipitation and solar radiation, and explored their impact on the outbreak of malaria. In doing so, we develop an integrated model that provides insight into which lacking pre-determined confounding effects could be identified as hidden ecological factors. In the third stage, we have used machine learning algorithms to identify a pattern/model that will be used to make an accurate prediction of malaria outbreak. We have evaluated the prediction of machine learning algorithms, and obtained a very high accuracy rate. Machine learning has been used for prediction and diagnosis of several diseases, e.g., Parkinson's [9], cancer [10] and heart disease [11]. Among machine learning methods, Support Vector Machines (SVM) [12] have been used in malaria incidence prediction [13]; but this study has several shortcomings:

(i) the dataset used was extremely small (the size is only 33), which makes accuracy of prediction questionable; (ii) the dataset was used without analysing ecological factors, which could result in the inclusion of statistically insignificant variables in the prediction model, and hence could cause overfitting; (iii) there is no systematic methodology to transform this predictor into a smart healthcare system.

In the fourth stage, we have developed a mobile application by embedding the best predictor generated in the previous stage. The application reads climatic information, i.e., temperature, relative humidity, wind speed, solar radiation and precipitation, from free weather and geographical Application Programming Interface (APIs). It then predicts the possibility of malaria outbreak several days in advance (based on available forecasting data).

The subsequent sections of this paper are presented as follows: In Section 2, we present the complete analysis of identification of hidden ecological factors for the incidence of malaria transmission and its health implications to the change in biodiversity. Section 3 presents the intelligent malaria outbreak warning system, comprising data pre-processing, generating a prediction model using a machine learning algorithm and deployment of an intelligent mobile application. Section 4 concludes the paper by providing the summary of our results and our future work.

2. Assessment of Hidden Ecological Factors

Climate factors are the drivers of malaria transmission [14]; however, a study analysing the causal ecological relationship among the climatic factors that affect the incidence of malaria is still lacking, particularly in Sub-Saharan African countries.

The malaria ecosystem comprises four main components: human host, mosquitoes vector, parasites and environmental condition (see Figure 1).

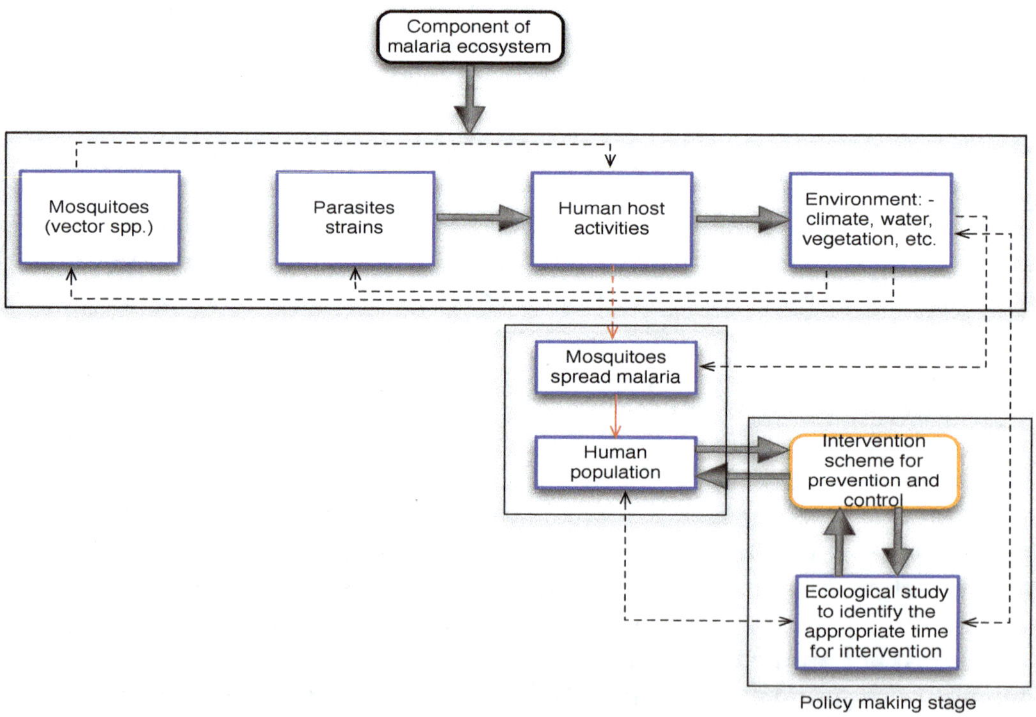

Figure 1. Conceptual framework of the malaria ecosystem describing the dynamic stages of malaria transmission from humans and mosquitoes under the influence of environmental factors. The boxes colored blue indicates the dynamics development of malaria parasite and its interaction between human host with mosquito vector and ecology. While the box colored red is the main scheme for malaria prevention and control indicating the intervention measure taken to mitigate the burden imposed on the human population.

These components are very dynamic in nature due to the inherent characteristics of ecology and the anticipatory change to biodiversity because of global warming. The works by [15–17] reported that ecological changes would adversely affect human health in some ways that are both obvious and obscure. However, the growing evidence also suggests that due to the rise in temperature as a result of the anticipated global warming, some previously unexposed regions of malaria transmission would have a 50% chance of experiencing it due to the link between malaria incidence and ecological factors [18]. The relationship between environmental changes and human health cannot be overemphasized because of the inherent variability and complexity of human nature. In many circumstances, grasslands and forest are converted for agriculture to reduce communicable disease, including wetland drainage for the prevention and control of malaria [17]. These activities can either lead to unintended negative health effects or succeed in the designed purpose. Also, transforming forest to augment food production may, in the long run, lead to the creation of a suitable environment for disease-causing agents such as mosquitoes for malaria transmission [19].

2.1. Study Site and Population

Ejisu-Juaben Municipal has a population of 143,762 [20], lies within latitudes $1°15'$ N and $1°45'$ N also with longitudes $6°15'$ W and $7°00'$ W, occupies a land area of 582.5 km^2 [21]. The vegetation of the municipal is a typical semi-deciduous forest (see Figure 2), with undulating topography and low altitude of about 240 m–300 m above sea level [21]. Also, the rainfall pattern of the area is bi-modal (i.e., two distinct seasons in a year), characterized by major and minor rainfall. The major rainfall begins from March to July with average annual rainfall between 1200 mm–1500 mm, while the minor rainfall begins in September and tapers off in November with annual average rainfall of 900 mm–1120 mm. Usually, December through February is hot, dry and dusty with mean annual temperature 25 °C–32 °C, and the relative humidity is moderately high during the rainy seasons [21]. Figure 2 presents the map of Ejisu-Juaben Municipal, which lies within the red-squared portion labelled Kumasi—the capital city of the Ashanti Region, in southern Ghana.

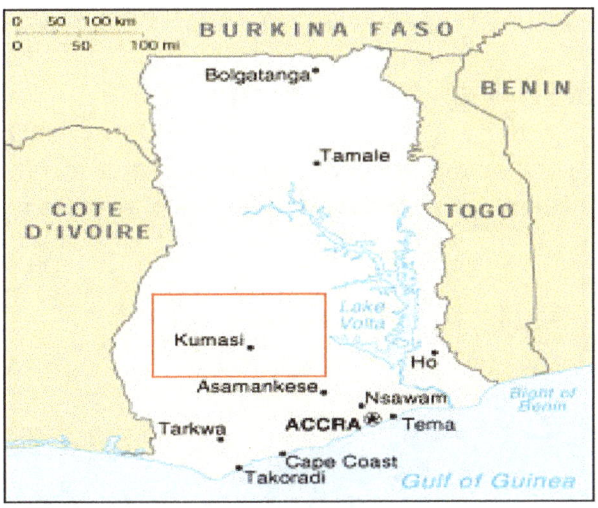

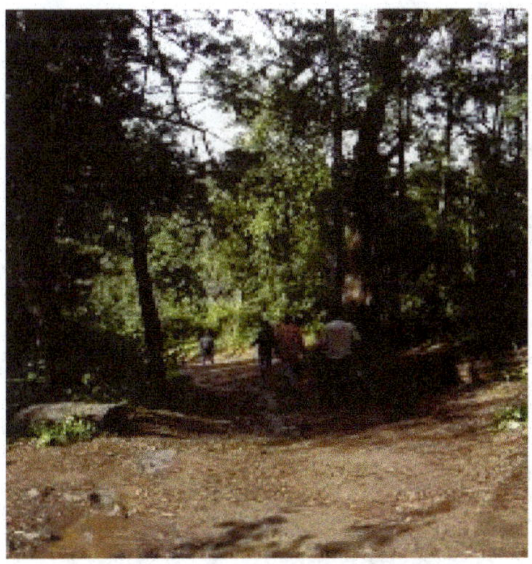

Figure 2. The picture on the left shows the map of Ghana and the portion of Kumasi city, where the study area within which Ejisu-Juaben lies. The picture on the right illustrates the climate vegetational belt characterized by a typical semi-deciduous forest.

2.2. Data Collection and Source

A total of 85,627 confirmed diagnosed cases of malaria incidence for the period of five years from 2009 to 2013, were retrieved in [22]. The distributional pattern of malaria cases reported in the study area shows an indication of high malaria incidence. We sought data on climate factors in the designated weather station of the study area location [20]; unfortunately, very few data are available and also a lot are missing. This is perhaps due to laxity of the weather station staff for not properly keeping up-to-date data. Since the data available is not sufficient for the analysis, we overcome this challenge by using satellite-based meteorological data obtained via [23]. We used the boundary metrics dimensions of [22] at latitude 6.7989° N to 6.6823° S and longitude −1.5656° W to −1.4186° E and demarcate the location of the study area on the satellite globe map. Within the demarcated area, we identify a weather station. We then generate the data of the climate variables of our interest. Moreover, the Ghana malaria incidence data is sufficient for the application of PLS-PM due to its suitability for handling small sample data, non-normality, multi-dimensions and multicollinearity [24,25]. However, the sample set is not sufficient to obtain high precision accuracy when applying machine learning algorithms. A small dataset might also cause the overfitting of data. For that reason, we coupled malaria incidence data used in [26] with [22] and proceed with the analysis.

2.3. Factor Analysis

Exploratory factor analysis (EFA) is one of the techniques for factor analysis (FA). It is primarily used in statistics to describe variance among observed correlated variables in terms of potentially a smaller number of unobserved variables, usually referred to as factors [27]. In this work, EFA was employed to search for confounding ecological factors that are latent [8,27] from the set of observed meteorological variables.

We demonstrate the FA technique using simple mathematical sketches; the observed variables can be expressed as linear combinations of the potential factors plus the residual terms. Consider the following observed variables $Y_1, Y_2, \cdots, Y_M$ of size M, and assume they are linearly related to a small number of unobservable (latent variables) factors $F_1, F_2, \cdots, F_N$, with $N \ll M$ such that:

$$\begin{aligned} Y_1 &= \psi_{10} + \psi_{11}F_1 + \cdots + \psi_{1N}F_N + e_1 \\ Y_2 &= \psi_{20} + \psi_{21}F_1 + \cdots + \psi_{1N}F_N + e_2 \\ &\vdots \\ Y_M &= \psi_{M0} + \psi_{M1}F_1 + \cdots + \psi_{MN}F_N + e_M \end{aligned} \tag{1}$$

where $e_1, \cdots, e_M$ are the residual terms, assuming that $E(e_i) = 0$, and $Var(e_i) = \delta_i^2$. While the unobservable factors F_i are independent from each other and $E(F_j) = 0$ and $Var(F_j) = 1$. These two assumptions stand as the robust pre-conditions for the application of structural equation modelling (SEM). The loading scores can be obtained from covariance and variance of any two observed variables using the following formula presented in Equation (2)

$$\begin{aligned} Cov(Y_i, Y_j) &= \sum_{i \neq j}^{N} \psi_{iN}\psi_{jN} \\ Var(Y_i) &= \sum_{i=1}^{N} \psi_{iK} + \delta_i^2 \end{aligned} \tag{2}$$

where the summation sign in Equation (2) denotes communality of the variables, the variance of which is explained by the common factors F_N.

2.4. Structural Equation Modelling

The SEM is a very popular technique that has multidisciplinary applications which combine together both the measurement and structural models [28–30]. In Figure 3a, we present a complex hypothetical SEM showing the causal relationship between malaria incidence and latent ecological factors together with their observed variables. We used ellipse shapes to represent latent factors, while the observed variables are represented by rectangular shapes.

The following system of Equation (3) describes the SEM technique in which the observed variables can be expressed as a linear combination of the potential factors plus residual terms. We therefore present SEM mathematical representations from Figure 3b as follows:

$$\begin{cases} \text{Factor I} = \lambda_{1,1}(\text{minimum temperature}) + \lambda_{1,2}(\text{relative humidity}) + \beta_{1,2}(\text{Factor II}) + \\ \gamma_1(\text{malaria incidence}) + e_1 \\ \text{Factor II} = \lambda_{2,1}(\text{maximum temperature}) + \lambda_{2,2}(\text{solar radiation}) + \beta_{2,3}(\text{Factor III}) + \\ \gamma_2(\text{malaria incidence}) + e_2 \\ \text{Factor III} = \lambda_{3,1}(\text{precipitation}) + \lambda_{3,2}(\text{wind speed}) + \gamma_3(\text{malaria incidence}) + e_3 \end{cases} \quad (3)$$

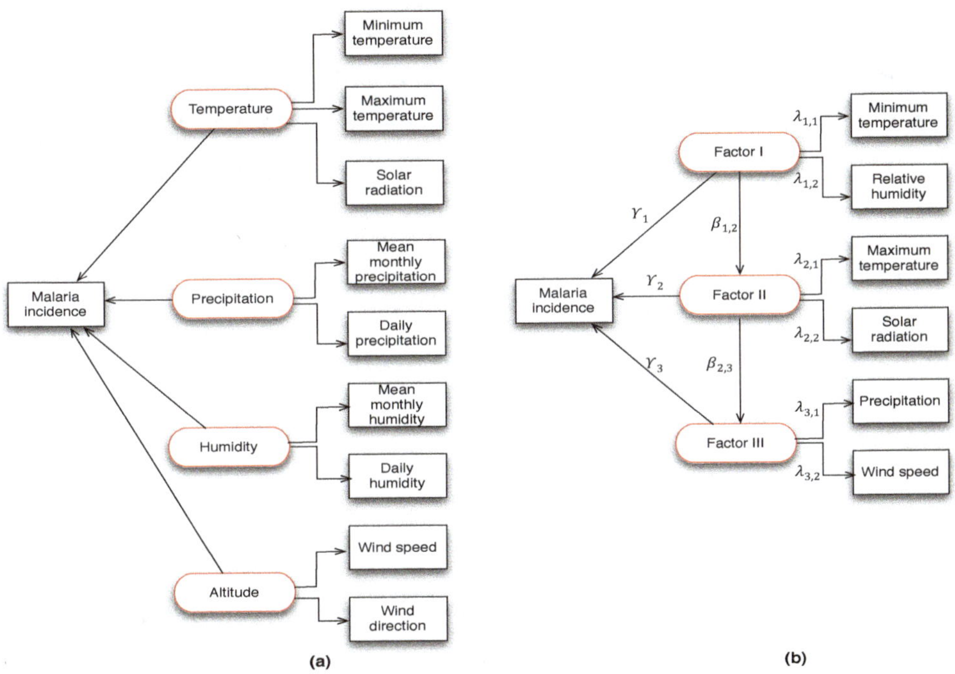

Figure 3. Structural equation model showing the relationship between malaria incidence and climate factors, the black colored rectangle indicating measurement variables while red colored ellipse is latent variables. (**a**) Showing the hypothetical causal relationship between malaria incidence and the climate factors. (**b**) Presenting the reduced causal relationship between malaria incidence and the climate factors after applying factor analysis to identify hidden factors and their dependent measurement variables.

2.5. Estimation of PLS-PM

The technique called PLS-PM or PLS-SEM was developed by [31] and chosen due to its characteristics in terms of small sample size, non-normality, multi-dimensions, and multicollinearity [23,24]. We have identified three hidden factors using EFA, and subsequently applied SEM for construction of the model (see Figure 3b). The PLS-PM is basically divided into three components: estimation of LVs, estimation of inner and outer models and estimation of the structural relations. The PLS algorithm is essentially represented as a sequence of regression in terms of weight vectors [32] and estimates the values of LVs (factor scores) iteratively until convergence is achieved. The fundamental PLS algorithm, as suggested by [30] (see Appendixes A.1–A.3 for detailed procedural descriptions). The PLS-PM is a component-based estimation technique that uses an iteration algorithm, separately analyzes the blocks of the measurement model and estimates the path coefficients in the structural model [33]. We used a package called semPLS in R for the estimation of PLS-SEM parameters including the analysis presented in Section 2.6.

For estimating parameters of SEM, we invoked the PLS technique, and further used 10,000 samples for the bootstrapping analysis instead of the default number of samples set to 500 selections [33]. Also, the PLS-PM latent variable scores were expressed as a linear combination of their observed variables and treated as an error-free substitute for the observed variables [33].

2.5.1. Measurement Model

The model, presented in Figure 3b, shows how observed Measurement Variables (MVs) are related to their Latent Variables (LVs). Hence without any loss of generality, for a good representation of the inner model, the following assumptions must hold:

- Matrix of MVs $\mathbf{Y}$ are scaled to have zero mean and unit variance.
- Each block of MVs $\mathbf{Y}_g$ is already transformed to be positively correlated for all LVs $\mathbf{x}_g, g = 1, \cdots, G$.

The measurement model is broadly classified as either reflective (Mode A) or formative (Mode B) [26], and this depends on the relation between LVs and MVs formation.

2.5.2. Mode A

In this form, each block of MVs reflects its LV and can be represented in multivariate regression form as:

$$\mathbf{Y}_g = \mathbf{x}_g \mathbf{w}_g^\top + \mathbf{F}_g \quad (4)$$

where the $\mathbf{w}_g^\top$ can be estimated using the least squares method.

2.5.3. Mode B

Also, in this form, the LV is considered to be formed by its MVs represented by a multiple regression as:

$$\mathbf{x}_g = \mathbf{Y}_g \mathbf{w}_g + \delta_g \quad (5)$$

using the same method of least squares, the estimate for $\mathbf{w}_g$ can be obtained.

2.6. *Presentation of Results*

In the application of PLS-SEM, three weighting schemes such as centroid weighting, factorial weighting and path weighting are conceptually used for model specifications and estimations. The conceptual SEM presented in Figure 3a shows the hypothetical causal relationship between latent (hidden) variables and observed meteorological (manifest) variables to the occurrence of malaria incidence. For the identification of confounding hidden variables, we performed factor analysis using exploratory factor analysis (EFA) [34]. From the results, three hidden factors were identified: Factor I (related to the minimum temperature and relative humidity), Factor II (related to the maximum temperature and solar radiation) and Factor III (related to precipitation and wind speed). The identified factors accounted for 64% of the total variance, and at α = 5% level of significance, χ^2 = 13.91, df = 8, Pvalue = 0.0841. This result provides sufficient evidence to explain malaria incidence in the study area.

We also explored the Guttman–Kaiser Criterion [35] and Cattell scree plots [36], to determine the number of factors to extract, the result of which reconfirmed the existence of three hidden ecological factors to the incidence of malaria. In the Guttman–Kaiser Criterion, we have the eigenvalues 2.71, 1.53, 1.02, 0.82, 0.57, 0.29, 0.05 computed using the correlation matrix (see Table 1); however, the rule for extraction is based on the factors whose eigenvalues are greater than unity. We then discard those factors that have eigenvalues less than unity, and are left with three eigenvalues indicating the number of factors to be considered. Similarly, the Cattell scree plot presented in (Figure 4) facilitates decisions regarding the number of factors to retain.

By analysing Table 1, we obtained the scree plot shown in Figure 4 which represents the relative proportion of variance accounted for by the components. In the scree plot, the eigenvalues of the first three components greater than unity can be seen from the parallel indicator, while the subsequent components below unity also line up beneath the parallel indicator. However, it is important to evaluate the variance accounted for by a few of the eigenvalues regarded as sufficient so that we can focus on them and discard the remaining insufficient factors as noise.

Table 1. Correlation matrix of climate drivers and malaria incidence.

	Mal. Incid.	Max. Temp.	Min. Temp.	Precip.	Rel. Humid	Solar Rad.	Wind Speed
Mal. Incid.	1.00	-	-	-	-	-	-
Max. Temp.	0.28	1.00	-	-	-	-	-
Min. Temp.	0.68	0.04	1.00	-	-	-	-
Precip.	−0.21	−0.36	0.22	1.00	-	-	-
Rel. Humid.	0.51	−0.24	0.90	0.38	1.00	-	-
Solar Rad.	0.19	0.54	−0.33	−0.10	−0.44	1.00	-
Wind Speed	−0.16	0.07	0.45	0.17	0.39	0.01	1.00

Note: (1) Malaria incidence, (2) Maximum temperature, (3) Minimum temperature, (4) Precipitation, (5) Relative humidity, (6) Solar radiation and (7) Wind speed.

In Table 2, we present Pearson's cross-correlation between meteorological variables and occurrence of malaria incidence at various lag effects from 0 to 3 months. The Lag 0, Lag 1 and Lag 2 (e.g., 0 month, 1 month and 2 month) presented in Table 2 which indicates the lagged correlation effects between climate variables and the incidence of malaria in the study area. We observed that at lag effects of 1 month, the minimum temperature, maximum temperature and relative humidity have positive association with malaria incidence as indicated by 0.321, 0.215 and 0.254 respectively. While the precipitation is negatively correlated with malaria incidence at lag effects of 1 month as indicated by −0.292. This explained that the climate drivers at lag of 1 month would be quite enough for the mosquitoes to reproduce and also complete their incubation periods (EIP) to becomes fully active in transmitting malaria infection. We found that the preceding result is consistent with other relevant studies on the influence of meteorological variables on the malaria incidence [37]. The 1 month time lag in the study area is sufficient to capture the pattern of malaria transmission for various strains of plasmodium parasites with definite lengths of EIP. This period usually takes about 10–15 days [38] and temporally varies over location, parasite species and climatic resolution. At Lag 0 and Lag 2, the minimum temperature, precipitation and relative humidity have negative lag effects at 0 month and 2 month except the maximum temperature which has effects of 0.284 and 0.092. These results revealed some clear indications that the malaria transmission in the study area at Lag 0 and Lag 2 suffered a negative effect, which might be attributed to the bi-annual rainfall pattern, low relative humidity—say less than 50%—and inability of mosquitoes completing the EIP cycle. In general, the result showed that maximum temperature, minimum temperature, and relative humidity were related to the malaria incidence at lagged effects of 1 month (i.e., a month in advance) except precipitation which has a negative association in the study area.

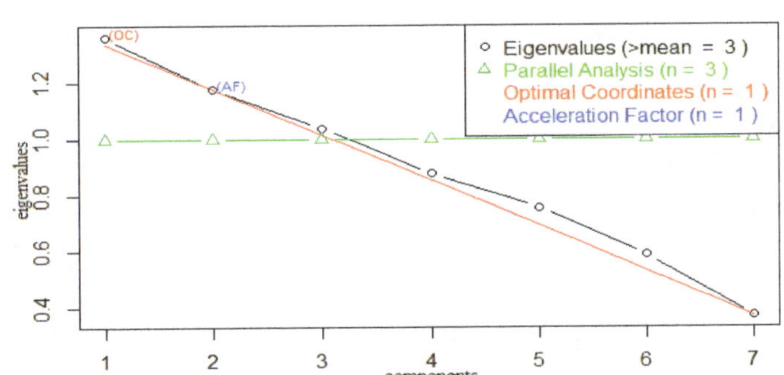

Figure 4. The Cattell scree plot presents the eigenvalues of the components and threshold for identifying the number of hidden ecological factors to be considered using the information in Table 1.

Table 2. Cross-correlation between meteorological variables and malaria incidence; VIF:variance inflated factor.

Variables	Lag 0	Lag 1	Lag 2	VIF	Kurtosis	Standard Error
Maximum temperature	0.284	0.321 [b]	0.092	2.4096	5.48	0.38
Minimum temperature	−0.122	0.215 [b]	−0.237	8.7919	2.07	0.33
Precipitation	−0.214	−0.292 [a]	−0.155	1.4194	20.73	0.27
Relative humidity	−0.134	0.254 [b]	−0.198	9.0065	1.42	0.02
Solar radiation	-	-	-	1.9000	6.73	0.50
Wind speed	-	-	-	1.3452	−0.58	0.04

[a] negative association at lag 1. [b] positive association at lag 1.

Some important summary statistics are presented in Table 2, which describe the distributional pattern of the climate indicators of malaria incidence and variance inflated factor (VIF). In factor analysis, multicollinearity can be used as a diagnostics check prior to application of regression analysis, whereby variables with high-factor loadings are typically multicollinear. We compute VIF of the climate variables to measure the degrees of multicollinearity and identify those factors that are independent of the magnitude of their VIF. In Table 2, the minimum temperature and relative humidity have VIF of 8.7919 and 9.0065 that gives a high degree of multicollinearity. The results revealed a high independent predictor of malaria incidence in the study area, and the degree to which they are independent gives evidence to accurately determine the major factors. However, the values of kurtosis (see Table 2) indicate a high peak of the climate variables with positive values across all the indicators except the wind speed which indicates a flat distribution. Positive values, generally listed in Table 2, indicate that the peakedness of distribution of the climate variables particularly influences the malaria incidence. Also, the standard error estimates provide information on the statistical accuracy of the climate variables; the larger the standard error, the wider the confidence interval of the statistic and vice-versa.

Non-normality of the dataset is one necessity for adopting PLS-SEM, and it is very robust when used on extremely non-normal data [39]. We examined the degree to which the data on malaria incidence are non-normal using the Shapiro–Wilk tests by invoking R software (3.4.1, University of Aukland, New Zealand). The results show that the null hypothesis (Ho) is rejected, indicating that the malaria incidence dataset is non-normal as suggested by the following indices $W = 0.9486$, p-value $= 0.0134$ and $\alpha = 0.05$, respectively. This method is particularly chosen and useful in smaller samples sizes, less than 2000 [40], and the null hypothesis is that the data are from a normal distribution. Similarly, we used a graphical approach called quantile–quantile (Q–Q) plot [41] and tested for normality of the dataset in similar fashion. The approach creates a plot from the ranked samples of the dataset against a similar number of ranked theoretical samples from a normal distribution. The plot shown in Figure 5, clearly indicates that the data points for malaria incidence are deviating from the straight line. Hence, the malaria incidence dataset is therefore not normally distributed using the Q–Q plot.

In Table 3, we show the results of the factor score estimates for path coefficients of SEM estimated using PLS path modelling, and three different structural model weighting schemes were analysed. We observed that Centroid (A) converges faster after 12 iterations, while factorial (B) and path weighting (C) converge after 15 iterations. The procedure of selecting the best weighting scheme is determined by the maximum number of iterations that will be used for calculating the PLS results and this algorithm did not stop until the maximum number of iterations is reached due to the stop criterion. From Table 3, we can observe that the B and C weighting schemes converge at the same maximum number of iterations in estimating the parameters of SEM. The weighting scheme provides the highest R^2 value for endogenous latent variables in the PLS path model specifications and estimations. This result shows that the C weighting scheme is better than A and B, as suggested by [42] in terms of robustness and also when the path model includes higher-order constructs.

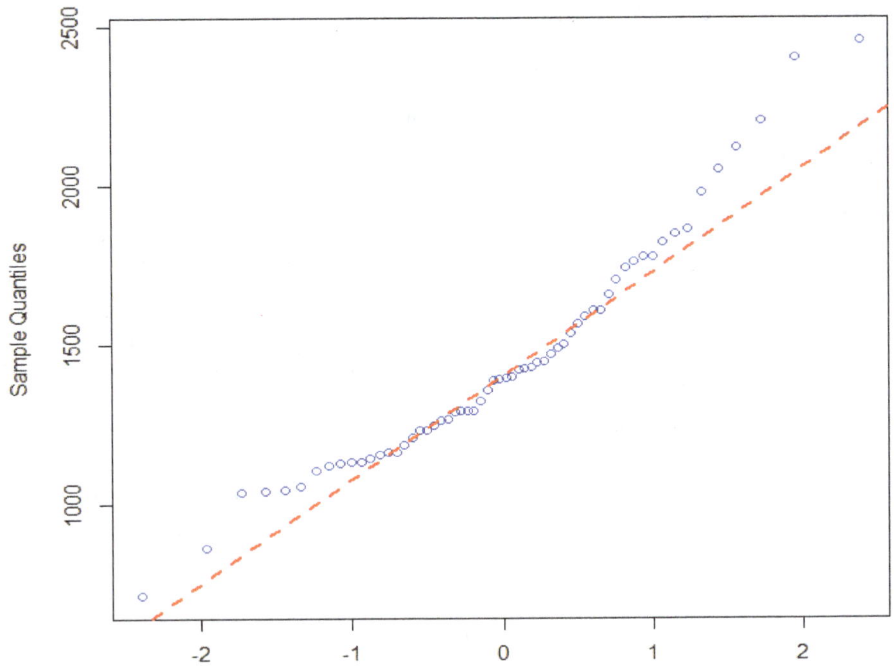

Figure 5. Graphical representation of quantile–quantile (Q–Q) plot normality tests.

Table 3. Factor scores for path coefficients in the PLS-PM using three weighting schemes.

Measurement/Structural Model	Parameter	Estimate	Centroid (A)	Factorial (B)	Path Weighting (C)
Minimum temperature ⟵ FactorI	$\lambda_{1,1}$	0.9479	0.9479	0.9495	0.9495
Relative humidity ⟵ FactorI	$\lambda_{1,2}$	0.9910	0.9910	0.9903	0.9903
Maximum temperature ⟵ FactorII	$\lambda_{2,1}$	0.8816	0.8816	0.8675	0.8675
Solar radiation ⟵ FactorII	$\lambda_{2,2}$	0.8735	0.8735	0.8873	0.8873
Precipitation ⟵ FactorIII	$\lambda_{3,1}$	0.9849	0.9849	0.9852	0.9852
Wind speed ⟵ FactorIII	$\lambda_{3,2}$	0.0017	0.0017	0.0031	0.0031
FactorI ⟶ FactorII	$\beta_{1,2}$	−0.3248	−0.3248	−0.3302	−0.3302
FactorII ⟶ FactorIII	$\beta_{2,3}$	−0.2774	−0.2774	−0.2690	−0.2690
FactorI ⟶ Malaria incidence	γ_1	0.9700	-	-	-
FactorII ⟶ Malaria incidence	γ_2	0.7700	-	-	-
FactorIII ⟶ Malaria incidence	γ_3	0.4900	-	-	-
Maximum number of iterations	-	-	12	15	15

Table 4 presents the results of bootstrapping sampling for outer loadings of the observed variables and path coefficient of the latent variables estimated using PLS-PM. The results also show that all outer loadings and path coefficients are significant at α = 5%, except for the solar radiation with Factor II and wind speed with Factor III that contains zero-point in the bootstrap confidence interval. Furthermore, the interaction effects of the Factors between I and II, II and III were also investigated and the results revealed that none of the Factor combinations is significant in the incidence of malaria in the study area. This result provides sufficient evidence that high malaria incidence in the study area was attributed to the occurrence of minimum temperature and relative humidity which are identified as Factor I.

The decision to select the most influential hidden ecological factor to the incidence of malaria is based on the communality and Dillon–Goldstein's indices. Furthermore, Table 5 summarizes the results, indicating some indices for selecting the hidden ecological factors to the high incidence of malaria in the study area. Among the three factors identified by EFA, we find that Factor I, indicated by minimum temperature and relative humidity, influences malaria transmission with communality index (0.94) and Dillon–Goldstein's ρ (0.97). This result is also consistent with the finding in [37], where a positive association exists between temperature and occurrence of dengue. Factor II and Factor III appear to have less influence on the malaria incidence.

Table 4. Bootstrapping test of the outer loadings and path coefficients in the PLS-PM with a 95% confidence interval.

Measurement/Structural Model	Parameter	Estimate	Bias	Standard Error	Lower	Upper
Minimum ⟵ FactorI	$\lambda_{1,1}$	0.9479	−0.0057	0.0467	0.8240	0.9890
Relative humidity ⟵ FactorI	$\lambda_{1,2}$	0.9910	−0.0055	0.0347	0.9823	1.0000
Maximum temperature ⟵ FactorII	$\lambda_{2,1}$	0.8816	−0.0329	0.1289	0.4769	0.9810
Solar radiation ⟵ FactorII	$\lambda_{2,2}$	0.8735	−0.0343	0.1748	−0.0705	0.9550
Precipitation ⟵ FactorIII	$\lambda_{3,1}$	0.9849	−0.1748	0.4044	0.7666	1.0000
Wind speed ⟵ FactorIII	$\lambda_{3,2}$	0.0017	0.1356	0.4059	−0.6593	0.7300
FactorI ⟶ FactorII	$\beta_{1,2}$	−0.3248	−0.0333	0.1692	−0.4974	0.4260
FactorII ⟶ FactorIII	$\beta_{2,3}$	−0.2774	−0.0264	0.2191	−0.4963	0.3810

Table 5. Indices for selecting the ecological hidden factor of high malaria incidence in the study area.

Factor	Reflective Variables	Communality	Dillon–Goldstein's ρ
I	2	0.94 [c] (94%)	0.97 [c] (97%)
II	2	0.77 (77%)	0.87 (87%)
III	2	0.49 (49%)	0.49 (49%)

[c] the most significant hidden factor.

3. Intelligent Malaria Outbreak Warning System

In the previous section, we identified the hidden ecological factors of malaria using partial least squares path modelling. In this section, we discuss, in detail, the implementation of the malaria outbreak system, based on the identified hidden ecological factors. The deployment comprises of three stages: data processing, generating the predictive model using machine learning and deployment of a mobile application.

3.1. Data Preprocessing

It was a tradition, prior to the application of machine learning algorithms, that datasets need to be pre-processed to enable a faster and more accurate learning process. The heuristic approach involves the discretization techniques most often used in data mining. This involves transforming continuous-valued datasets to discrete datasets by creating a set of contiguous intervals [43]. In this paper, we are making use of a dataset on climate variables as the input while the output variable is malaria incidence data. Our concern is the development of a predictive model using supervised machine learning algorithms that will predict the likelihood of malaria incidence. The output variable appeared to have high-magnitude in-terms of reported number of malaria cases; hence using it directly may cause over-fitting to the predictive model. Therefore, it is pertinent to transform the dataset using some techniques for discretization to enable us to build efficient models.

We have therefore discretized the output variable to form a target variable using the k-means clustering algorithm [44]. This methodology is chosen over equal width (EW) and equal frequency (EF) because it is less sensitive to outliers and also the number of clusters (partitions) can be optimized by analysis rather than pre-determination. In general, the choice of discretization method and choice of k can be guided by the objectives of the discretization task. By invoking R software, we can determine the optimum number of clusters to enable us to partition the output variable.

From the analysis, the optimum number of clusters obtained is k = 4 and the algorithm converges after nine iterations with 89.9% variation. Also, we observed that for k = 5, the number of iterations exceeded the maximum number of tolerable iterations supposed to achieve convergence and in this case it diverges even though the percentage of variation is still good at 93%. For k = 2 and 3, the algorithm converges after three and four iterations with 66.4% and 82% variation, respectively. This gives sufficient evidence to choose the optimum number of clusters as k = 4. Similarly, we have also tried the "NbClust" package in R software for determining the optimal number of clusters. Using the values of k ranging from two to five allows the algorithm to select the optimum number of clusters to be used in order to partition the output variable. The algorithm run and selected k = 4 as the optimum number of clusters to partition the output variables. Hence, both methodologies give the same number of optimum clusters to consider and subsequently prove to be consistent. We then partitioned the output variable into four classes according to the results of k-means algorithm and re-labeled them as: low, medium, high and very high incidence status of malaria. We present, in Table 6, the summary analysis of k-means algorithm clustering.

Table 6. Summary of data discretization using the k-means algorithm. SSB: The sum of squares of errors between the clusters; SST: The total sum of squares of the entire clusters.

Number of Clusters (k)	2	3	4	5
iteration	3	4	9	6
convergence	yes	yes	yes	no
$\frac{SSB}{SST}$	66.4%	82%	89.9%	93%

3.2. Machine Learning

The next stage is to identify a pattern/model from the data processed in Section 3.1 that will be used to make an accurate prediction of malaria incidence. Evolved from traditional pattern recognition approaches, machine learning methods explore the algorithms that can learn from the data and overcome prediction tasks by building a mathematical model with a data sample input. A learning algorithm will mark each given Malaria epidemic data sample as one category, then after being trained using the training dataset, it will build a model to predict which category a forthcoming data sample falls into.

We have applied several machine learning algorithms, including Support Vector Machine (SVM), K-Nearest Neighbours (KNN), Naive Bayes and Decision Trees, to find the best predicting algorithm from the scikit framework [45] in Python.

To evaluate the prediction of machine learning algorithms on the training set, we have used the 10-fold cross-validation technique by selecting a training set and test sets that are mutually independent. Table 7 shows the prediction results in comparison to seven different Machine Learning methods.

Table 7. Comparison of the accuracy of model checking algorithms. LiR: Linear Regression; LoR: Logistic Regression; DT: Decision Tree; SVM: Support Vector Machine; SVM (o): Optimized Support Vector Machine; NB: Naive Bayes; KNN: K-Nearest Neighbours; K-M: K-Means.

Algorithm	LiR	LoR	DT	SVM	SVM (o)	NB	KNN1	KNN5	KNN10	K-M (3)
Accuracy	83.8%	75.0%	63.8%	80.6%	99.0%	63.9%	58.3%	80.6%	80.6%	47.2%

- Linear Regression (LiR) method gives overall good prediction results, but it seems that the method failed to produce any medium predictions.
- Logistic Regression (LoR) method predicts the probability of occurrence of an event by fitting the dataset, as a set of independent variables, into a logic function. In other words, for a correlated data set, LoR may not be able to find the intrinsic-relationships between events.
- Decision Tree (DT) works very well for both categorical and continuous dependent variables; however, this dataset cannot be separated as distinct groups since the edges of the samples are fuzzy. Therefore, DT gave a bad prediction after all.

- Support Vector Machine (SVM) is one of the most efficient supervised machine learning algorithms, which is mainly used for solving classification and regression problems. The best part of this algorithm is that training and testing data can be plotted as a point in a n-dimensional plane, with a feature being the value of a particular coordinate. Without optimisation of the parameters, SVM gave a 80.56% predicting result. After parameter optimisation, especially on the penalty parameter and gamma coefficient adjustment, SVM (o) gave a 99.0% predicting result.
- Naive Bayes (NB) is a well-known classification method, which is based on Bayes' Theorem with an oversimplified assumption of independence between classifiers. Moreover, NB is a conditional probability model, which means that the method needs to be assigned a series of certain events. For this data set, NB did not produce a good prediction overall.
- K-Nearest Neighbours (KNN) method is able to deal with both classification and regression problems. In comparison to KNN5 (where k = 5) and KNN10 (where k = 10), KNN1 (where k = 1) failed to make a good prediction. It means that the data may need to do more pre-process and/or noise removal in a theory; however, most of data from the real world are incomplete; that is why KNN5 and KNN10 make a better prediction.
- K-Means (K-M) is a type of un-supervised method for clustering. In this case, three clusters have been set at the beginning; however, a convergence did not perfectly land; therefore, it cannot give a good overall prediction.

The results, presented in Table 7, show that the best performing algorithm is SVM. We therefore integrate the SVM model into our system.

3.3. Mobile Application

We have developed a mobile application, Malaria Outbreak Warning System, with a built-in SVM model, published at Google Play. The tool can be accessed via [46].

The application is based on the theoretical experiences and practical experiments of the SVM algorithm and model, which has been tested for developing systematic and effective strategies to predict the outbreak of a Malaria epidemic. Meanwhile, the parameters of the model kernel have been optimised and set into this application.

The application consists of three processes: pre-processing the weather forecasting data, processing the data by applying them into the model and implementing the model's interface, and post-processing the prediction data by presenting results on the app's UI front layer. It is a well-suited implementation for location detection.

Figure 6 shows a screen shot of the tool. The application not only supports the automatic gathering of weather forecasting data, but also supports manual data input. The application reads climatic information, i.e., temperature, relative humidity, wind speed, solar radiation and precipitation, from the weather and geographical APIs. When the units of the weather and atmosphere are different from the data set used to construct the predictor, we carry out the required normalisation or feature scaling or similar pre-processing. The tool then predicts the Malaria outbreak a couple of days in advance based on available forecast information acquired from the APIs. The user can slide the screen to see the available outbreak predictions for the current and future days. The additional button on the bottom of the screen is to let the user manually enter a set of weather measurements to make a prediction for customised parameters.

The trained SVM model has been implemented in Java by taking advantage of the LIBSVM (2.88, University of California, Berkeley, CA, USA) [47]. LIBSVM is an integrated software for SVM, regression and distribution estimation. The mobile application has been developed for Android using Android Studio. The weather forecasting data is powered by OpenWeatherMap API (3.0, Riga, Latvia) [48], which is an online service provider for weather data. OpenWeatherMap provides API for searching forecasting data for up to 5 days by coordinates; and the responses served as JavaScript Object Notation (JSON), Extensible Markup Language (XML) and HyperText Markup Language (HTML) endpoints. All of the data provided is under CC BY-SA 4.0 license.

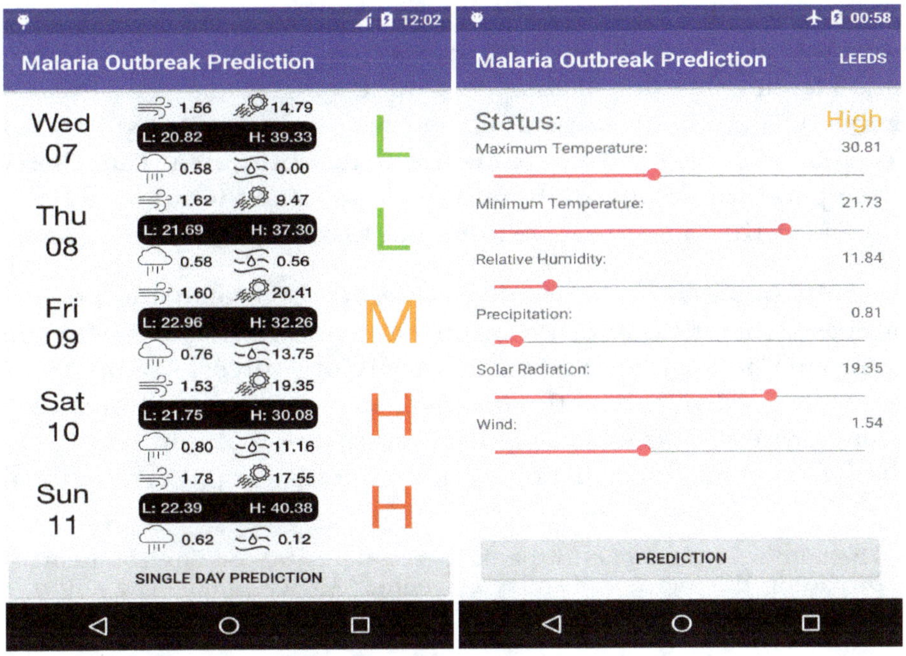

Figure 6. A screen shot of the mobile application.

3.4. Discussion

The current prototype of the intelligent malaria outbreak warning system relies on a batch machine learning process. That is, the learning algorithm is trained and tested offline using the available dataset, and the prediction model is embedded within the tool. Hence, the prediction process relies on the prediction model trained offline at once.

A more effective approach is to make the learning process online. That is, whenever new data is available, the data is automatically updated, and the learning process is run again to encapsulate the new data. This will not only allow an automatic and dynamic learning process, but also increase the accuracy of the prediction by adapting to new patterns in the data.

The online learning approach requires a mechanistic data collection mechanism, which is very challenging to perform as hospitals and health service providers do not make the relevant data available online. Even acquiring permission to have access to the available data is a long and bureaucratic process. On the other hand, as discussed in Section 2.2, most available data cannot be directly used in this system as they are incomplete and/or not processed.

To alleviate these issues and to support the online learning process, the Malaria outbreak warning application can be extended to collect online data from its users. Namely, the users, e.g., hospitals, healthcare providers, individuals etc., report a Malaria case to the system. Using the geographical location of the incident, the application will acquire all the necessary information for the ecological factors. In this way, new data will be collected at run time, and the learning process will be instantiated each time new data is available. We are currently working on the development of this approach.

4. Conclusions

In this study, we have deployed an intelligent malaria outbreak early warning system, predicting malaria outbreaks based on climatic factors using machine learning algorithms. The system will help hospitals, healthcare providers, and health organizations take precautions in time and utilize their resources in case of emergency. To our best knowledge, the system developed in this paper is the first publicly available application.

We have also provided an ecosystem overview for malaria modelling and proposed a new framework for the study of a malaria transmission ecosystem to prevent and control its effects. We have assessed and identified hidden factors that lead to a high malaria outbreak. Our data analysis results have shown that the minimum temperature and relative humidity, which are related to Factor I, have a positive association with the incidence of malaria in the study area. The other observed variables such as maximum temperature, solar radiation, precipitation and wind speed, which are related to hidden Factor II and Factor III, appear to have mildly influenced malaria incidence.

The primary results obtained in this study have demonstrated the power of the proposed predicative analytics-based malaria outbreak warning system. The further development of the system will incorporate automatic data gathering from a variety of sources. We are currently working on further development of our system and methodology to support automatic data collection at run time, and the online learning process. This will not only allow an automatic and dynamic learning process, but also increase the accuracy of the prediction by adapting to new patterns in the data.

Acknowledgments: The authors would like to thank National Centre for Environmental Prediction (NCEP), for their support in providing this work with relevant meteorological data. The author B.M. would like to thank Tertiary Education Trust Fund (tetFund), Nigeria for sponsoring his Ph.D. programme at the University of Bradford, UK. Y.L and S.K. acknowledge Innovate UK KTP010551 grant.

Author Contributions: Savas Konur, Nereida Polovina, Yang Lan, A. Taufiq Asyhari and Yonghong Peng designed the experiments; Babagana Modu performed the experiments; Babagana Modu analysed the data; Babagana Modu, Savas Konur, Nereida Polovina, Yang Lan, A. Taufiq Asyhari and Yonghong Peng contributed reagents/materials/analysis tools; Babagana Modu wrote the paper.

Abbreviations

The following abbreviations are used in this manuscript:

SEM	Structural Equation Modelling
EFA	Exploratory Factor Analysis
PLS-PM	Partial Least Squares Path Modelling
LVs	Latent Variables
MVs	Measurement Variables
FA	Factor Analysis
API	Application Programming Interface
SVM	Support Vector Machine
LiR	Linear Regression
LoR	Logistic Regression
DT	Decision Tree
NB	Naive Bayes
KNN	K-Nearest Neighbours
K-M	K-Means
CFSR	Climate Forecast System Reanalysis
NCEP	National Centre for Environmental Prediction
JSON	JavaScript Object Notation
XML	Extensible Markup Language
HTML	HyperText Markup Language

Appendix A

Appendix A.1. Estimation of Parameters

Step 1 Initialization: Suppose $\mathbf{Y}_1, \cdots, \mathbf{Y}_K$ are the respective MVs, and are scaled such that $\mathbf{E}(\mathbf{Y}_i) = 0$ and $\mathbf{V}(\mathbf{Y}_i) = 1$. We are interested in expressing each LV as a linear combination of MVs, represented in compact form:

$$\hat{\mathbf{X}} = \mathbf{YM}$$
$$\hat{\mathbf{x}}_g = \frac{\hat{x}_g}{\sqrt{VAR(\hat{x}_g)}}, g = 1, \cdots, G \quad \text{(A1)}$$

Hence, the LVs are initialized as: $\hat{\mathbf{X}} = \hat{\mathbf{x}}_1, \cdots, \hat{\mathbf{x}}_G$.

Step 2 Inner approximation

Within the inner model domain, the estimation of the path parameter of each LV can be mathematically represented as the weighted sum of its neighbouring LVs.

$$\tilde{\mathbf{X}} = \hat{\mathbf{X}}\mathbf{E}$$
$$\tilde{\mathbf{x}}_g = \frac{\tilde{x}_g}{\sqrt{(VAR(\tilde{\mathbf{x}}_g))}}, g = 1, \cdots, G \quad \text{(A2)}$$

The approximate estimation of the inner model path parameter takes: $\tilde{\mathbf{X}} = (\tilde{\mathbf{x}}_1, \cdots, \tilde{\mathbf{x}}_G)$.

Step 3 Outer approximation

The outer approximation is computed based on the weight of the LV loads from the inner approximation. This comes in two forms, Mode A and Mode B. For Mode A, a multivariate regression coefficient with the block of MVs as the response and the LV as the regressor:

$$\hat{\mathbf{w}}_g^\top = (\tilde{\mathbf{x}}_g^\top \tilde{\mathbf{x}}_g)^{-1} \tilde{\mathbf{x}}_g^\top \mathbf{Y}_g \quad \text{(A3)}$$

Mode B is a multiple regression coefficient with the block of MVs as the response and its block of MVs as the regressor:

$$\hat{\mathbf{w}}_g = (\mathbf{Y}_g^\top \mathbf{Y}_g)^{-1} \mathbf{Y}_g^t \tilde{\mathbf{x}}_g \quad \text{(A4)}$$

Step 4 Outer weight vector

Let $k_g = \{k \in \{1, \cdots, K\} | y_k \, x_g\}$ be a set of indices for MVs related to LV x_g; then, w_g, $g = 1, \cdots, g$, is a column vector of length $|k_g|$. We can write down the matrix of outer weights, W as:

$$W = \begin{pmatrix} w_1 & 0 & \cdots & 0 \\ 0 & w_2 & \cdots & 0 \\ \vdots & \vdots & \ddots & \vdots \\ 0 & 0 & \cdots & w_G \end{pmatrix}$$

The outer weight vectors, $w_1, \cdots, w_G$, in an outer weights matrix W, which we are using now to estimate the factor scores by means of the MVs, are

$$\hat{\mathbf{X}} = \mathbf{YW}$$
$$\hat{\mathbf{X}}_g = \frac{\hat{\mathbf{X}}_g}{\sqrt{VAR(\hat{\mathbf{X}}_g)}}, g = 1, \cdots, G, \quad \text{(A5)}$$

resulting in the outer estimation: $\mathbf{X} = (\hat{\mathbf{x}}_1, \cdots, \hat{\mathbf{x}}_G)$.

Step 5 Iteration

If the relative change of all the outer weights from one iteration to the next are smaller than a predefined tolerance,

$$\left|\frac{\hat{w}_{kg}^{old} - \hat{w}_{kg}^{new}}{\hat{w}_{kg}^{new}}\right| < \epsilon, \forall, k = 1, \cdots, K \wedge g = 1, \cdots, G, \tag{A6}$$

the estimation of factor scores done in (A5) is taken to be final. Otherwise, go back to (A2).

Appendix A.2. Weighting Scheme

The weighting schemes are used to estimate the inner weight in (A2) of the PLS algorithm. Generally, there are three weighting schemes, centroid [49], and later [42] introduced the factorial and path weighting schemes.

Appendix A.2.1. Centroid (A)

The centroid weighting scheme takes the form:

$$e_{ij} = \begin{cases} sign(r_{ij}), & \text{for } c_{ij} = 1, i, j = 1, \cdots, G \\ 0, & \text{else} \end{cases} \tag{A7}$$

where $\mathbf{E}$ denotes the matrix of inner weights.

Appendix A.2.2. Factorial (B)

The factorial weighting scheme also takes the form:

$$e_{ij} = \begin{cases} r_{ij}, & \text{for } c_{ij} = 1, i, j = 1, \cdots, G \\ 0, & \text{else} \end{cases} \tag{A8}$$

Appendix A.2.3. Path Weighting (C)

In this weighting scheme, the predecessor and successor of a LV play a different role in the relation. The relation between one specific LV $\mathbf{x}_i$ and its successor is determined by their correlation; for the predecessors it is determined by a multiple regression

$$\begin{aligned} \mathbf{x}_i &= \mathbf{x}_i^{pred}\gamma + \mathbf{z}_i \\ \mathbf{E}[\mathbf{z}_i] &= 0, i = 1, \cdots, G \end{aligned} \tag{A9}$$

where $\mathbf{x}_i^{pred}$ is the predecessor set of the LV $\mathbf{x}_i$. Denoting $\mathbf{x}_i^{succ}$ as the successor set of the LV $\mathbf{x}_i$; the elements of the inner weight matrix are denoted $\mathbf{E}$ as

$$e_{ij} = \begin{cases} \gamma_j, & \text{for } j \in \mathbf{x}_i^{pred}, \\ COR(\mathbf{y}_i, \mathbf{x}_j), & \text{for } j \in \mathbf{x}_i^{succ}, \\ 0, & \text{else} \end{cases} \tag{A10}$$

Appendix A.3. Discriminant Validity Check

In the structural equation model, the factor scores are estimated by the PLS algorithm, while the path coefficients are also estimated using ordinary least squares (OLS). Now, for each LV $\hat{\mathbf{x}}_g$, $g = 1, \cdots, G$, the path coefficient is the regression coefficient in its predecessor set $\hat{\mathbf{x}}_g^{pred}$ defined as:

$$\hat{\beta}_g = (\hat{\mathbf{x}}_g^{pred\top} \hat{\mathbf{x}}_g^{pred})^{-1} \hat{\mathbf{x}}_g^{pred\top} \hat{\mathbf{x}}_g \tag{A11}$$

Using (A11), we can compute the element $\hat{\mathbf{b}}_{ij}, i, j = 1, \cdots, G$, of the estimated matrix of path coefficients $\hat{\beta}$.

Appendix A.3.1. Path Coefficients

$$\hat{\beta}_{ij} = \begin{cases} \hat{\beta}_{gj}, & \text{for } j \in \mathbf{x}_i^{pred}, \\ 0, & \text{else} \end{cases} \tag{A12}$$

Therefore, matrix $\hat{\mathbf{B}}$ denotes a transition matrix for the structural equation model.

Appendix A.3.2. Total Effects

We can calculate the matrix of the total effects $\hat{\mathbf{T}}$ as the sum of the 1 to **G** step transition matrices:

$$\hat{\mathbf{T}} = \sum_{g=1}^{G} \hat{\mathbf{B}}_g \tag{A13}$$

Note that $\hat{\mathbf{B}}^g$ expands to $\overbrace{\hat{\mathbf{B}} \cdot \hat{\mathbf{B}} \cdot \cdots \cdot \hat{\mathbf{B}}}^{g-times}$, e.g., $\hat{\mathbf{B}}^2$ contains all the indirect effects mediated by only one LV.

Appendix A.3.3. Outer Loadings

The cross and outer loadings are estimated as:

$$\hat{\lambda}^{cross} = COR(\mathbf{Y}, \hat{\mathbf{X}}) \tag{A14}$$

$$\hat{\lambda}_{kg}^{outer} = \begin{cases} \hat{\lambda}_{kg}^{cross}, & \text{if } m_{kg} = 1 \\ 0, & \text{else} \end{cases} \tag{A15}$$

References

1. World Health Organization. *Malaria Rapid Diagnostic Test Performance: Results of WHO Product Testing of Malaria RDTs: Round 6*; World Health Organization: Geneva, Switzerland, 2015.
2. Haque, U.; Hashizume, M.; Glass, G.E.; Dewan, A.M.; Overgaard, H.J.; Yamamoto, T. The role of climate variability in the spread of malaria in Bangladeshi highlands. *PLoS ONE* **2010**, *5*, e14341.
3. Bonan, G.B.; Shugart, H.H. Environmental factors and ecological processes in boreal forests. *Annu. Rev. Ecol. Syst.* **1989**, *20*, 1–28.
4. Kumar, V.; Mangal, A.; Panesar, S.; Yadav, G.; Talwar, R.; Raut, D.; Singh, S. Forecasting malaria cases using climatic factors in Delhi, India: A time series analysis. *Malar. Res. Treat.* **2014**, doi:10.1155/2014/482851.
5. Ngarakana-Gwasira, E.T.; Bhunu, C.P.; Masocha, M.; Mashonjowa, E. Assessing the Role of Climate Change in Malaria Transmission in Africa. *Malar. Res. Treat.* **2016**, doi:10.1155/2016/7104291.
6. Nath, D.C.; Mwchahary, D.D. Association between Climatic Variables and Malaria Incidence: A Study in Kokrajhar District of Assam, India: Climatic Variables and Malaria Incidence in Kokrajhar District. *Glob. J. Health Sci.* **2013**, *5*, 90.
7. Modu, B.; Asyhari, A.T.; Peng, Y. Data Analytics of climatic factor influence on the impact of malaria incidence. In Proceedings of the 2016 IEEE Symposium Series on Computational Intelligence (SSCI), Athens, Greece, 6–9 December 2016; pp. 1–8.
8. Tenenhaus, M.; Vinzi, V.E.; Chatelin, Y.M.; Lauro, C. PLS path modeling. *Comput. Stat. Data Anal.* **2005**, *48*, 159–205.

9. Sriram, T.; Rao, V.; Narayana, S.; Dowluru, K. Intelligent Parkinson disease prediction using machine learning algorithms. *Int. J. Eng. Innov. Technol.* **2013**, *3*, 212–215.
10. Ganesan, N.; Venkatesh, K.; Rama, M.A. Application of Neural Networks in diagnosing cancer disease using demographic data. *Int. J. Comput. Appl.* **2010**, *1*, 76–85.
11. Aditya, M.; Prince, K.; Himanshu, A.; Pankaj, K. Early heart disease prediction using data mining techniques. *Comput. Sci. Inf. Technol.* **2014**, 53–59, doi:10.5121/csit.2014.4807.
12. Wang, L. (Ed.) *Support Vector Machines: Theory and Applications*; Springer: Berlin, Germany, 2005; Volume 177.
13. Sharma, V.; Kumar, A.; Panat, L.; Karajkhede, G.; Lele, A. Malaria outbreak prediction model using machine learning. *Int. J. Adv. Res. Comput. Eng. Technol.* **2015**, *4*, 4415–4419.
14. Parham, P.E.; Michael, E. Modelling the effects of weather and climate change on malaria transmission. *Environ. Health Perspect.* **2010**, *118*, 620.
15. Myers, S.S.; Patz, J.A. Emerging threats to human health from global environmental change. *Annu. Rev. Environ. Resour.* **2009**, *34*, 223–252.
16. Myers, S.S.; Gaffikin, L.; Golden, C.D.; Ostfeld, R.S.; Redford, K.H.; Ricketts, T.H.; Osofsky, S.A. Human health impacts of ecosystem alteration. *Proc. Natl. Acad. Sci. USA* **2013**, *110*, 18753–18760.
17. Bayles, B.R.; Brauman, K.A.; Adkins, J.N.; Allan, B.F.; Ellis, A.M.; Goldberg, T.L.; Ricketts, T.H. Ecosystem Services Connect Environmental Change to Human Health Outcomes. *EcoHealth* **2016**, *13*, 443–449.
18. The Potsdam Institute for Climate Impact Research and Climate Analytics. *Turn-Down the Heat—Why a 4 Degree Warmer World Must Be Avoided*; International Bank for Reconstruction and Development and World Bank: Washington, DC, USA, 2012.
19. De Castro, M.C.; Monte-Mór, R.L.; Sawyer, D.O.; Singer, B.H. Malaria risk on the Amazon frontier. *Proc. Natl. Acad. Sci. USA* **2006**, *103*, 2452–2457.
20. Nyarko, P. Population and Housing Census, District Analytical Report, Ejisu-Juaben Municipal. Available online: https://www.citypopulation.de/php/ghana-admin.php?adm2id=0117. (accessed on 12 January 2017).
21. Addai, G.; Anyatewon Kwesi, D. *2010 Population and Housing Census: District Analytical Report*, 1st ed.; Ghana Statistical Service: Accra, Ghana, 2014
22. Takyi Appiah, S.; Otoo, H.; Nabubie, I.B. Times Series Analysis Of Malaria Cases In Ejisu-Juaben Municipality. *Int. J. Sci. Technol. Res.* **2015**, *4*, 220–226.
23. Global Weather Data for SWAT. Available online: http://globalweather.tamu.edu (accessed on 24 June 2017).
24. Nitzl, C.; Chin, W.W. The case of partial least squares (PLS) path modeling in managerial accounting research. *J. Manag. Control* **2017**, *28*, 137–156.
25. Bagozzi, R.P.; Yi, Y. Specification, evaluation, and interpretation of structural equation models. *J. Acad. Mark. Sci.* **2012**, *40*, 8–34.
26. Dan, E.D.; Jude, O.; Idochi, O. Modelling and forecasting malaria mortality rate using SARIMA models (a case study of Aboh Mbaise general hospital, Imo State Nigeria). *Sci. J. Appl. Math. Stat.* **2014**, *2*, 31–41.
27. Ruscio, J.; Roche, B. Determining the number of factors to retain in an exploratory factor analysis using comparison data of known factorial structure. *Psychol. Assess.* **2012**, *24*, 282.
28. Kline, R.B. *Principles and Practice of Structural Equation Modelling*; Guilford Publications: New York, NY, USA, 2015.
29. Kelloway, E.K.; Santor, D.A. Using LISREL for Structural Equation Modelling: A Researcher's Guide. *Can. Psychol.* **1999**, *40*, 381.
30. Monecke, A.; Leisch, F. SemPLS: Structural Equation Modeling Using Partial Least Squares. *J. Stat. Softw.* **2012**, *48*, 1–32.
31. Wold, H. Soft Modeling: The Basic Design and Some Extensions. In *Systems under Indirect Observation: Causality– Structure– Prediction*; Part 2; Jöreskog, K.G., Wold, H., Eds.; North-Holland Publishing Company: Amsterdam, The Netherlands, 1982; pp. 1–54.
32. Dijkstra, T.K. Latent variables and indices: Herman Wold's basic design and partial least squares. In *Handbook of Partial Least Squares*; Springer: Berlin, Germany, 2010; pp. 23–46.
33. Byrne, B.M. *Structural Equation Modelling with LISREL, PRELIS, and SIMPLIS: Basic Concepts, Applications, and Programming*; Psychology Press: Hove, UK, 2013.

34. Li, X.X.; Wang, L.X.; Zhang, J.; Liu, Y.X.; Zhang, H.; Jiang, S.W.; Zhou, X.N. Exploration of ecological factors related to the spatial heterogeneity of tuberculosis prevalence in PR China. *Glob. Health Action* **2014**, *7*, doi:10.3402/gha.v7.23620.
35. Yeomans, K.A.; Golder, P.A. The Guttman-Kaiser criterion as a predictor of the number of common factors. *Statistician* **1982**, *31*, 221–229.
36. Ledesma, R.D.; Valero-Mora, P.; Macbeth, G. The scree test and the number of factors: A dynamic graphics approach. *Span. J. Psychol.* **2015**, *18*, doi:10.1017/sjp.2015.13.
37. Xu, L.; Stige, L.C.; Chan, K.S.; Zhou, J.; Yang, J.; Sang, S.; Lu, L. Climate variation drives dengue dynamics. *Proc. Natl. Acad. Sci. USA* **2016**, *114*, 113–118.
38. Srinivasulu, N.; Gujju Gandhi, B.; Naik, R.; Daravath, S. Influence of Climate Change on Malaria Incidence in Mahaboobnagar District of Andhra Pradesh, India. Available online: https://www.ijcmas.com/Archives/vol-2-5/N.%20Srinivasulu,%20et%20al.pdf (accessed on 24 June 2017).
39. Hair, J.F.; Sarstedt, M.; Pieper, T.M.; Ringle, C.M. The use of partial least squares structural equation modelling in strategic management research: A review of past practices and recommendations for future applications. *Long Range Plan.* **2012**, *45*, 320–340.
40. Jarque, C.M.; Bera, A.K. A test for normality of observations and regression residuals. *Int. Stat. Rev./Rev. Int. Stat.* **1987**, *55*, 163–172.
41. Wilk, M.B.; Gnanadesikan, R. Probability plotting methods for the analysis for the analysis of data. *Biometrika* **1968**, *55*, 1–17.
42. Lohmöller, J.B. *Latent Variable Path Analysis with Partial Least Squares*; Physica-Verlag: Heidelberg, Germany, 1989.
43. Lustgarten, J.L.; Gopalakrishnan, V.; Grover, H.; Visweswaran, S. Improving classification performance with discretization on biomedical datasets. In Proceedings of the AMIA Annual Symposium, Hilton Washington and Tower, Washington, DC, USA, 8 November 2008.
44. Maslove, D.M.; Podchiyska, T.; Lowe, H.J. Discretization of continuous features in clinical datasets. *J. Am. Med. Inf. Assoc.* **2013**, *20*, 544–553.
45. Scikit-Learn. Available online: http://www.scikit-learn.org (accessed on 24 June 2017).
46. MLSVM for Research. Available online: https://play.google.com/store/apps/details?id=project.lanydr.mlsvm&hl=en (accessed on 24 June 2017).
47. LIBSVM-A Library for Support Vector Machines. Available online: www.csie.ntu.edu.tw/~cjlin/libsvm/ (accessed on 24 June 2017).
48. Weather API. Available online: http://openweathermap.org/api) (accessed on 24 June 2017).
49. Gang, S. Soft modeling: Intermediate between traditional model building and data analysis. In *Mathematical Statistics*; Polish Scientific Publishers: Warsaw, Poland, 1980; Volume 6, pp. 333–346.

6

Reformulation-Linearization Technique Approach for Kidney Exchange Program IT Healthcare Platforms

Junsang Yuh [1,2], Seokhyun Chung [2] and Taesu Cheong [2,*]

1 R&D Center, Begas, Seoul 06179, Korea; yuhjunsang@gmail.com
2 School of Industrial Management Engineering, Korea University, Seoul 02841, Korea; csh98016@gmail.com
* Correspondence: tcheong@korea.ac.kr; Tel.: +82-2-3290-3382

Abstract: Kidney exchange allows a potential living donor whose kidney is incompatible with his intended recipient to donate a kidney to another patient so that the donor's intended recipient can receive a compatible kidney from another donor. These exchanges can include cycles of longer than two donor–patient pairs and chains produced by altruistic donors. Kidney exchange programs (KEPs) can be modeled as a maximum-weight cycle-packing problem in a directed graph. This paper develops a new integer programming model for KEPs by applying the reformulation-linearization technique (RLT) to enhance a lower bound obtained by its linear programming (LP) relaxation. Given the results obtained from the proposed model, the model is expected to be utilized in the integrated KEP IT (Information Technology) healthcare platform to obtain plans for optimized kidney exchanges.

Keywords: kidney exchange program; integer programming; reformulation-linearization technique; IT healthcare platform

1. Introduction

Kidney transplants are essential for many end-stage renal disease sufferers. However, finding compatible kidneys may be difficult because of blood or tissue incompatibilities between donors and their intended recipients. The issue of incompatibility can be overcome by establishing a kidney exchange program (KEP). The first of these was performed in South Korea [1–3] in 1991 and they have since been widely performed in many countries, including the United States of America [4–9], the United Kingdom [10–12] and Australia [13]. A KEP helps a potential living donor to donate his or her kidney, which is incompatible with the intended recipient, to another recipient so that the donor's intended recipient can also receive a compatible kidney from another donor. The Korea Centers for Disease Control & Prevention (KCDC), the government ministry that maintains a unified administration to avoid disease and to improve public health welfare in South Korea, has recently paid attention to the contribution of the KEP, which increases the number of renal disease sufferers able to receive kidney transplants. The KCDC has pushed ahead with a plan for the development of an integrated IT healthcare platform for the KEP. On the platform, hospitals can register the essential information for verifying the compatibility of their renal disease sufferers. Then, the proposed KEP platform would provide matching plans to maximize the number of possible kidney exchanges in the program. Hence, it is important to establish an efficient optimization model for KEPs that can provide optimized kidney exchange plans within a reasonable time, and, in this paper, we intend to provide a high-performance mathematical programming model easily solvable by commercial optimization solvers (e.g., Cplex, Gurobi) to support the integrated KEP IT healthcare platform of South Korea. We remark that, as in our case, operations research (OR) techniques have been applied and utilized to tackle many important and challenging optimization issues in healthcare (e.g., [14] for an overview of recent research on several OR applications in healthcare, and [15,16] for medical resident scheduling problems and sensor-based patient monitoring problems, respectively).

Figure 1 illustrates two-way and three-way KEPs. Figure 1a illustrates a case consisting of only two pairs. Within each pair, the patient and donor are incompatible. However, the patient in pair 1 is compatible with the donor in pair 2 and the patient in pair 2 is compatible with the donor in pair 1. We note that in precedent times, when exchanges between pairs were not allowed, there was no way to perform the transplants. However, with the KEP, exchanges between the pairs become possible, and the two transplants can be performed. As we will explain in detail below, the KEP can be expressed as a digraph for which a node corresponds to an incompatible donor–recipient pair and a directed arc is introduced if a donor in an initial node is compatible with a recipient in the terminal node of the arc (see the graph in Figure 1a). In practice, three-way exchanges are the most complicated exchanges performed because one of all the operations on an exchange cycle must be performed simultaneously to avoid the risk of one of the donors reneging, and it is technically difficult to simultaneously reserve operation rooms for more than six patients in a hospital. Figure 1b illustrates three-way kidney exchanges.

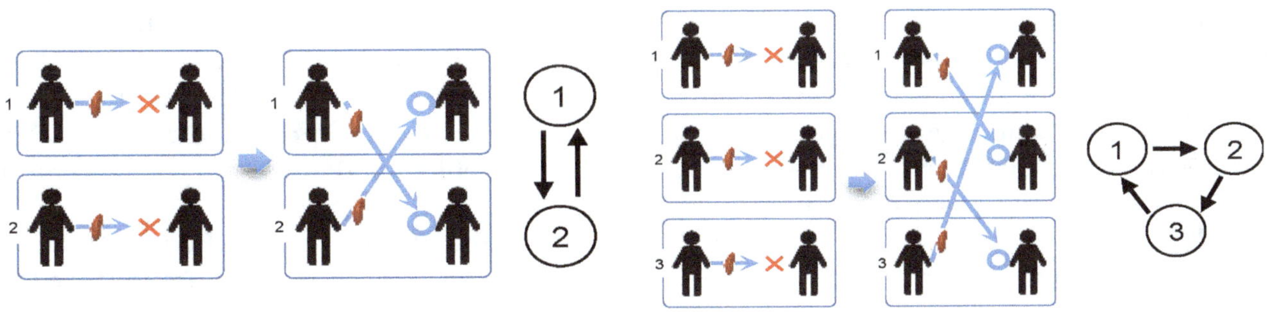

(a) (b)

Figure 1. Illustration of (**a**) two-way and (**b**) three-way kidney exchange program (KEP).

As we briefly mentioned before, the KEP model can be expressed by a digraph $G(V, A)$, called a *KEP graph* in this paper, where V and A indicate the set of vertices and arcs of the graph G, respectively. Figure 2 presents an example of G and a solution to the model (i.e., possible kidney exchanges on a KEP graph). In Figure 2a, a vertex $i \in V$ corresponds to a current incompatible pair consisting of a patient i and a donor i, and an arc $(i, j) \in A$ indicates the compatibility between donor i and patient j, which means that donor i can provide his or her kidney to patient j. Figure 2b demonstrates an example of a feasible solution. The thick arrows represent an exchange cycle among pairs 1, 2, and 4.

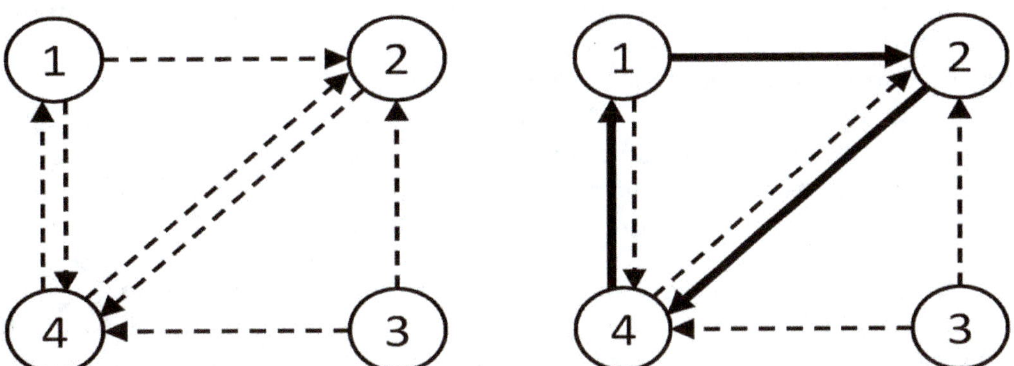

(a) (b)

Figure 2. Kidney exchange program (KEP) graph (**a**) and its feasible solution (**b**).

We now discuss the optimization problem for a KEP, given a KEP graph G. The objective of the optimization of a KEP is generally to maximize the number of possible kidney exchanges in a given pool of candidates, and the KEP can be mathematically modeled as an integer programming problem, which is the main focus of this paper. Roth et al. [17] proposed an edge formulation and a cycle formulation for KEPs, and Abraham et al. [7] developed a solution algorithm for those formulations. Furthermore, Constantino et al. [18] proposed two compact formulations—that is, an edge-assignment (EA) formulation and an extended edge (EE) formulation. Manlove and O'Malley [19] presented how the cycle formulation by Roth et al. [17] can be extended to find optimal solutions for the KEP in the United Kingdom, which are compatible with U.K. National Living Donor Kidney Sharing Schemes (NLDKSS).

The reformulation-linearization technique (RLT), which we intend to utilize in this paper, is a procedure that can be used to generate a tight linear programming (LP) relaxation for a discrete optimization problem. Various strong formulations on several classes of structured problems are generated by the RLT. Sherali et al. [20] developed a new integer programming model for the traveling salesman problem (TSP) by applying the RLT to the Miller–Tucker–Zemlin (MTZ) formulation. Moreover, they showed that the resulting formulation dominates the lifted-MTZ formulation of Desrochers and Laporte [21]. Sherali et al. [22] applied the RLT to the path-based TSP model using logical restrictions. They proposed a variety of new formulations for the TSP, and exploited several dominance relationships between them. Park et al. [23] dealt with a two-level facility location–allocation problem arising from the access network design of a telecommunication network. They developed a mixed-integer program for the problem and applied the RLT to improve computational effectiveness.

In this paper, we focus on the best-known compact formulations for the KEP in the literature, which are the EA and EE formulations proposed by Constantino et al. [18]. We first induce the EE formulation by applying the partial level 1 RLT to the EA formulation. After that, we further strengthen the formulation via the level 1 RLT and propose a new integer programming model that dominates existing formulations. Computational results are provided to demonstrate the effectiveness of our formulation compared to that of those previous. Therefore, the contribution of our study can be summarized as below.

- We propose a new integer programming model, which is proved to be more compact and effective than previous optimization models through computational experiments. Although our new formulation gives a solution that allows only one more patient to have a kidney transplant than the matching solutions made by existing formulations, this is a meaningful result because a kidney transplant is immediately related to the precious life of a patient. Furthermore, our proposed model would be directly related to the performance of the KEP IT healthcare platform.
- We derive the EE formulation from the EA formulation by applying a systematic approach, the RLT. As presented by Constantino et al. [18], establishing a more compact integer programming formulation requires the exploitation of the special structures inherent to the problem of interest. On the other hand, by using our approach, such a formulation can be derived by a simple and systematic application of the RLT independent of the problem-specific structures. This difference suggests the possibility that our approach can be applied to other real-world optimization problems to obtain more significant formulations.

This paper is organized as follows: Section 2 briefly provides the overview of the RLT for the reference. Section 3 reviews the two representative integer programming models (i.e., the EE and EA formulations) for the KEP in literature. Section 4 presents how the EE formulation can be derived from the EA formulation by applying the RLT and how we could further strengthen the EE formulation. Section 5 presents the computational results. Finally, we conclude the discussion in Section 6.

2. Reformulation-Linearization Technique

In this section, we briefly describe the concept of the RLT process in the context of zero-one integer problems. Let us define the feasible region of a zero-one integer problem as

$$X = \{x : \mathbf{A}x \leq b,\ x \in \mathbb{B}^r\}$$

where $\mathbf{A}$ is a $q \times r$ matrix, b is a q vector, and $N = \{1, 2, \ldots, r\}$ is the index set of all variables. Without loss of generality, we assume that every component of $\mathbf{A}$ and b is an integer. Additionally, the inequalities accommodate the upper bounds of $x_j \leq 1$ for $j \in N$. As usual, $\mathbb{B}$ and $\mathbb{R}$ denote the sets of binary and real numbers, respectively.

The RLT process by Sherali and Adams [24] to construct relaxation X_d at any level $d \in \{1, \ldots, r\}$ in higher dimensional space consists of two steps, as follows:

Step 1. (Reformulation) Multiply each constraint defining the feasible region with every product factor of the form $\prod_{i\in J_1} x_i \prod_{i\in J_2}(1-x_i)$, where $J_1, J_2 \subseteq N$, $J_1 \cap J_2 = \emptyset$, and $|J_1 \cup J_2| = d$, and then apply the identity $x_i^2 = x_i$ for all $i \in N$.
Step 2. (Linearization) Linearize the resulting polynomial system by substituting a variable λ_J for every distinct product term $\prod_{i\in J} x_i$, where $J \subseteq N$.

The results of Sherali and Adams [24] show that, by denoting the projection of X_d onto the space of the original variables x by $X_{P_d} = \{x : (x, \lambda) \in X_d\}$, we obtain the hierarchy of relaxations

$$X_{P_0} \equiv X_0 \supseteq X_{P_1} \supseteq X_{P_2} \supseteq \cdots \supseteq X_{P_r} \equiv conv(X)$$

where $X_{P_0} \equiv X_0$ denotes the linear programming relaxation of X. The results above imply that we can theoretically obtain the convex hull of the feasible solution set X via the level r RLT and can hence obtain the optimal solution by solving the linear programming problem over X_{P_r}.

For a better understanding, we illustrate the RLT process through the following example [25].

Example 1. *Consider the following polytope:*

$$X = \{x \in \mathbb{R}^2 : 2x_1 + 3x_2 \leq 4,\ x_j \in \{0, 1\},\ j = 1, 2\}.$$

The linear programming of this polytope is given as $X_0 = \{x \in R^2 : 2x_1 + 3x_2 \leq 4,\ 0 \leq x_1 \leq 1,\ 0 \leq x_2 \leq 1\}$, *and the convex hull of* X *is given as* $conv(X) = \{x \in R^2 : x_1 + x_2 \leq 1,\ x_1 \geq 0,\ x_2 \geq 0\}$ *(see Figure 3).*

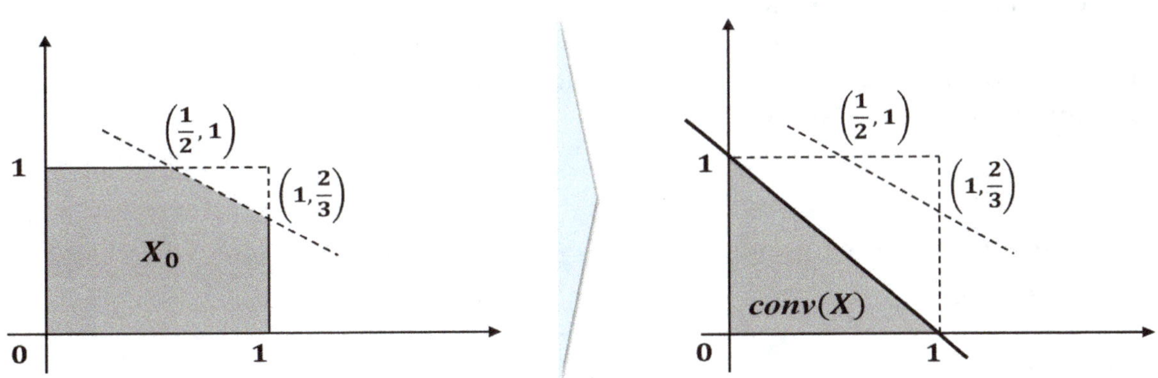

Figure 3. Illustration of polytope X_0 (**left**) and its convex hull $conv(X)$ (**right**).

Now, we apply the level 2 RLT to X_0 to illustrate how $conv(X)$ can be obtained by the RLT process.

Step 1. *(Reformulation) Multiply each constraint of X_0 by each of the factors x_1x_2, $x_1(1-x_2)$, $(1-x_1)x_2$, and $(1-x_1)(1-x_2)$. This process generates various duplicated or redundant inequalities; thus, we summarize the valid inequalities only, as follows:*

$$
\begin{array}{rcl}
(2x_1+3x_2 \le 4) \times x_1x_2 & \rightarrow & 2x_1x_2+3x_1x_2 \le 4x_1x_2 \\
 & \hookrightarrow & x_1x_2 \le 0 \\
(2x_1+3x_2 \le 4) \times (1-x_1)(1-x_2) & \rightarrow & 0 \le 4(1-x_1)(1-x_2) \\
 & \hookrightarrow & x_1+x_2 \le 1+x_1x_2 \\
(x_1 \ge 0) \times x_1x_2 & \rightarrow & x_1x_2 \ge 0 \\
(x_1 \ge 0) \times x_1(1-x_2) & \rightarrow & x_1 - x_1x_2 \ge 0 \\
(x_2 \ge 0) \times (1-x_1)x_2 & \rightarrow & x_2 - x_1x_2 \ge 0
\end{array}
$$

Step 2. *(Linearization) After linearizing the resulting polynomial system by substituting a variable z_{12} for the product term x_1x_2, we have*

$$
\begin{aligned}
& z_{12} \le 0 \\
& x_1+x_2 \le 1+z_{12} \\
& z_{12} \ge 0 \\
& x_1 - z_{12} \ge 0 \\
& x_2 - z_{12} \ge 0
\end{aligned}
$$

By $z_{12} \le 0$ and $z_{12} \ge 0$, we have $z_{12} = 0$. Therefore, the last set of inequalities produces

$$\{x \in R^2 : \ x_1+x_2 \le 1, \ x_1 \ge 0, \ x_2 \ge 0\}$$

which is $conv(X)$.

3. Two Representative Models for the KEP: EA and EE Formulations

In this section, we present two compact formulations, the EA and EE formulations, which were proposed by Constantino et al. [18] as reference models. In these formulations, the possible cycles in G and L are considered to be defined as a set composed of indices $\{1, ..., l_u\}$, where l_u indicates the upper bound on the possible number of cycles in G. The additional parameters and decision variables used in the formulation are given as follows:

Parameters

w_{ij}: Weight of edge $(i,j) \in A$, representing the level of compatibility between donor i and recipient j.
k: Maximum cycle length.

Decision Variables

x_{ij}: 1 if a kidney is transplanted from donor i to patient j, and 0 otherwise.
y_i^l: 1 if node i is included in cycle l, and 0 otherwise.

Then, the EA formulation is given as follows:

$$\text{EA}: \text{ Maximize } \sum_{(i,j)\in A} w_{ij}x_{ij} \tag{1a}$$

$$\text{subject to } \sum_{j:\,(j,\,i)\in A} x_{ji} = \sum_{j:\,(i,\,j)\in A} x_{ij}, \qquad \forall i \in V \tag{1b}$$

$$\sum_{j:\,(i,\,j)\in A} x_{ij} \le 1, \qquad \forall i \in V \tag{1c}$$

$$\sum_{i\in V} y_i^l \le k, \qquad \forall l \in L \tag{1d}$$

$$\sum_{l\in L} y_i^l = \sum_{j:\,(i,\,j)\in A} x_{ij}, \qquad \forall i \in V \tag{1e}$$

$$y_i^l + x_{ij} \le 1 + y_j^l, \qquad \forall (i,\,j) \in A,\ \forall l \in L \tag{1f}$$

$$x_{ij} \in \{0,\,1\}, \qquad \forall (i,\,j) \in A \tag{1g}$$

$$y_i^l \in \{0,\,1\}, \qquad \forall i \in V,\ l \in L \tag{1h}$$

The objective function of Equation (1a) is to maximize the sum of weights of the transplantations. Because the weight of each edge indicates the appropriateness of the corresponding transplantation, the KEP maximizing the total appropriateness of all transplantations is planned. We note that setting w_{ij} to the same value for all $(i,j) \in A$ allows the maximum number of possible kidney exchanges in a given pool of candidates to be obtained. Constraint (1b) indicates that if a donor in pair i donates his or her kidney to a patient in another pair, then the patient in pair i must receive a kidney. This constraint further implies that if a donor does not participate in transplantation, the paired patient would not receive a kidney. Constraint (1c) implies that a donor cannot donate more than one kidney. Constraint (1d) ensures that the length of each cycle cannot be greater than k. Constraint (1e) assigns a pair to a cycle if it takes part in kidney exchanges. We note that because $\sum_{j:(i,j)\in A} x_{ij} \le 1$, a pair has to be assigned to one of the cycles. Constraint (1f) implies that if a donor in pair i gives his or her kidney to a patient in pair j and if the pair i is assigned to a cycle l, then pair j also has to be included in cycle l. Constraints (1g) and (1h) indicate that all the decision variables in the model are binary variables.

We now present the EE formulation. We suppose that there are copies of graph G and we let the index of each copy be $l \in L$, where L is a set of the copies of G. Then, the EE formulation requires the additional decision variables x_{ij}^l, as follows:

Decision Variable

x_{ij}^l: 1 if a kidney is transplanted from donor i to patient j in copy l, and 0 otherwise.

Then, the EE formulation is given as follows:

$$\text{EE}: \text{ Maximize } \sum_{l\in L}\sum_{(i,j)\in A} w_{ij}x_{ij}^l \tag{2a}$$

$$\text{Subject to } \sum_{j:\,(j,\,i)\in A} x_{ji}^l = \sum_{j:\,(i,\,j)\in A} x_{ij}^l, \qquad \forall i \in V, \forall l \in L \tag{2b}$$

$$\sum_{l\in L}\sum_{j:\,(i,\,j)\in A} x_{ij}^l \le 1, \qquad \forall i \in V \tag{2c}$$

$$\sum_{(i,j)\in A} x_{ij}^l \le k, \qquad \forall l \in L \tag{2d}$$

$$x_{ij} \in \{0,\,1\}, \qquad \forall (i,\,j) \in A \tag{2e}$$

The objective function of Equation (2a) indicates that the model maximizes the total weight of arcs among all copies of G. Constraint (2b) ensures that the number of kidneys given by donor i and received by patient i should be same at each pair i for each copy l. Constraint (2c) indicates that a pair can donate or receive at most one kidney. We note that the constraint holds for all copies $l \in L$ and that an arc cannot be selected for more than two copies of G. Constraint (2d) restricts the length of exchange cycles to less than or equal to k.

In addition, in order to have further simplified formulations, symmetry elimination constraints were applied, as discussed by Constantino et al. [18]:

$$y_i^l \leq y_l^l, \qquad \forall i \in V,\ l \in L,\ i > l \tag{3}$$

for the EA formulation, and

$$\sum_{j:\ (i,\ j) \in A} x_{ij}^l \leq \sum_{j:\ (l,\ j) \in A} x_{lj}^l, \qquad \forall i > l$$

for the EE formulation. These inequalities enforce node l to be in cycle l and enforce all other nodes in the cycle to have indices larger than l. For further details, we refer the readers to Constantino et al. [18].

4. RLT Applications

In this section, we will present the application of the RLT to two existing compact formulations (i.e., the EA and EE formulations). We first show that the EE formulation can be derived by applying the RLT to the EA formulation systemically without relying on any problem-specific structures or insights. After that, we derive a new compact formulation that dominates the EE formulation by further applying the RLT to it.

4.1. Derivation of the EE Formulation from the EA Formulation

We now apply a specialized version of the RLT to the EA formulation by following the discussion by Sherali and Adams [24,26]. To contain the size of the resulting relaxation, we apply only a partial first-level version of this approach. Our approach is to first reformulate the EA formulation by generating the additional (nonlinear) implied constraints. By applying a linearization, which substitutes variables in place of each distinct nonlinear term, we can expose the useful relationships between the new and original variables that intend to enforce the nonlinear relationships. Specifically, we perform the following operations:

- **Reformulation Phase.** Construct additional sets of constraints via (R1)–(R5) stated below.

(R1) Similarly to Constraint (1f), construct the following valid inequalities:

$$y_j^l + x_{ij} \leq 1 + y_i^l, \qquad \forall (i,\ j) \in A,\ \forall l \in L \tag{4}$$

Using Constraints (1f) and (4), construct the valid inequalities

$$x_{ij}(y_i^l + x_{ij} - 1 - y_j^l) \leq 0 \quad \text{for} \quad (i,\ j) \in A,\ l \in L$$

and

$$x_{ij}(y_j^l + x_{ij} - 1 - y_i^l) \leq 0 \quad \text{for} \quad (i,\ j) \in A,\ l \in L.$$

(R2) For each $i \in V$, multiply the equation $\sum_{j:\ (j,\ i) \in A} x_{ji} = \sum_{j:\ (i,\ j) \in A} x_{ij}$ of Constraint (1b) by $y_i^l \geq 0$ for each $i \in V,\ l \in L$.

(R3) For each $i \in V$, multiply the inequality $\sum_{j:\ (i,\ j) \in A} x_{ij} \leq 1$ of Constraint (1c) by $y_i^l \geq 0$ for each $i \in V,\ l \in L$.

(R4) From Constraints (1c) and (1e), we can derive $\sum_{l \in L} y_i^l \leq 1$ for $i \in V$. For each $i \in V$, multiply $\sum_{l \in L} y_i^l \leq 1$ and $\sum_{l \in L} y_i^l = \sum_{j:\ (i,\ j) \in A} x_{ij}$ by $y_i^{l'}$ for each $i \in V, l' \in L$.

(R5) For each $i \in V$, multiply the inequality $\sum_{j:\,(i,\,j)\in A} x_{ij} \leq 1$ of Constraint (1c) by $x_{ij'}$ for each $(i,\, j') \in A$, and for each $i \in V$, multiply the equation $\sum_{l\in L} y_i^l = \sum_{j:\,(i,\,j)\in A} x_{ij}$ by $x_{ij'}$ for each $(i,\, j') \in A$.

- **Linearization Phase.** Linearize the new classes of constraints generated by (R1)–(R5) above by using the substitutions

$$u_{ij}^l = y_i^l x_{ij} \qquad \text{and} \qquad v_{ij}^l = y_j^l x_{ij} \qquad \forall (i,\, j) \in A,\ \forall l \in L.$$

Reformulation step (R1) produces $u_{ij}^l \leq v_{ij}^l$ for $(i,\, j) \in A,\ l \in L$ and $v_{ij}^l \leq u_{ij}^l$ for $(i,\, j) \in A,\ l \in L$. Therefore, we have $u_{ij}^l = v_{ij}^l$ for $(i,\, j) \in A,\ l \in L$ and we only use u variables for the linearization. Step (R2) produces $\sum_{j:\,(j,\,i)\in A} u_{ji}^l = \sum_{j:\,(i,\,j)\in A} u_{ij}^l$ for $i \in V,\ l \in L$. Step (R3) gives $\sum_{j:\,(i,\,j)\in A} u_{ij}^l \leq y_i^l$ for $i \in V,\ l \in L$, and surrogates them for each $l \in L$, which results in $\sum_{l\in L}\sum_{j:\,(i,\,j)\in A} u_{ij}^l \leq \sum_{l\in L} y_i^l$ for $i \in V$. By Constraints (1c) and (1e), we have $\sum_{l\in L}\sum_{j:\,(i,\,j)\in A} u_{ij}^l \leq 1$ for $i \in V$. Reformulation step (R4) generates $y_i^{l'} + \sum_{l(\neq l')\in L} y_i^l y_i^{l'} \leq y_i^{l'}$ for $i \in V$, which leads to $\sum_{l(\neq l')\in L} y_i^l y_i^{l'} = 0$. Therefore, $\sum_{l\in L} y_i^l = \sum_{j:\,(i,\,j)\in A} x_{ij}$ multiplied by $y_i^{l'}$ for each $i \in V, l' \in L$ yields $y_i^l = \sum_{j:\,(i,\,j)\in A} u_{ij}^l$ for $i \in V,\ l \in L$ (l' is substituted by l for convenience). Next, surrogating $y_i^l = \sum_{j:\,(i,\,j)\in A} u_{ij}^l$ for each $i \in V$ gives $\sum_{i\in V} y_i^l = \sum_{(i,\,j)\in A} u_{ij}^l$ for $l \in L$. Hence, by Constraint (1d), we have $\sum_{(i,\,j)\in A} u_{ij}^l \leq k$ for $l \in L$. According to the first statement of step (R5) along with $x_{ij} \geq 0$ for $(i,\, j) \in A$, we can obtain $\sum_{j\neq j':\,(i,\,j)\in A} x_{ij}x_{ij'} = 0$ for $i \in V$. The next statement along with the first result produces $x_{ij} = \sum_{l\in L} u_{ij}^l$ for $i \in V$. Therefore, we can replace the objective function of Equation (1a) with $\sum_{l\in L}\sum_{(i,\,j)\in A} w_{ij}u_{ij}^l$. Consequently, after substituting x_{ij}^l for u_{ij}^l, the RLT application constructs the EE formulation. We again emphasize that the aforementioned procedures do not rely on any problem-specific structures or insights, but they derive the same compact formulation, the EE formulation, from the EA formulation.

4.2. Extended Formulation Derived from the EE Formulation

In this subsection, we further strengthen the EE formulation by applying the RLT while maintaining the y variables. The specific RLT procedure we perform is explained in detail below.

- **Reformulation Phase.** Construct the additional set of constraints via (R6)–(R9) stated below.

(R6) For each $i \in V$, multiply the inequality $\sum_{j:\,(i,\,j)\in A} x_{ij} \leq 1$ of Constraint (1c) by $y_i^l \geq 0$ for each $i \in V,\ l \in L$.

(R7) For each $(i,\, j) \in A$ and $l \in L$, multiply the inequality $y_i^l + x_{ij} \leq 1 + y_j^l$ of Constraint (1f) by $y_i^l \geq 0$ and y_j^l. Similarly, for each $(i,\, j) \in A$ and $l \in L$, multiply the inequality $y_j^l + x_{ij} \leq 1 + y_i^l$ by $y_i^l \geq 0$.

(R8) For each $l \in L$, multiply the inequality $\sum_{i\in V} y_i^l \leq k$ of Constraint (1d) by $y_j^l \geq 0$ for each $j \in V$.

(R9) For each $i \in V,\ l \in L,\ i > l$, multiply the inequality $y_i^l \leq y_l^l$ of the symmetry elimination constraints (3) by $y_i^l \geq 0$, $y_l^l \geq 0$, and $y_j^l \geq 0$ for each $j \in V$.

- **Linearization Phase.** Linearize the new classes of constraints generated by (R6)–(R9) above by using the substitutions

$$x_{ij}^l = y_i^l x_{ij} = y_j^l x_{ij} \qquad \forall (i,\, j) \in A,\ \forall l \in L \qquad \text{and} \qquad z_{(ij)}^l = y_i^l y_j^l \qquad \forall i,\, j \in V,\ \forall l \in L.$$

Reformulation step (R6) produces $\sum_{j:\,(i,\,j)\in A} x_{ij}^l \leq y_i^l$ for $i \in V,\ l \in L$. Step (R7) gives three classes of valid inequalities $x_{ij}^l \leq z_{(ij)}^l$, $z_{(ij)}^l + x_{ij}^l \leq 2y_j^l$, and $z_{(ij)}^l + x_{ij}^l \leq 2y_i^l$ for $(i,\, j) \in A,\ l \in L$. Step (R8) generates $\sum_{j(\neq i)\in V} z^l_{(ij)} \leq (k-1)y^l_i$ for $i \in V,\ l \in L$. The last step (R9) produces $y^l_i \leq z^l_{il} \leq y^l_l$ for $i \in V,\ l \in L$, and $z^l_{(ij)} \leq z^l_{jl}$ for $i,\ j \in V,\ l \in L$.

We summarize the overall RLT process above to derive a new compact formulation from the EE formulation in Figure 4. By augmenting the valid inequalities generated above to some set of constraints from the EE and EA formulations, we derive a new integer programming model for the KEP, which is more compact and tighter than the EE formulation, as follows:

$$\text{RLT}: \text{ Maximize} \sum_{l\in L}\sum_{(i,\,j)\in A} w_{ij}x^l_{ij} \tag{5a}$$

Subject to Constraints (2b), (2c), (2d), (2e), (1h)

$$\sum_{j:\,(i,\,j)\in A} x^l_{ij} \leq y^l_i, \qquad \forall i \in V,\ l \in L \tag{5b}$$

$$x^l_{ij} \leq z^l_{(ij)}, \qquad \forall (i,\ j) \in A,\ l \in L \tag{5c}$$

$$z^l_{(ij)} + x^l_{ij} \leq 2y^l_j, \qquad \forall (i,\ j) \in A,\ l \in L \tag{5d}$$

$$z^l_{(ij)} + x^l_{ij} \leq 2y^l_i, \qquad \forall (i,\ j) \in A,\ l \in L \tag{5e}$$

$$\sum_{j(\neq i)\in V} z^l_{(ij)} \leq (k-1)y^l_i, \qquad \forall i \in V,\ l \in L \tag{5f}$$

$$y^l_i \leq z^l_{il} \leq y^l_l, \qquad \forall i \in V,\ l \in L \tag{5g}$$

$$z^l_{(ij)} \leq z^l_{jl}, \qquad \forall i,\ j \in V,\ l \in L \tag{5h}$$

$$z^l_{(ij)} \in \{0,\ 1\}, \qquad \forall i,\ j \in V,\ l \in L. \tag{5i}$$

Reformulation

$\left(\sum_{j:(i,j)\in A} x_{ij} \leq 1\right) \times y^l_i$

$(y^l_i + x_{ij} \leq 1 + y^l_j) \times y^l_i$

$(y^l_i + x_{ij} \leq 1 + y^l_j) \times y^l_j$

$(y^l_j + x_{ij} \leq 1 + y^l_i) \times y^l_i$

$\left(\sum_{i\in V} y^l_i \leq k\right) \times y^l_j$

$(y^l_i \leq y^l_l) \times y^l_i$

$(y^l_i \leq y^l_l) \times y^l_l$

$(y^l_i \leq y^l_l) \times y^l_j$

Linearization

$z^l_{(ij)} \equiv y^l_i \times y^l_j$

$z^l_{(ij)} = \begin{cases} z^l_{ij}, & i < j \\ z^l_{ji}, & i > j \end{cases}$

Resulting valid inequalities

$\sum_{j:(i,j)\in A} x^l_{ij} \leq y^l_i, \quad \forall i \in V, l \in L$

$x^l_{ij} \leq z^l_{(ij)}, \quad \forall (i,j) \in A, l \in L$

$z^l_{(ij)} + x^l_{ij} \leq 2y^l_j, \quad \forall (i,j) \in A, l \in L$

$z^l_{(ij)} + x^l_{ij} \leq 2y^l_i, \quad \forall (i,j) \in A, l \in L$

$\sum_{j(\neq i)\in V} z^l_{(ij)} \leq (k-1)y^l_i, \quad \forall i \in V, l \in L$

$y^l_i \leq z^l_{il} \leq y^l_l, \quad \forall i \in V, l \in L$

$z^l_{(ij)} \leq z^l_{jl}, \quad \forall i,j \in V, l \in L$

Figure 4. Illustration of the reformulation-linearization technique (RLT) for deriving new valid inequalities.

5. Computational Results

In this section, we present the results of the computational experiments for the KEP. The experiments were performed using an Intel(R) Core(TM) i7-4770 CPU @ 3.40 GHz, and CPLEX 12.4 as a LP/MIP (mixed integer programming) optimization solver. The experiments were designed to compare the EA, EE, and RLT formulations in terms of performance. Problem instances were constructed as by Constantino et al. [18]. A random generator that created random KEP graphs of chosen certain arc densities was used. To be specific, on each position of the node adjacency matrix of a graph, a probability p is used to determine whether the element equals 1 or 0. Constantino et al. [18] used values of 0.2, 0.5, and 0.7 for the probability p. However, it was found that with probabilities of 0.5 and 0.7, almost every instance had an optimal objective n equal to the number of nodes. Because n is the trivial upper bound of these KEP problems, no formulation can improve the linear relaxation bound of such problem instances. Thus, because an important goal of this paper is to compare the tightness of KEP formulations, p was set to 0.1, 0.2, and 0.5 for low-, medium-, and high-density instances, respectively. For each density, we generated the problem instances with the input parameter $k = 3, 4, 5, 6$. In addition, n, the number of pairs, was further set to 10, 20, and 30 for each k. For each n and k, 10 instances were generated and tested. All the cases were executed within a time limit of 3600 s. The formulations were compared in terms of the optimality gap (GAP) and the execution time. The GAP is calculated by $(Z_{LP} - Z_{IP})/Z_{IP}$, where Z_{IP} is the best objective function value of the integer programming model and Z_{LP} is the optimal objective function value of the corresponding linear programming relaxation. Hence, the lower the GAP obtained, the better the solution (i.e., closer to the optimal solution). On the other hand, T_{IP} and T_{LP} are the average elapsed time of the integer programming model and its linear programming relaxation, respectively.

Table 1. Computational results for low-density instances. EA: edge-assignment; EE: extended edge; RLT: reformulation-linearization technique; GAP: optimality gap.

Problem Instances		**EA**			**EE**			**RLT**		
		T_{LP}	T_{IP}	GAP	T_{LP}	T_{IP}	GAP	T_{LP}	T_{IP}	GAP
$k = 3$	$n = 10$	0.00	0.00	10.7%	0.00	0.00	8.7%	0.00	0.01	6.7%
	$n = 20$	0.00	0.01	87.5%	0.00	0.00	68.2%	0.02	0.03	67.8%
	$n = 30$	0.02	0.53	98.1%	0.01	0.01	84.2%	0.29	0.11	83.9%
$k = 4$	$n = 10$	0.00	0.00	4.3%	0.00	0.00	3.3%	0.00	0.00	3.0%
	$n = 20$	0.00	0.01	45.1%	0.00	0.00	39.0%	0.00	0.00	38.1%
	$n = 30$	0.02	1.68	37.3%	0.01	0.02	33.2%	0.22	0.05	33.1%
$k = 5$	$n = 10$	0.00	0.00	4.7%	0.00	0.00	4.2%	0.00	0.00	3.8%
	$n = 20$	0.00	0.01	17.9%	0.00	0.01	14.8%	0.02	0.03	14.1%
	$n = 30$	0.02	0.76	18.0%	0.01	0.07	15.9%	0.34	0.10	14.9%
$k = 6$	$n = 10$	0.00	0.00	0.0%	0.00	0.00	0.0%	0.00	0.00	0.0%
	$n = 20$	0.00	0.01	10.5%	0.00	0.01	9.6%	0.02	0.04	9.5%
	$n = 30$	0.01	0.59	10.9%	0.01	0.12	9.6%	0.59	0.27	9.6%

Table 1 summarizes the computational results for low-density instances. The EE formulation found the optimal upper bound for 43 out of 120 low-density instances. Of the remaining 77 instances for which the EE formulation could not find the optimal solution, the upper bounds of 36 instances were improved by our RLT model. Subsequently, the average value of the GAP was improved by our RLT formulation. On the other hand, the improvement in the GAP obtained by the RLT formulation tended to be smaller as k grew.

Figure 5 presents box plots of the GAPs (%) produced by each formulation from problem instances for each combination of (n, k). From the figure, we can observe that our RLT formulation yielded the lowest average GAPs, and that furthermore, the variability of the GAPs produced by our RLT formulation was also lower than that of the best-known compact formulations. Specifically, both the maximum and minimum GAPs, as well as the difference between the lower and upper quartiles, significantly dropped from the EA formulation to the EE formulation, and then further again to the RLT formulation. Moreover, such observations were consistent for every combination of (n, k). The results imply that the EA formulation is highly dominated by the EE and RLT formulations, and moreover, that our proposed RLT formulation is more reliable than the EE formulation in terms of solution quality—that is, our approach produces more reliable and higher quality solutions than the best-known compact formulations, without compromising computational time.

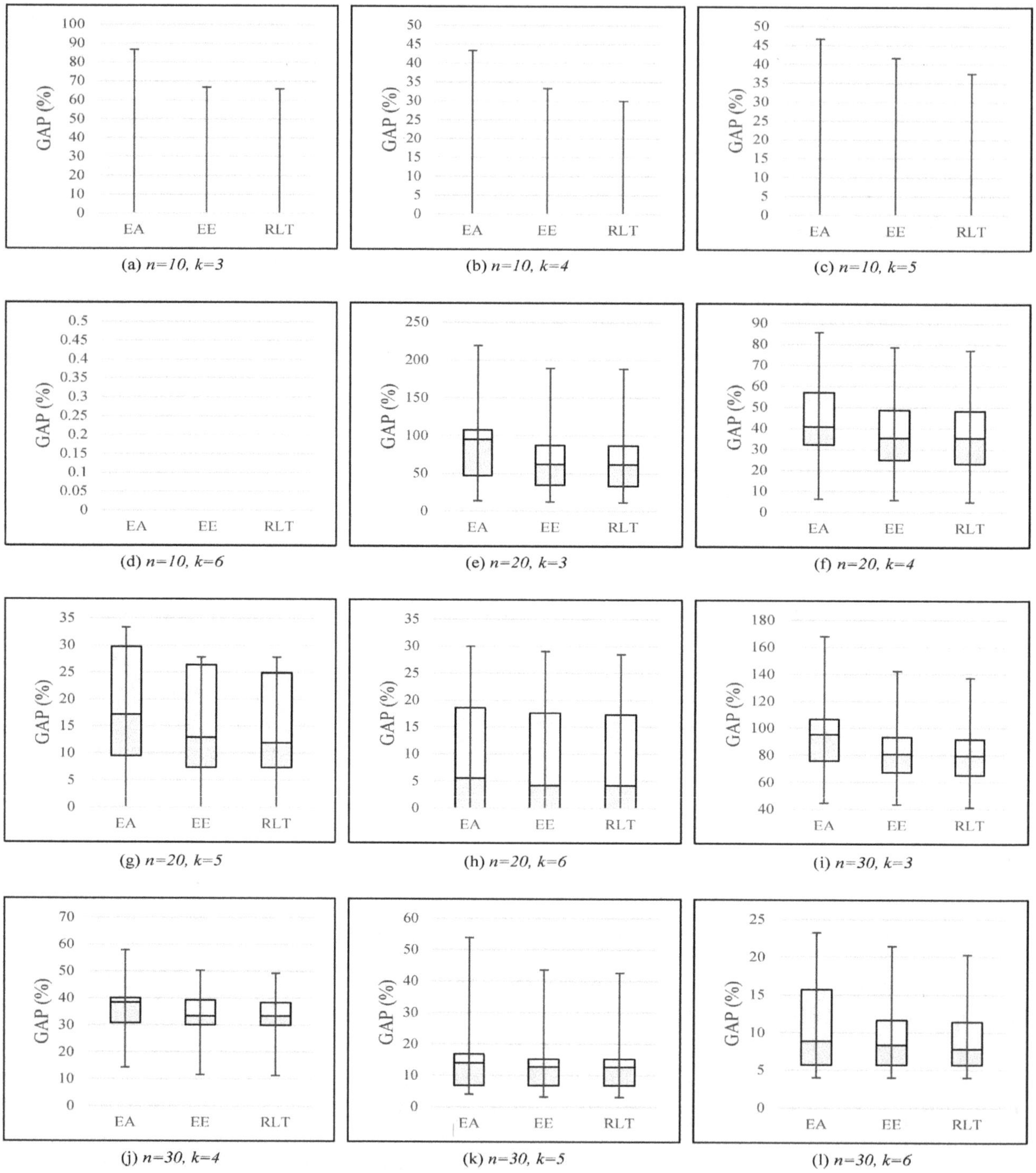

Figure 5. Box plots of optimality gaps (GAPs) for low-density instances.

Similarly, Table 2 demonstrates the computational results for medium-density instances. According to the results, the average GAP was smaller than for the low-density instances for all the formulations. Having such a result is intuitive because the medium-density graph had more arcs representing compatibility; thus, feasible solutions could be more easily found than in the low-density cases. In the experiments, the EE formulation found the optimal upper bounds for 83 out of 120 instances. Our RLT formulation improved the upper bounds of 17 out of the remaining

37 instances whose optimal solutions were not obtained by the EE formulation. When it comes to the box plots of the GAPs for the medium-density problem instances, we are able to make similar observations to those for the low-density instances as presented in Figure 6. As mentioned previously, compared to the low-density case, there were more combinations of (n, k) for which the GAPs of all the problem instances were equal to zero (i.e., (j), (k) and (l) in Figure 6).

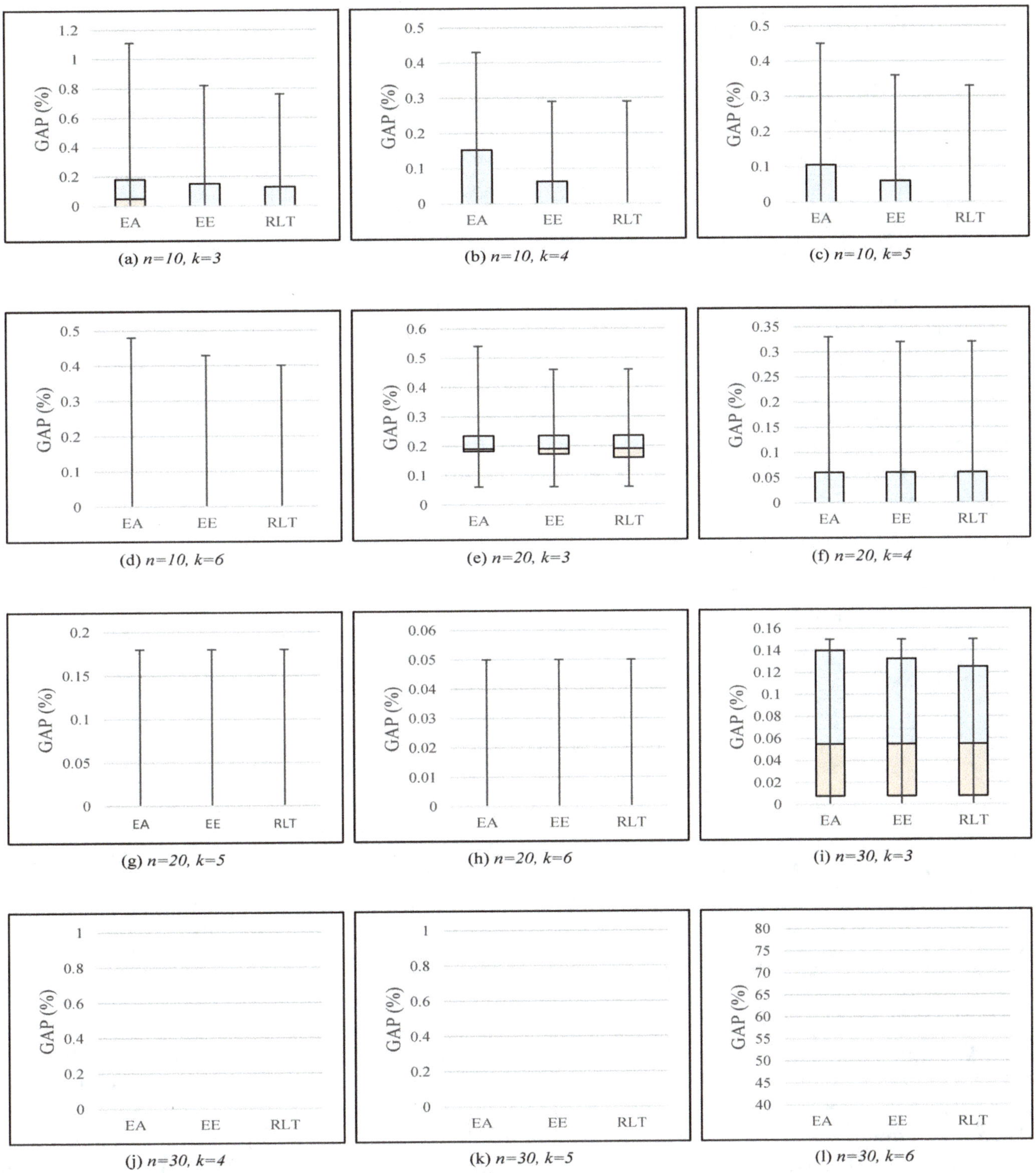

Figure 6. Box plots of optimality gaps (GAPs) for medium-density instances.

Table 2. Computational results for medium-density instances.

Problem Instances		EA			EE			RLT		
		T_{LP}	T_{IP}	GAP	T_{LP}	T_{IP}	GAP	T_{LP}	T_{IP}	GAP
$k=3$	$n=10$	0.00	0.00	22.0%	0.00	0.00	16.2%	0.00	0.00	16.0%
	$n=20$	0.01	0.95	22.2%	0.00	0.01	20.8%	0.05	0.07	20.5%
	$n=30$	0.03	238.11	7.1%	0.03	0.09	7.0%	0.05	0.12	6.9%
$k=4$	$n=10$	0.00	0.00	9.7%	0.00	0.02	6.3%	0.00	0.01	5.1%
	$n=20$	0.01	0.41	6.2%	0.00	0.06	6.0%	0.53	0.41	6.0%
	$n=30$	0.02	100.95	0.0%	0.03	0.93	0.0%	0.68	1.55	0.0%
$k=5$	$n=10$	0.00	0.00	7.8%	0.00	0.00	5.7%	0.00	0.01	3.8%
	$n=20$	0.01	0.22	2.9%	0.00	0.07	2.9%	0.40	0.58	2.9%
	$n=30$	0.02	12.55	0.0%	0.02	0.38	0.0%	0.29	0.67	0.0%
$k=6$	$n=10$	0.00	0.00	6.3%	0.00	0.00	5.5%	0.00	0.01	4.8%
	$n=20$	0.01	0.11	1.1%	0.00	0.07	1.1%	0.27	0.76	1.1%
	$n=30$	0.02	3.91	0.0%	0.03	0.25	0.0%	0.19	0.42	0.0%

Finally, the computational results for the high-density instances are presented in Table 3. We observe that the GAPs of all the formulations were equal to 0 for all the instances; hence, we here compare them in terms of the computational time only. As presented in Table 3, in terms of computational time, the RLT formulation outperformed the EA formulation, but the EE formulation performed slightly better than the RLT formulation. However, both cases were reasonably acceptable for practical-size problems. We remark that high-density instances rarely appear in real-world situations, as a donor is unlikely to find as many compatible patients as in high-density cases in a given pool of candidates.

Table 3. Computational results for high-density instances.

Problem Instances		EA			EE			RLT		
		T_{LP}	T_{IP}	GAP	T_{LP}	T_{IP}	GAP	T_{LP}	T_{IP}	GAP
$k=3$	$n=10$	0.00	0.02	0.0%	0.00	0.01	0.0%	0.02	0.03	0.0%
	$n=20$	0.01	1.20	0.0%	0.01	0.14	0.0%	0.96	0.31	0.0%
	$n=30$	0.03	57.15	0.0%	0.03	0.71	0.0%	0.86	1.87	0.0%
$k=4$	$n=10$	0.00	0.03	0.0%	0.00	0.01	0.0%	0.01	0.03	0.0%
	$n=20$	0.01	0.32	0.0%	0.01	0.09	0.0%	0.68	0.49	0.0%
	$n=30$	0.03	35.29	0.0%	0.04	0.43	0.0%	0.82	0.99	0.0%
$k=5$	$n=10$	0.00	0.01	0.0%	0.00	0.01	0.0%	0.01	0.02	0.0%
	$n=20$	0.01	0.23	0.0%	0.01	0.08	0.0%	0.65	0.48	0.0%
	$n=30$	0.03	10.02	0.0%	0.04	0.29	0.0%	0.57	0.88	0.0%
$k=6$	$n=10$	0.00	0.01	0.0%	0.00	0.01	0.0%	0.01	0.02	0.0%
	$n=20$	0.01	0.17	0.0%	0.01	0.07	0.0%	0.51	0.46	0.0%
	$n=30$	0.02	2.53	0.0%	0.04	0.26	0.0%	1.04	0.82	0.0%

6. Conclusions

In this paper, we first show that the EE formulation, until now considered to be the most compact formulation, can be systematically derived from the EA formulation through the RLT process. A previous study developed the EE formulation by exploiting special structures inherent to the problem. However, we show that we can readily apply the RLT procedure to the EA formulation to obtain the same EE formulation. Furthermore, we apply the RLT to the EA and EE formulations and thereby derive a tighter and more compact formulation. Computational results show that the proposed RLT model outperforms the existing EA and EE formulations in terms of solution quality as well as computational time. Specifically, the RLT model provides improved GAPs in several instances for which the EE formulation could not find the optimal solutions within the time limit—especially for low- and medium-density graphs. For high-density instances, although the RLT model does not significantly reduce the execution time, it can produce the same high-quality solutions as the existing formulations. We believe that, given the results obtained by the proposed model, it could be utilized in the integrated KEP IT healthcare platform to obtain optimized KEP exchange plans.

As extended research, several models derived from that proposed in this paper can be considered. For example, firstly, a problem dealing with fair allocations, such as in terms of donor and patient age and health, among the pairs in the candidate pool may be interesting. Indeed, some problems of fairness in kidney transplantation or kidney exchange are discussed by Bertsimas et al. [27] and by Anderson [15] respectively in literature. Secondly, some limitations of this study include that all data (e.g., w_{ij}) were considered to be certain. When a KEP solution is actually implemented, it may be possible to have several unexpected events, including last-minute incompatibility and unavailability of either donors or recipients [28,29]. To handle the data or event uncertainty in KEPs, Alvelos et al. [29], for example, examined an optimization problem whose objective was to maximize the expected number of transplants in a KEP given that all the arcs and vertices in a KEP graph have equal probabilities of failure, and there are some attempts to apply robust optimization theory [30,31] to a KEP [28]. Thus, we can extend our model to incorporate the aforementioned uncertainties and take the solution approaches, such as stochastic optimization or robust optimization techniques, into account. Finally, proposing an efficient heuristic-based approach for solving highly large-scale problems more generally would be the topic for future research.

Acknowledgments: This work was supported by the National Research Foundation of Korea(NRF) grant funded by the Korea government(Ministry of Science, ICT & Future Planning) (No. NRF-2015R1C1A1A02036682).

Author Contributions: Junsang Yuh developed the mathematical programming models and performed the experiments. Seokhyun Chung contributed to the literature review, experimental part and result analysis. Taesu Cheong guided the whole research, supported the structure of the paper and prepared the manuscript. All authors read and approved the final manuscript.

References

1. Kwak, J.Y.; Kwon, O.J.; Lee, K.S.; Kang, C.M.; Park, H.Y.; Kim, J.H. Exchange-donor program in renal transplantation: A single-center experience. *Transplant. Proc.* **1999**, *31*, 344–345.
2. Park, K.; Lee, J.H.; Huh, K.H.; Kim, S.I.; Kim, Y.S. Exchange living-donor kidney transplantation: Diminution of donor organ shortage. *Transplant. Proc.* **2004**, *36*, 2949–2951.
3. Huh, K.H.; Kim, M.S.; Ju, M.K.; Chang, H.K.; Ahn, H.J.; Lee, S.H.; Park, K. Exchange living-donor kidney transplantation: Merits and limitations. *Transplantation* **2008**, *86*, 430–435.
4. Ellison, M.D.; McBride, M.A.; Taranto, S.E.; Delmonico, F.L.; Kauffman, H.M. Living kidney donors in need of kidney transplants: A report from the organ procurement and transplantation network. *Transplantation* **2002**, *74*, 1349–1351.
5. Segev, D.L.; Gentry, S.E.; Warren, D.S.; Reeb, B.; Montgomery, R.A. Kidney paired donation and optimizing the use of live donor organs. *JAMA* **2005**, *293*, 1883–1890.
6. Saidman, S.L.; Roth, A.E.; Sönmez, T.; Ünver, M.U.; Delmonico, F.L. Increasing the opportunity of live kidney donation by matching for two- and three-way exchanges. *Transplantation* **2006**, *81*, 773–782.
7. Abraham, D.J.; Blum, A.; Sandholm, T. Clearing algorithms for barter exchange markets: Enabling nationwide kidney exchanges. In Proceedings of the 8th ACM Conference on Electronic Commerce, San Diego, CA, USA, 11–15 June 2007; pp. 295–304.
8. Veale, J.; Hil, G. National Kidney Registry: 213 transplants in three years. *Clin. Transpl.* **2010**, 333–344. Available online: http://www.kidneyregistry.org/docs/nkr_transplants_2010_chain_chapter.pdf (accessed on 10 April 2017).
9. Wallis, C.; Samy, K.; Roth, A.; Rees, M. Kidney paired donation. *Nephrol. Dial. Transplant.* **2011**, *26*, 2091–2099, doi:10.1093/ndt/gfr155.

10. Johnson, R.; Collett, D.; Birch, R.; Fuggle, S.; Rudge, C. Kidney donation and transplantation in the UK from 1998 to 2007. *Clin. Transpl.* **2008**, 75–88, doi:10.1201/9781420086423.ch10.
11. Johnson, R.J.; Allen, J.E.; Fuggle, S.V.; Bradley, J.A.; Rudge, C. Early experience of paired living kidney donation in the United Kingdom. *Transplantation* **2008**, *86*, 1672–1677.
12. Biro, P.; Manlove, D.F.; Rizzi, R. Maximum weight cycle packing in directed graphs, with application to kidney exchange programs. *Discret. Math. Algorithms Appl.* **2009**, *1*, 499–517.
13. Ferrari, P.; Woodroffe, C.; Christiansen, F.T. Paired kidney donations to expand the living donor pool: The Western Australian experience. *Med. J. Australia* **2009**, *190*, 700.
14. Rais, A.; Viana, A. Operations Research in Healthcare: A Survey. *Int. Trans. Oper. Res.* **2011**, *18*, 1–31.
15. Anderson, R.M. Stochastic Models and Data Driven Simulations for Healthcare Operations. Ph.D. Thesis, Massachusetts Institute of Technology, Cambridge, MA, USA, 2014.
16. D'Andreagiovanni, F.; Nardin, A. Towards the Fast and Robust Optimal Design of Wireless Body Area Networks. *Appl. Soft Comput.* **2015**, *37*, 971–982.
17. Roth, A.E.; Sönmez, T.; Ünver, M.U. Efficient Kidney Exchange: Coincidence of Wants in Markets with Compatibility-Based Preferences. *Am. Econ. Rev.* **2007**, *97*, 828–851.
18. Constantino, M.; Klimentova, X.; Viana, A.; Rais, A. New insights on integer-programming models for the kidney exchange problem. *Eur. J. Oper. Res.* **2013**, *231*, 57–68.
19. Manlove, D.F.; O'Malley, G. Paired and Altruistic Kidney Donation in the UK: Algorithms and Experimentation. *ACM J. Exp. Algorithmics* **2015**, *19*, doi:10.1145/2670129.
20. Sherali, H.D.; Driscoll, P.J. On Tightening the Relaxations of Miller-Tucker-Zemlin Formulations for Asymmetric Traveling Salesman Problems. *Oper. Res.* **2002**, *50*, 656–669.
21. Desrochers, M.; Laporte, G. Improvements and Extensions to the Miller-Tucker-Zemlin Subtour Elimination Constraints. *Oper. Res. Lett.* **1991**, *10*, 27–36.
22. Sherali, H.D.; Sarin, S.C.; Tsai, P. A Class of Lifted Path and Flow-Based Formulations for the Asymmetric Traveling Salesman Problem with and without Precedence Constraints. *Discret. Optim.* **2006**, *3*, 20–32.
23. Park, G.; Lee, Y.; Han, J. A Two-Level Location-Allocation Problem in Designing Local Access Fiber Optic Networks. *Comput. Oper. Res.* **2014**, *51*, 52–63.
24. Sherali, H.D.; Adams, W.P. A hierarchy of relaxations and convex hull characterizations for mixed-integer zero-one programming problems. *Discret. Appl. Math.* **1994**, *52*, 83–106.
25. Sherali, H.D.; Lee, Y.; Kim, Y. Partial convexification cuts for 0–1 mixed-integer programs. *Eur. J. Oper. Res.* **2005**, *165*, 625–648.
26. Sherali, H.D.; Adams, W.P. A hierarchy of relaxations between the continuous and convex hull representations for zero-one programming problems. *SIAM J. Discret. Math.* **1990**, *3*, 411–430.
27. Bertsimas, D.; Farias, V.F.; Trichakis, N. Fairness, Efficiency, and Flexibility in Organ Allocation for Kidney Transplantation. *Oper. Res.* **2013**, *61*, 73–87.
28. Dickerson, J.P. Robust Dynamic Optimization with Application to Kidney Exchange. In Proceedings of the 13th International Conference on Autonomous Agents and Multiagent Systems, Paris, France, 5–9 May 2014; pp. 1701–1702.
29. Alvelos, F.; Klimentova, X.; Rais, A. A Compact Formulation for Maximizing the Expected Number of Transplants in Kidney Exchange Programs. *J. Phys. Conf. Ser.* **2015**, *616*, 012011.
30. Bertsimas, D.; Sim, M. The Price of Robustness. *Oper. Res.* **2004**, *52*, 35–53.
31. Büsing, C.; D'Andreagiovanni, F. New Results about Multi-Band Uncertainty in Robust Optimization. In *Experimental Algorithms—SEA 2012, Lecture Notes in Computer Science*; Klasing, R., Ed.; Springer: Berlin/Heidelberg, Germany, 2012; Volume 7276, 63–74.

7

Learning-Based Screening of Endothelial Dysfunction from Photoplethysmographic Signals

Chiara Calamanti *, Sara Moccia, Lucia Migliorelli, Marina Paolanti and Emanuele Frontoni

Department of Information Engineering, Universitá Politecnica delle Marche, 60121 Ancona, Italy; s.moccia@univpm.it (S.M.); l.migliorelli@pm.univpm.it (L.M.); m.paolanti@univpm.it (M.P.); e.frontoni@univpm.it (E.F.)

* Correspondence: c.calamanti@pm.univpm.it

Abstract: Endothelial-Dysfunction (ED) screening is of primary importance to early diagnosis cardiovascular diseases. Recently, approaches to ED screening are focusing more and more on photoplethysmography (PPG)-signal analysis, which is performed in a threshold-sensitive way and may not be suitable for tackling the high variability of PPG signals. The goal of this work was to present an innovative machine-learning (ML) approach to ED screening that could tackle such variability. Two research hypotheses guided this work: (H1) ML can support ED screening by classifying PPG features; and (H2) classification performance can be improved when including also anthropometric features. To investigate H1 and H2, a new dataset was built from 59 subject. The dataset is balanced in terms of subjects with and without ED. Support vector machine (SVM), random forest (RF) and k-nearest neighbors (KNN) classifiers were investigated for feature classification. With the leave-one-out evaluation protocol, the best classification results for H1 were obtained with SVM (accuracy = 71%, recall = 59%). When testing H2, the recall was further improved to 67%. Such results are a promising step for developing a novel and intelligent PPG device to assist clinicians in performing large scale and low cost ED screening.

Keywords: endothelial dysfunction; photoplethysmography; machine learning; computer-assisted screening

---

1. Introduction

Cardiovascular Diseases (CVDs) refer to a class of cardiac disorders that, according to the European Heart Network, cause every year 3.9 million deaths in Europe, with estimated costs up to 210 billion euro per year [1]. As reported in the guidelines of the World Health Organization (https://www.who.int/cardiovascular_diseases/guidelines/Pocket_GL_information/en/) for the assessment and management of cardiovascular risks, several factors (e.g., physical inactivity, tobacco use, and obesity) have been shown to influence CVD onset.

Moreover, when these factors are present, there is also a high probability of Endothelial Dysfunction (ED), which is actually recognized to be of primary importance to early diagnosis of CVDs [2–4]. In physiological conditions, the endothelial tissue regulates many functions, among which the most important are to maintain vascular homeostasis and modulate the vascular tone by balancing the production of vasodilators, including nitric oxide, and vasoconstrictors. In presence of ED, the endothelium is liable to anatomical alteration (e.g., smooth muscle cell proliferation and migration, leukocyte adhesion and migration) and its regulation mechanisms are compromised [5,6].

The current gold standard technique for ED diagnosis is the Flow Mediated Dilatation (FMD), which uses high-resolution UltraSound (US) signals acquired on subject arm. FMD is measured after a 5-min arm compression followed by relaxation and measured as the percentage increase of the resulted maximum brachial-artery diameter with respect to the baseline diameter [7]. FMD computation is, however, operator dependent, expensive and requires an expert clinician, thus not suitable for screening purposes.

To overcome these limitations, studies in the clinical literature highlight the efficacy of PhotoPlethysmoGraphy (PPG) in assessing ED [8–12]. PPG is a noninvasive optical technique in which PPG sensors are applied on subject's fingers to measure changes in blood volume as a function of time [13,14]. From the PPG signal, similar to US-based analysis, the incremental ratio of the PPG signal amplitude (with respect to its baseline) is evaluated by clinicians in a sensitive, threshold-based way (not being compatible with the high variability of the PPG signals).

To successfully tackle data variability, different researchers in similar contexts exploited Machine-Learning (ML) techniques. For example, Weng et al. [15] adopted Random Forest (RF), Logistic Regression (LR), Gradient Boosting Machines (GBM) and Neural Networks (NN) with 30 features extracted from electronic health records (EHRs) (such as blood pressure, Body Mass Index (BMI), gender, etc.) to identify patients at risk of developing CVDs. They obtained overall classification recalls of 65.3% (RF), 67.1% (LR), 67.5% (GBM), and 67.5% (NN). Similarly, Boursalie et al. [16] used Support Vector Machines (SVMs) to classify features from wearable sensors and EHRs, achieving a classification accuracy of 90.5%. Work similar to that proposed in this paper is reported in [17], where several ML classifiers (such as SVM and RF) are investigated for the specific task of ED classification, although it focuses on features extracted from FMD data.

Considering the clinical relevance of early-diagnosing ED from PPG data (over the FMD ones), the goal of this research was to test if ML methodologies are suitable for ED classification starting from PPG-signal analysis, by providing a fast and low cost approach to the problem. Specifically, we investigated the following two hypotheses:

Hypothesis 1 (H1). *ML techniques can classify ED by PPG features.*

Hypothesis 2 (H2). *Including anthropometric features may improve classification results.*

Due to the lack of work in this field of research to test H1 and H2, a new publicly available dataset, the PPG Endothelial Dysfunction Dataset (ppgEDD), was collected (http://vrai.dii.univpm.it/content/ppgEDD-dataset).

The paper is organized as follows: Section 2 gives details on the EDD and the features used for endothelial dysfunction classification. Results and conclusions are presented in Sections 3 and 4, respectively.

2. Methods

This section presents the proposed approach to ED screening from PPG data (Section 2.1) and the experimental protocol used to investigate H1 and H2 (Section 2.2).

2.1. Endothelial-Dysfunction screening methodology

The proposed method consists of the following steps: (i) data collection (Section 2.1.1); (ii) feature extraction (Section 2.1.2); and (iii) classification (Section 2.1.3). The workflow of the approach is shown in Figure 1.

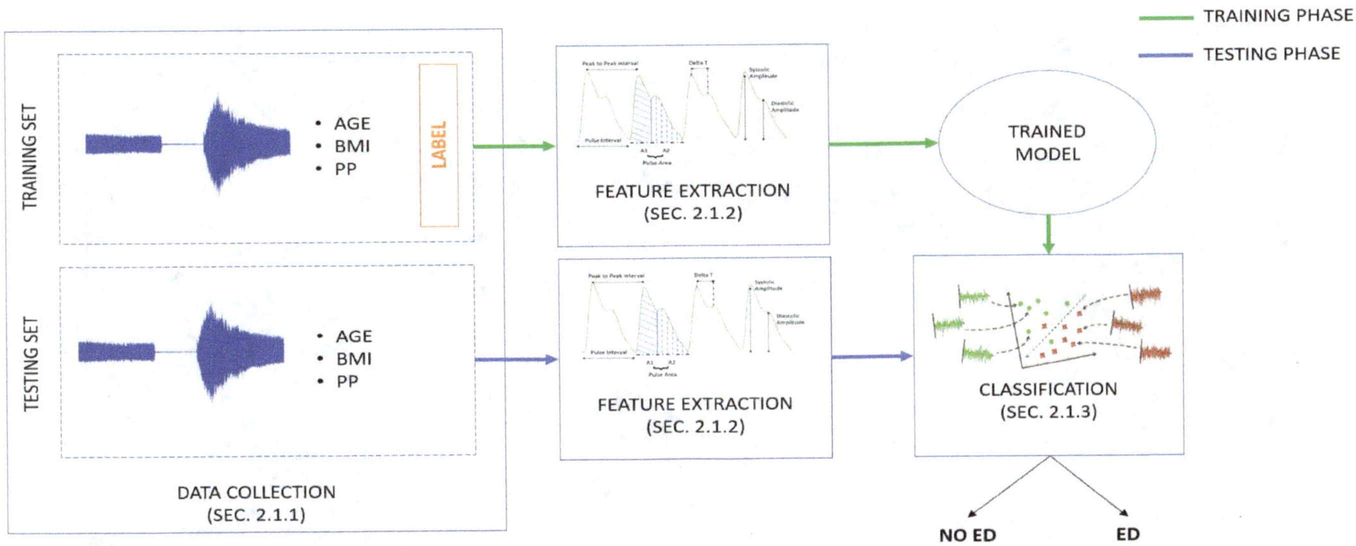

Figure 1. Workflow of the proposed learning-based approach to endothelial dysfunction (ED) screening from photoplethysmographic and anthropometric data.

2.1.1. PPG Endothelial-Dysfunction-Dataset Collection

The ppgEDD was built from 59 voluntary patients. Thirty-one subjects (F/M = 28/31, age = 39 ± 16 years) were healthy and the remaining ones had ED. The PPG-signal acquisition was carried out in the morning, in an environment with comfortable temperature and in absence of noise. Each subject was in the room at least half an hour before the exam to let his/her body to adapt to the temperature. All subjects respected the following instructions:

- Fasting for at least 8 h
- No drug consumption in the previous 6 h
- No smoking in the previous 6 h
- No intense physical activity in the hours immediately preceding the exam
- No nail polish

All participants were informed and provided a written agreement in accordance with the Declaration of Helsinki.

As shown in Figure 2, the medical equipment used to measure the PPG signal included:

- **VenoScreen®** (medis). VenoScreen was connected via a USB interface to a computer equipped with the CardioVascular Lab software package (MEDIS company, Ilmenau). The software verified, evaluated and displayed the measured PPG signals.
- **Prakticus II aneroid sphygmomanometer®** (Friedrich Bosch GmbH & Co. KG). The sphygmomanometer, applied above the elbow on the subject's left arm, was used to induce blood-flow blockage while measuring the blood pressure.

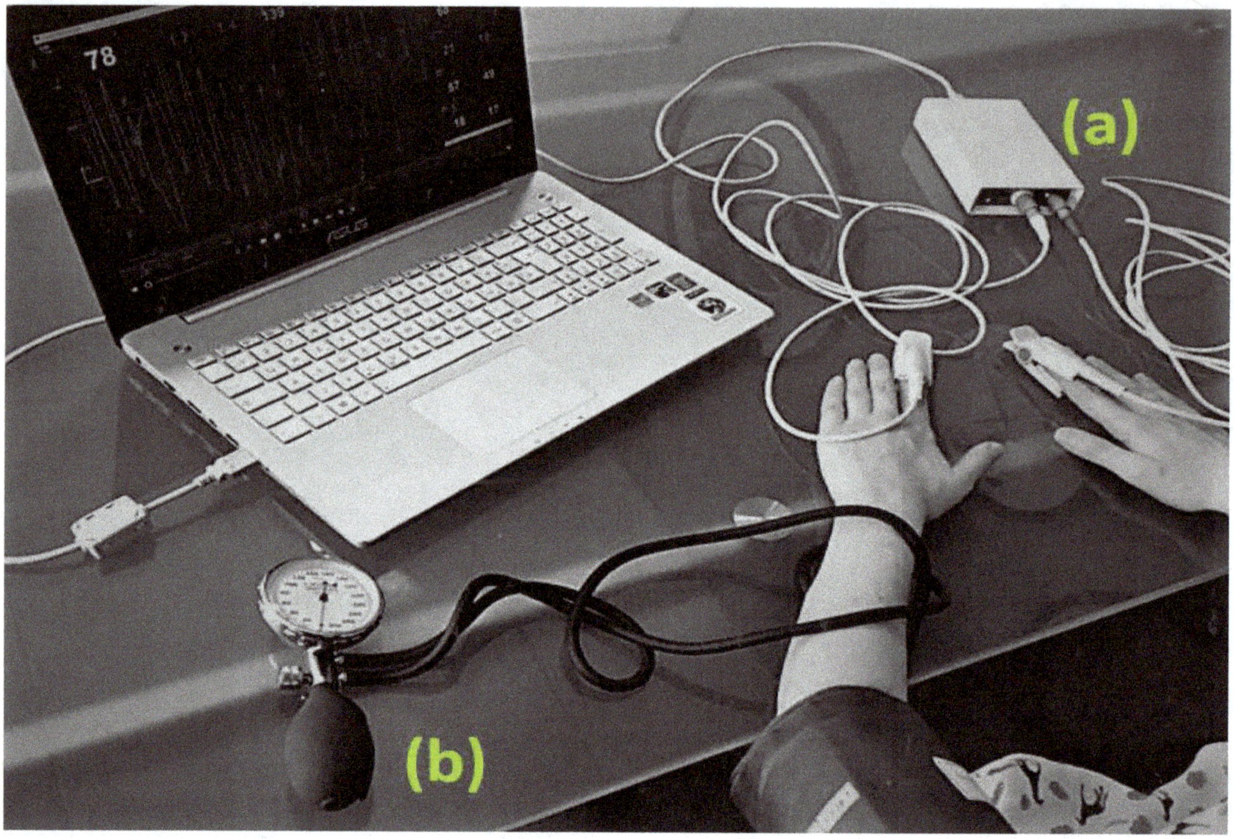

Figure 2. PPG-signal acquisition setup: (**a**) VenoScreen®(medis) with two photoplethysmography sensors; and (**b**) sphygmomanometer with cuff. Acquired signals were processed by the VenoScreen® (medis) software.

PPG processing

The PPG signal was obtained by measuring infrared light passing through finger skin. A LED light is diffused through the human tissue and then detected by a photo-detector located at the opposite side of the LED. The transmittance varies over time in accordance with variations in the blood volume. The device that records the PPG signal provides two different type of information: the signal that represents the light that is detected by a photo-detector (light transmitted) and the transmittance, which is the proportion of the incident (approaching) light that travels through the tissue to the photo-detector. The PPG signal is modulated by each cardiac cycle and may be influenced by several factors, such as breathing and movements. Moreover, the PPG signals may vary according to blood-oxygen saturation, skin temperatures, skin structure and external factors such as light in the environment. The aim of the pre-processing phase is reducing the PPG distortions, which may be observed in the wave profiles and may influence the features extraction, thus negatively impacting the subsequent phases of signal processing and the final diagnosis. For this reason, the following filters were applied on the PPG signal:

- **Noise**: Inevitably, the PPG signal contained high-frequency noise, which resulted from ambient light, thermal noise and other unclassified noise. The power line represented another noise source characterized by 50 Hz sinusoidal interference, probably accompanied by a number of harmonics [18]. To remove this noise, a simple filtering approach was applied, i.e., low-pass filter with 20 dB attenuation at 8 Hz [19].
- **Baseline wander**: Baseline wander filtering was required in order to minimize changes in beat morphology, which did not have cardiac origin [18]. The technique used for baseline wander

filtering consisted in down-sampling the PPG signal to 2 Hz, followed by forward/backwards filtering using a second-order low-pass Butterworth filter with a cut-off frequency of 0.5 Hz [20]. After that, the signal was unsampled and subtracted from the original PPG signal.

- **Outliers**: To remove outliers, the "isoutlier" function (The MathWorks, Inc., Natick, MA, USA), was applied to the PPG signal. A point was considered outlier when its value was more than three scaled median absolute deviations (MAD) away from the PPG signal median. The outliers were detected every 10 s and they were replaced by the mean value calculated in the same interval.

The sampling frequency of the PPG signal recorded by the VenoScreen device was 200 Hz.

ED gold standard classification was obtained by evaluating the PPG signal as in the actual clinical practice (Section 1).

2.1.2. Feature Extraction

PPG features

Inspired by the authors of [21,22], who proved the heart rate and augmentation index correlate with ED, and considering the work in [23], where a set of PPG features are shown to be potentially related to CVDs, in this work, we identified the following as features:

1. Systolic Amplitude (SA):
$$SA = M_{S_1} - M_{F_1} \tag{1}$$
where M_{S_1} and M_{F_1} are the PPG signal amplitude in S_1 (systolic peak) and F_1 (dicrotic point before the systolic peak).
2. Inflection Point Area ratio (IPA):
$$IPA = \frac{A2}{A1} \tag{2}$$
where area A1 and area A2 are obtained by dividing the pulse area into two areas at the dicrotic notch.
3. Pulse Interval (PI):
$$PI = t_{F2} - t_{F1} \tag{3}$$
4. Hearth Rate (HR):
$$HR = \frac{1}{t_{S_2} - t_{S_1}} \tag{4}$$
where t_{S_2} is the time at which the second systolic peak occurred.
5. $Delta_T$, which is the time between the systolic and diastolic peaks:
$$Delta_T = t_{E_1} - t_{S_1} \tag{5}$$
where t_{E_1} is the time of diastolic peak.
6. Stiffness Index (SI):
$$SI = \frac{H_P}{(t_{E_1} - t_{S_1})} \tag{6}$$
where H_P is the subject's height.
7. Augmentation Index (AI):
$$AI = \frac{(M_{S_2} - M_{F_2}) - (M_{E_2} - M_{F_2})}{Delta_T} \tag{7}$$
where M_{S_2} and M_{F_2} are the PPG signal amplitude in S_2 (systolic peak) and F_2 (dicrotic point before the systolic peak), and M_{E_2} is the PPG signal amplitude in E_2 (diastolic peak).

8. Recovery Time (*RT*). *RT* indicates how many seconds, from the maximum value of the PPG during the post-occlusion phase, are required to return to PPG pre-occlusion condition (Figure 3a).

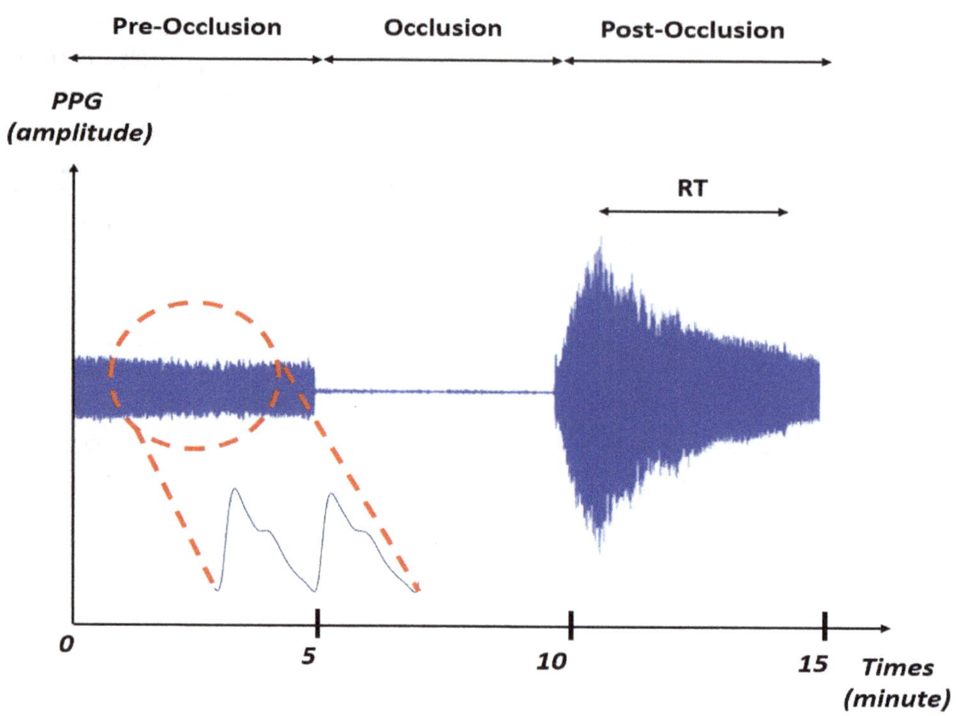

(a) PPG signal sample.

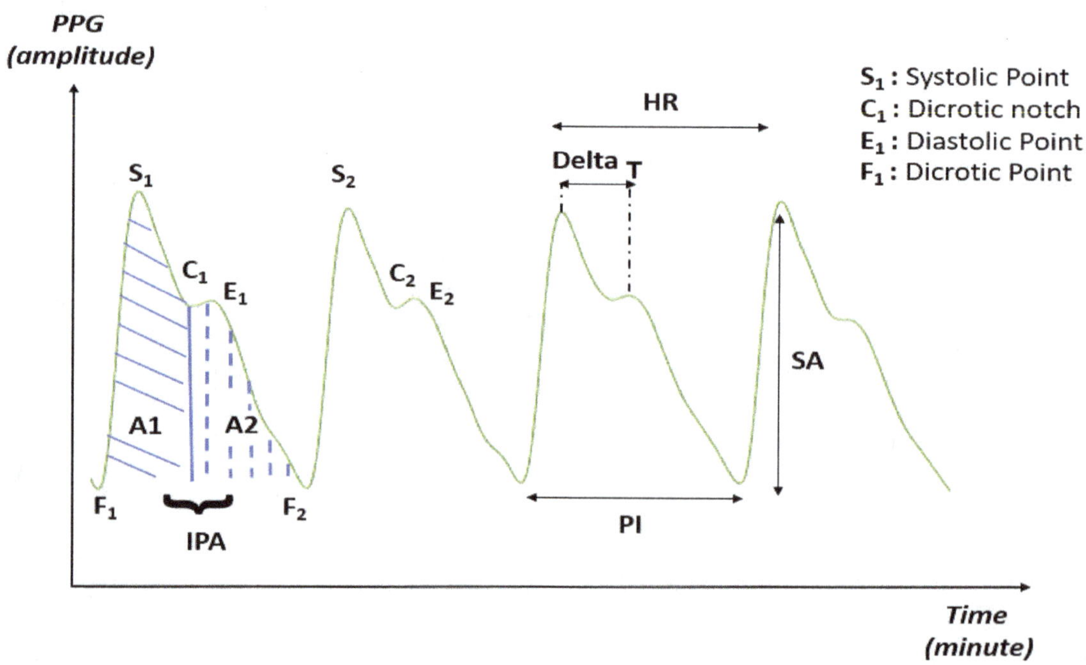

(b) Parameters for PPG-feature computation.

Figure 3. (**a**) The three phases of the photoplethysmography (PPG) signal acquisition: pre-occlusion (normal blood flow), occlusion (occluded flow), and post-occlusion (restored flow). Dotted lines highlights a zoomed signal portion. (**b**) From the zoomed signal portion, the parameters useful for computing PPG features are highlighted.

For the extraction of the features from the PPG signal, ten beats were selected randomly during the pre-occlusion phase. The fiducial points were identified for each beat (C1, C2, E1, E2, F1, F2, S1, and S2) to identify and quantify the parameters. Finally, the mean for each feature was calculated.

Anthropometric features

Considering our previous experience in this field [17], the following anthropometric features were investigated: age, BMI and pulse pressure (PP), (i.e., the difference between systolic and diastolic blood pressure at rests measured with the sphygmomanometer) [24].

2.1.3. Classification

To perform feature classification, SVMs were implemented [25]. Indeed, SVM decisions are only determined by the support vectors, which makes SVM robust to noise in training data. Here, SVM with the Gaussian kernel (Ψ) was used to prevent parameter proliferation while lowering computational complexity and limiting overfitting. For our binary classification problem, given a training set of N data $\{y_k, \mathbf{x_k}\}_{k=1}^{N}$, where $\mathbf{x_k}$ is the kth input feature vector and y_k is the kth output label, the SVM decision function takes the form of as follows:

$$f(\mathbf{x}) = sign\Big[\sum_{k=1}^{N} a_k^* y_k \Psi(\mathbf{x}, \mathbf{x_k}) + b\Big] \tag{8}$$

where

$$\Psi(\mathbf{x}, \mathbf{x_k}) = exp\{-\gamma||\mathbf{x} - \mathbf{x_k}||_2^2/\sigma^2\}, \qquad \gamma > 0 \tag{9}$$

b is a real constant and a_k^* is retrieved as follow:

$$a_k^* = \max\Big\{-\frac{1}{2}\sum_{k,l=1}^{N} y_k y_l \Psi(\mathbf{x_k}, \mathbf{x_l}) a_k a_l + \sum_{k=1}^{N} a_k\Big\} \tag{10}$$

with

$$\sum_{k=1}^{N} a_k y_k = 0, \qquad 0 \leq a_k \leq C, \qquad k = 1, ..., N \tag{11}$$

γ and C were retrieved with grid search, as explained more in detail in Section 2.2.

For the sake of completeness, the performance of other classifiers, i.e., k-nearest neighbors (KNN) [26] and RF [27], were investigated too.

Prior to classification, the feature matrices were normalized within each feature dimension.

2.2. Experimental protocol

To investigate the two hypotheses mentioned in Section 1, different set of features were considered (as introduced in Section 2.1.2):

- For H1, eight PPG features were used (Table 1).
- For H2, 11 features (three anthropometric features (Table 2) as well as eight PPG features) were used.

Table 1. PPG feature mean (±Standard Deviation (SD)) of the PPG endothelial dysfunction dataset (ppgEDD).

Features	Mean ± SD
SA	7.91 ± 5.68
IPA	0.61 ± 0.28
PI	172.92 ± 22.98
HR	69.19 ± 9.67
$Delta_T$	202.48 ± 40.29
SI	0.87 ± 0.18
AI	1.45 ± 0.38
RT	5.05 ± 0.66

Table 2. Anthropometric feature mean (±Standard Deviation (SD)) of the PPG endothelial dysfunction dataset (ppgEDD).

Features	Mean ± SD
Age (years)	39.0 ± 16.0
BMI (Kg/m^2)	25.7 ± 4.9
PP (mmHg)	44.15 ± 12.1

Considering the limited size of ppgEDD, Leave-One-Out (LOO) cross validation (CV) was implemented for testing purposes, as suggested in the ML literature (e.g., [28]). LOO-CV implies that, each time, 58 patients were used for training and the remaining one for testing.

During the training phase, classifier–hyperparameter tuning was implemented using a grid-search and LOO-CV approach. For SVMs, the grid-search space for γ and C was set to [1, 0.1, 0.001, 0.0001] and [1, 10, 100, 1000], respectively. The grid-search space for KNN number of neighbors was [1, 3, 5, 7, 9] and that for the number of trees for RF was [5, 10, 15, 20, 30, 40].

The performance of each classifier was evaluated in terms of accuracy (Acc), recall (Rec) and precision ($Prec$):

$$Acc = \frac{TP + TN}{TP + TN + FP + FN} \tag{12}$$

$$Rec = \frac{TP}{TP + FN} \tag{13}$$

$$Prec = \frac{TP}{TP + FP} \tag{14}$$

where TP and FN refer to subjects with ED that were and were not classified correctly, respectively, and TN and FP refer to subjects without ED that were and were not classified correctly, respectively.

All the experiments were implemented using scikit-learn Python libraries https://scikit-learn.org/stable/index.html.

3. Results

We tested our approach on the ppgEDD dataset to compare the endothelial function differences between patient with ED (n = 28) and patient without the disease (n = 31) based on the PPG signal. A full leave-one-out cross-validation was performed in our experiments procedure described in Section 2.2. In Tables 3 and 4, the performance of each classifier is shown for H1 and H2, respectively. For H1, the best performance in terms of accuracy (Acc = 71%) was obtained with SVM, with a recall of 59% and a precision of 73%. The confusion matrices for KNN, RF and SVM are shown in Figure 4a–c.

When investigating H2, as shown in Table 4, the SVM classification results were still the best, with a further improvement to 67% (Rec) and 69% ($Prec$). The normalized confusion matrices for KNN, RF and SVM are shown in Figure 4d.

The tested classifiers achieved encouraging results, with the best performance achieved by SVM (accuracy = 71%, recall = 67%). As reported in the literature [29]), similarity in performance metrics among the ML methods may be due to the fact that the analyzed dataset and the feature space were small.

Table 3. Investigation of H1: Classification performance obtained when classifying PPG features with K-Nearest Neighbor (KNN), Random Forest (RF) and Support Vector Machine (SVM) classifiers. Classification accuracy (*Acc*), recall (*Rec*) and precision (*Prec*) are reported.

Classifier	*Acc*	*Rec*	*Prec*
KNN	0.64	0.59	0.62
RF	0.66	0.63	0.63
SVM	**0.71**	**0.59**	**0.73**

Table 4. Investigation of H2: Classification performance obtained when classifying photoplethysmography and anthropometric features with KNN, Random Forest (RF) and SVM classifiers. Classification accuracy (*Acc*), recall (*Rec*) and precision (*Prec*) are reported.

Classifier	*Acc*	*Rec*	*Prec*
KNN	0.64	0.52	0.64
RF	0.49	0.44	0.44
SVM	**0.71**	**0.67**	**0.69**

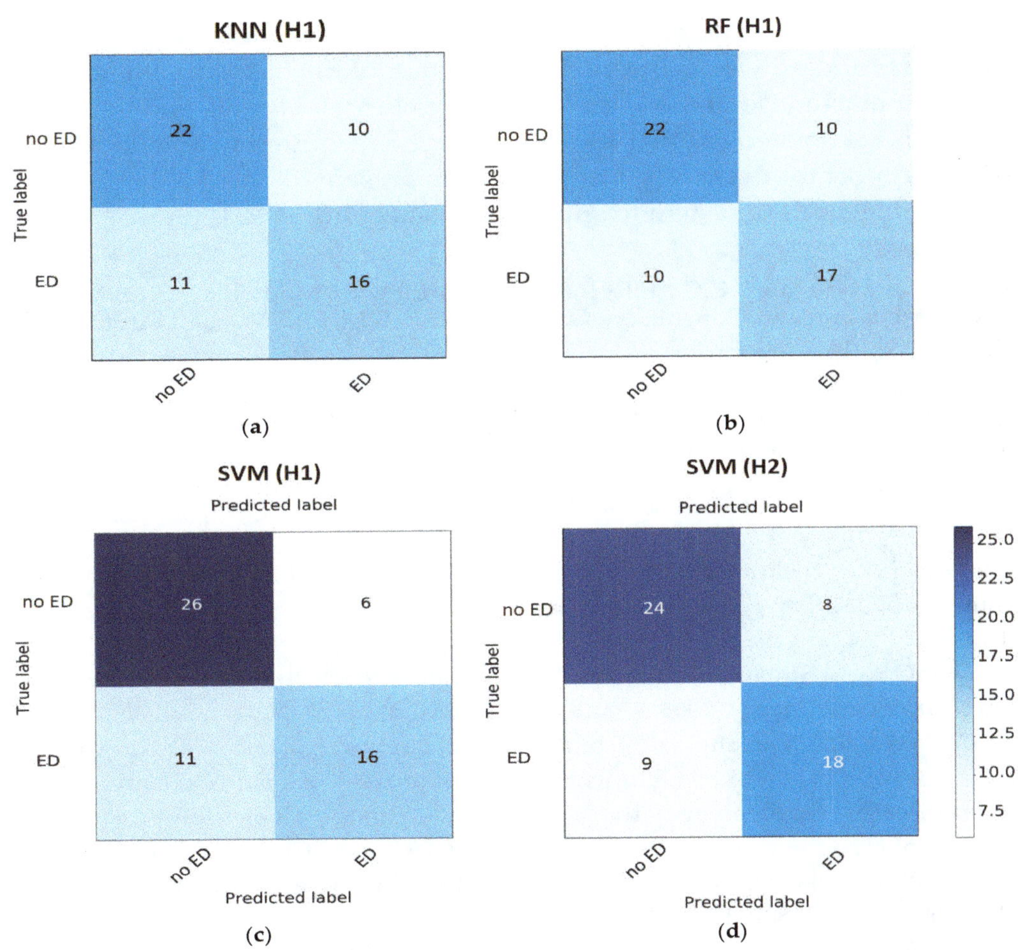

Figure 4. Confusion matrices (CMs) obtained when classifying photoplethysmography features (H1) with: **(a)** K-Nearest Neighbor (KNN); **(b)** Random Forest (RF); and **(c)** Support Vector Machine (SVM) classifier. **(d)** CM for SVM obtained when testing H2 (both photoplethysmography and anthropometric features).

4. Discussion and Conclusions

In this study, we presented and evaluated an innovative learning-based approach to ED screening from PPG data. Two different hypotheses were investigated for ED classification, i.e., using (H1) only PPG features and (H2) including also anthropometric features. Three ML classifiers (i.e., SVM, KNN and RF) were tested.

With H1 and H2, we showed that the proposed feature set can be promising for ED screening, even though further investigation is needed, e.g., to increase the ppgEDD dataset size numerosity. Results achieved when investigating H2 suggest that including anthropometric features is useful, as in accord with previous work in the literature (e.g., [17]).

The experimental results show that SVM outperformed KNN and RF. This is probably due to the SVM's ability to tackle: (1) the dimension of our feature space, which was high when compared with the number of ppgEDD subjects; and (2) the noise present in the PPG data.

The main novelty of this study relies on the fact that PPG features were used in combination with anthropometric ones to classify ED. The results verify that the ED SVM classification method significantly improved the generalization capability achievable with the SVM classifier. Another advantage of the SVM approach was found in its high sparseness, explained by the fact that the adopted optimization criterion was based on minimizing the number of support vectors.

As future work, we would like to investigate other anthropometric features, such as dyslipidemia and smoking habits, integrating PPG data with data coming from structured electronic-health-record datasets. Furthermore, we will investigate other features extracted from the PPG signal, such as those proposed in [30] to compute the diastolic and systolic pressure, and in [31,32] to analyze the ECG waveform. Our expectation is that research on this new ML approach based on PPG features will be empowered by the proposed work. Surely the prediction of ED based on this approach should be further explored using machine learning with other large clinical datasets and in other populations.

In conclusion, it is acknowledged that further research is required to ameliorate the algorithm as to offer all possible support for diagnosis, but the results presented here are surely a promising step towards a helpful intelligent PPG system to support the screening of ED.

Author Contributions: Introduction, C.C., E.F., S.M., L.M. and M.P.; Methods,C.C., S.M. and L.M.; Results, C.C., S.M. and L.M.; Discussion and Conclusion, C.C., E.F., S.M., L.M. and M.P. All authors contributed to the development and set up of the general idea.

Acknowledgments: The work described in this paper was supported by STRUMEDICAL srl that provided us with the VenoScreen devices used in our studies.

References

1. Wilkins, E.; Wilson, L.; Wickramasinghe, K.; Bhatnagar, P.; Leal, J.; Luengo-Fernandez, R.; Burns, R.; Rayner, M.; Townsend, N. *European Cardiovascular Disease Statistics 2017*; European Heart Network: Brussels, Belgium, 2017.
2. Hadi, H.A.; Carr, C.S.; Al Suwaidi, J. Endothelial dysfunction: Cardiovascular risk factors, therapy, and outcome. *Vasc. Health Risk Manag.* **2005**, *1*, 183–198. [PubMed]
3. Brunner, H.; Cockcroft, J.R.; Deanfield, J.; Donald, A.; Ferrannini, E.; Halcox, J.; Kiowski, W.; Lüscher, T.F.; Mancia, G.; Natali, A.; et al. Endothelial function and dysfunction. Part II: Association with cardiovascular risk factors and diseases. A statement by the Working Group on Endothelins and Endothelial Factors of the European Society of Hypertension. *J. Hypertens.* **2005**, *23*, 233–246. [CrossRef] [PubMed]
4. Anderson, T.J. Arterial stiffness or endothelial dysfunction as a surrogate marker of vascular risk. *Can. J. Cardiol.* **2006**, *22*, 72B–80B. [CrossRef]
5. Félétou, M. The endothelium, Part I: Multiple functions of the endothelial cells—Focus on endothelium-derived vasoactive mediators. Colloquium Series on Integrated Systems Physiology: From Molecule to Function. *Morgan Claypool Life Sci.* **2011**, *3*, 1–306.

6. van Hinsbergh, V.W. Endothelium role in regulation of coagulation and inflammation. In *Seminars in Immunopathology*; Springer: Berlin, Germany, 2012; Volume 34, pp. 93–106.
7. Corretti, M.C.; Anderson, T.J.; Benjamin, E.J.; Celermajer, D.; Charbonneau, F.; Creager, M.A.; Deanfield, J.; Drexler, H.; Gerhard-Herman, M.; Herrington, D.; et al. Guidelines for the ultrasound assessment of endothelial-dependent flow-mediated vasodilation of the brachial artery: A report of the International Brachial Artery Reactivity Task Force. *J. Am. Coll. Cardiol.* **2002**, *39*, 257–265. [CrossRef]
8. Zahedi, E.; Jaafar, R.; Ali, M.M.; Mohamed, A.; Maskon, O. Finger photoplethysmogram pulse amplitude changes induced by flow-mediated dilation. *Physiol. Meas.* **2008**, *29*, 625–637. [CrossRef] [PubMed]
9. Flammer, A.J.; Anderson, T.; Celermajer, D.S.; Creager, M.A.; Deanfield, J.; Ganz, P.; Hamburg, N.M.; Lüscher, T.F.; Shechter, M.; Taddei, S.; et al. The assessment of endothelial function: From research into clinical practice. *Circulation* **2012**, *126*, 753–767. [CrossRef] [PubMed]
10. Kuznetsova, T.; Van Vlierberghe, E.; Knez, J.; Szczesny, G.; Thijs, L.; Jozeau, D.; Balestra, C.; Dhooge, J.; Staessen, J.A. Association of digital vascular function with cardiovascular risk factors: A population study. *Br. Med J. Open* **2014**, *4*, e004399. [CrossRef] [PubMed]
11. Mashayekhi, G.; Zahedi, E.; Attar, H.M.; Sharifi, F. Flow mediated dilation with photoplethysmography as a substitute for ultrasonic imaging. *Physiol. Meas.* **2015**, *36*, 1551–1571. [CrossRef] [PubMed]
12. Moerland, M.; Kales, A.; Schrier, L.; Van Dongen, M.; Bradnock, D.; Burggraaf, J. Evaluation of the EndoPAT as a tool to assess endothelial function. *Int. J. Vasc. Med.* **2012**, *2012*, 1–8. [CrossRef] [PubMed]
13. Allen, J. Photoplethysmography and its application in clinical physiological measurement. *Physiol. Meas.* **2007**, *28*, 1–39. [CrossRef] [PubMed]
14. Moraes, J.; Rocha, M.; Vasconcelos, G.; Vasconcelos Filho, J.; de Albuquerque, V. Advances in photopletysmography signal analysis for biomedical applications. *Sensors* **2018**, *18*, 1894. [CrossRef] [PubMed]
15. Weng, S.F.; Reps, J.; Kai, J.; Garibaldi, J.M.; Qureshi, N. Can machine-learning improve cardiovascular risk prediction using routine clinical data? *PLoS ONE* **2017**, *12*, e0174944. [CrossRef] [PubMed]
16. Boursalie, O.; Samavi, R.; Doyle, T.E. M4CVD: Mobile machine learning model for monitoring cardiovascular disease. *Procedia Comput. Sci.* **2015**, *63*, 384–391. [CrossRef]
17. Calamanti, C.; Paolanti, M.; Romeo, L.; Bernardini, M.; Frontoni, E. Machine learning-based approaches to analyse and improve the diagnosis of endothelial dysfunction. In Proceedings of the IEEE/ASME International Conference on Mechatronic and Embedded Systems and Applications, New York, NY, USA, 2–4 July 2018; pp. 1–6.
18. Sörnmo, L.; Laguna, P. *Bioelectrical Signal Processing in Cardiac and Neurological Applications*; Academic Press: Cambridge, MA, USA, 2005; Volume 8,
19. Peng, F.; Zhang, Z.; Gou, X.; Liu, H.; Wang, W. Motion artifact removal from photoplethysmographic signals by combining temporally constrained independent component analysis and adaptive filter. *Biomed. Eng. Online* **2014**, *13*, 50. [CrossRef] [PubMed]
20. Solem, K.; Olde, B.; Sornmo, L. Prediction of intradialytic hypotension using photoplethysmography. *IEEE Trans. Biomed. Eng.* **2010**, *57*, 1611–1619. [CrossRef] [PubMed]
21. Maio, R.; Miceli, S.; Sciacqua, A.; Leone, G.G.; Bruni, R.; Naccarato, P.; Martino, F.; Sesti, G.; Perticone, F. Heart rate affects endothelial function in essential hypertension. *Intern. Emerg. Med.* **2013**, *8*, 211–219. [CrossRef] [PubMed]
22. McEniery, C.M.; Wallace, S.; Mackenzie, I.S.; McDonnell, B.; Yasmin.; Newby, D.E.; Cockcroft, J.R.; Wilkinson, I.B. Endothelial function is associated with pulse pressure, pulse wave velocity, and augmentation index in healthy humans. *Hypertension* **2006**, *48*, 602–608. [CrossRef] [PubMed]
23. Elgendi, M. On the analysis of fingertip photoplethysmogram signals. *Curr. Cardiol. Rev.* **2012**, *8*, 14–25. [CrossRef] [PubMed]
24. Beigel, R.; Dvir, D.; Arbel, Y.; Shechter, A.; Feinberg, M.S.; Shechter, M. Pulse pressure is a predictor of vascular endothelial function in middle-aged subjects with no apparent heart disease. *Vasc. Med.* **2010**, *15*, 299–305. [CrossRef] [PubMed]
25. Burges, C.J. A tutorial on support vector machines for pattern recognition. *Data Min. Knowl. Discov.* **1998**, *2*, 121–167. [CrossRef]
26. Keller, J.M.; Gray, M.R.; Givens, J.A. A fuzzy k-nearest neighbor algorithm. *IEEE Trans. Syst. Man Cybern.* **1985**, *SMC-15*, 580–585. [CrossRef]
27. Breiman, L. Random forests. *Mach. Learn.* **2001**, *45*, 5–32. [CrossRef]

28. Wong, T.T. Performance evaluation of classification algorithms by k-fold and leave-one-out cross validation. *Pattern Recognit.* **2015**, *48*, 2839–2846. [CrossRef]
29. Nasrabadi, N.M. Pattern recognition and machine learning. *J. Electron. Imaging* **2007**, *16*, 049901.
30. Rundo, F.; Ortis, A.; Battiato, S.; Conoci, S. Advanced bio-inspired system for noninvasive cuff-less blood pressure estimation from physiological signal analysis. *Computation* **2018**, *6*, 46. [CrossRef]
31. Rundo, F.; Conoci, S.; Ortis, A.; Battiato, S. An advanced bio-inspired PhotoPlethysmoGraphy (PPG) and ECG pattern recognition system for medical assessment. *Sensors* **2018**, *18*, 405. [CrossRef] [PubMed]
32. Dutt, D.N.; Shruthi, S. Digital processing of ECG and PPG signals for study of arterial parameters for cardiovascular risk assessment. In Proceedings of the 2015 International Conference on Communications and Signal Processing (ICCSP), Melmaruvathur, India, 2–4 April 2015; pp. 1506–1510.

8

Parallel K-Means Clustering for Brain Cancer Detection Using Hyperspectral Images

Emanuele Torti [1,*], Giordana Florimbi [1], Francesca Castelli [1], Samuel Ortega [2], Himar Fabelo [2], Gustavo Marrero Callicó [2], Margarita Marrero-Martin [2] and Francesco Leporati [1]

1. Department of Electrical, Computer and Biomedical Engineering, University of Pavia, I-27100 Pavia, Italy; giordana.florimbi01@ateneopv.it (G.F.); francesca.castelli02@ateneopv.it (F.C.); francesco.leporati@unipv.it (F.L.)
2. Institute for Applied Microelectronics (IUMA), University of Las Palmas de Gran Canaria (ULPGC), 35017 Las Palmas de Gran Canaria, Spain; sortega@iuma.ulpgc.es (S.O.); hfabelo@iuma.ulpgc.es (H.F.); gustavo@iuma.ulpgc.es (G.M.C.); margarita@iuma.ulpgc.es (M.M.-M.)

* Correspondence: emanuele.torti@unipv.it

Abstract: The precise delineation of brain cancer is a crucial task during surgery. There are several techniques employed during surgical procedures to guide neurosurgeons in the tumor resection. However, hyperspectral imaging (HSI) is a promising non-invasive and non-ionizing imaging technique that could improve and complement the currently used methods. The HypErspectraL Imaging Cancer Detection (HELICoiD) European project has addressed the development of a methodology for tumor tissue detection and delineation exploiting HSI techniques. In this approach, the K-means algorithm emerged in the delimitation of tumor borders, which is of crucial importance. The main drawback is the computational complexity of this algorithm. This paper describes the development of the K-means clustering algorithm on different parallel architectures, in order to provide real-time processing during surgical procedures. This algorithm will generate an unsupervised segmentation map that, combined with a supervised classification map, will offer guidance to the neurosurgeon during the tumor resection task. We present parallel K-means clustering based on OpenMP, CUDA and OpenCL paradigms. These algorithms have been validated through an in-vivo hyperspectral human brain image database. Experimental results show that the CUDA version can achieve a speed-up of ~150× with respect to a sequential processing. The remarkable result obtained in this paper makes possible the development of a real-time classification system.

Keywords: Graphics Processing Units (GPUs); CUDA; OpenMP; OpenCL; K-means; brain cancer detection; hyperspectral imaging; unsupervised clustering

---

1. Introduction

One of the most diffused types of cancer is the brain tumor, which has an estimated incidence of 3.4 per 100,000 subjects [1]. There are different types of brain tumors; the most common one concerns the *glial* cells of the brain and is called *glioma*. It accounts from the 30% to the 50% of the cases. In particular, in the 85% of these cases, it is a malignant tumor called *glioblastoma*. Moreover, these kind of *gliomas* are characterized by fast-growing invasiveness, which is locally very aggressive, in most cases unicentric and rarely metastasizing [2].

Typically, the first diagnosis is performed through the Magnetic Resonance Imaging (MRI) and the Computed Tomography (CT). Those techniques are capable to highlight possible lesions. However, it is not always possible to use them, since they can, for example, make interference with pacemakers or other implantable devices. Moreover, the certainty of the diagnosis only comes from the histological and pathological analyses, which require samples of the tissue. In order to obtain this tissue, an *excisional biopsy* is necessary, which consists in the removal of tissue from the living body through surgical cutting. It is important to notice that all those approaches have some disadvantages; in particular they are not capable of providing a real-time response and, most important, they are invasive and/or ionizing.

The clinical practice for brain cancers is the tumor resection, which can cure the lowest grade tumors and prolongs the life of the patient in the most aggressive cases. The main issue about this approach is the inaccuracy of the human eye in distinguishing between healthy tissue and cancer. This is because the cancer often infiltrates and diffuses into the surrounding healthy tissue and this is particularly critical for brain cancers. As a consequence, the surgeon can unintentionally leave behind tumor tissue during a surgery routine potentially causing tumor recurrence. On the other hand, if the surgeon removes too much healthy tissue, a permanent disability to the patient can be provoked [3].

The HELICoiD European project aims at providing to the surgeon a system which can accurately discriminate between tumor and healthy tissue in real-time during surgery routines [4,5]. Traditional imaging techniques feature a low grade of sensitivity and often cannot clearly determine the tumor region and its boundaries. Therefore, the HELICoiD project exploits Hyperspectral Imaging (HSI) techniques in order to solve this critical issue. Hyperspectral images (HS) can be acquired over a wide range of the electromagnetic spectrum, from visible to near-infrared frequencies and beyond. Hyperspectral sensors acquire the so-called *HS cube* where the spatial information is in the x-axis and in the y-axis, while the spectral information is in the z-axis. Thus, a single hyperspectral pixel can be seen as a mono-dimensional vector, which contains the spectral response across the different wavelengths. Moreover, it is important to notice that the spectral information is strictly correlated with the chemical composition of the specific material. It is possible to say that each hyperspectral pixel contains the so-called *spectral signature* of a certain substance. Thus, different substances can be distinguished by properly analyzing those images [6].

A previous study [4,7] proposed a processing chain for hyperspectral image analysis acquired during brain surgery. The framework developed in this work is depicted in Figure 1.

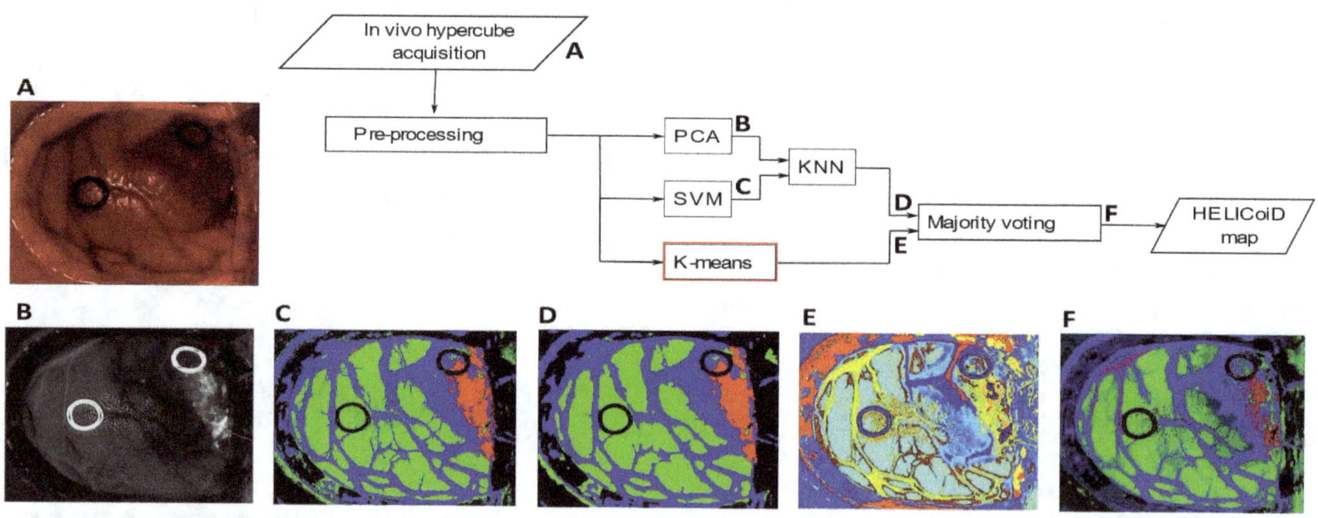

Figure 1. Hyperspectral brain cancer detection algorithm proposed in [7]. After acquiring (**A**) and pre-processing the image, the system performs a supervised classification through Principal Component Analysis (PCA) (**B**), Support Vector Machine (SVM) (**C**) and K-Nearest Neighbor (KNN) (**D**). Moreover, it generates a segmentation map through the K-means (**E**). The (**D**,**E**) maps are merged using the majority voting (**F**).

First, the acquired HS cube (Figure 1A) is pre-processed in order to perform a radiometric calibration, reduce the noise and the dimensionality of the HS image and normalize it. After this preparatory step, the image is analyzed using the supervised and unsupervised classification. The former is performed exploiting the Principal Component Analysis (PCA), the Support Vector

Machine (SVM) and the K-Nearest Neighbor (KNN). The KNN filters the spatial information given by the PCA (Figure 1B) and the classification map generated by the SVM (Figure 1C). Its output (Figure 1D) is a map where tissues are displayed with different colors representing the associated classes. The unsupervised classification is based on the K-means algorithm. Despite the supervised classification output, the unsupervised result is a segmentation map (Figure 1E), whose clusters are semantically meaningless. However, the K-means provides a good delimitation of the different areas present in the scene. Since the goal of the system is to accurately delineate the tumor borders, the K-means plays a crucial role for its ability to clearly separate different areas. For these reasons, it is important to merge the two outputs in order to exploit the benefits of the two approaches. The majority voting provides the final output combining the supervised and unsupervised classifications (Figure 1F).

While the PCA, the SVM and the KNN filter are executed through a fixed number of steps, the K-means algorithm iterates until a certain condition is satisfied. In order to provide the real-time classification during surgery, parallel computing is required, since the computational load of the algorithms is extremely high. The other algorithms of this framework have been already developed in parallel, in particular the SVM [8] and the KNN filtering [9] have been recently proposed in the literature. Those works target Graphics Processing Units (GPUs) technology since the considered algorithms have an intrinsically parallel structure. Previously, other parallel technologies have been evaluated in order to provide faster implementations of the PCA [10], SVM [11] and KNN [12] compared to the serial ones. Despite this, in our work we choose to exploit GPUs since they assure higher performance. Moreover, GPUs are going to be increasingly used for real-time image processing [13–15], together with other scientific applications related to simulation and modeling or machine learning in biomedical applications [16,17].

In this paper, we present the parallelization of the K-means algorithm on different parallel architectures in order to evaluate which one is more suitable for real-time processing. In particular, we consider multi-core CPUs through the OpenMP API and the GPU technology using NVIDIA CUDA framework. We also propose OpenCL-based implementations in order to address code portability.

In other words, the work performed allows identifying the best suitable parallel approach between one that could be more appealing since it requires low programming effort and another one more efficient but also more demanding in terms of optimization and tuning. A tool that allows intra-architectures portability (OpenCL) was also considered but due to its lower performance it is not competitive with the other two approaches.

The paper is organized as follows: Section 2 describes the K-means algorithm for hyperspectral images, while Section 3 details the different parallel versions. Section 4 contains the experimental results and their discussion, making comparisons between the different approaches described in this paper. Section 5 concludes the papers and addresses some possible future research lines.

2. K-Means Algorithm for Hyperspectral Images

As already said, the K-means algorithm, unlike the other ones of the hyperspectral brain cancer detection algorithm, is not performed through a fixed number of steps. It performs an unsupervised learning since no previous knowledge of the data is needed. The algorithm separates the input data into K different clusters with a K value fixed a priori. Data are grouped together on the basis of feature similarity. The first step of the algorithm is the definition of K *centroids*, one for each cluster. Using those centroids, a first grouping is performed on the basis of the distance of each point to the centroids. A point is associate to the cluster represented by the nearest centroid. At this moment, each k *centroid* is updated as the baricenter of the group it represents. This process iterates until the difference between the centroids of two consecutive iterations are smaller than a fixed threshold or if the maximum number of iterations is reached.

The pseudo-code of the K-means algorithm is shown in Algorithm 1, where Y indicates a hyperspectral image made up of N pixels and L bands. Therefore, the hyperspectral image can be seen as an $N \times L$ matrix. The number of clusters to produce is determined by K, the threshold error by min_error and the maximum number of iterations by max_iter. The K-means algorithm produces as a result a $K \times L$ array containing the centroids, which will be referred as cluster_centroids in Algorithm 1 and an N-dimensional array containing the label of the cluster assigned to each pixel. This array is denoted by assigned_cluster.

Algorithm 1 K-means

```
Input: Y, K, min_error, max_iter

1: Pseudo-random initialization of cluster_centroids
2: Initialize previous_centroids at 0        ▷ previous_centroids is an K × L array
3: n_iter ← 0                                ▷ initialize the iteration counter to 0
4: Initialize actual_error with a huge value
5: while actual_error > min_error and n_iter < max_iter do
6:     for i:=1 to N do
7:         Initialize centroid_distances to 0   ▷ centroid_distances is a K-dimensional array
8:         for j:=1 to K do
9:             centroid_distance_j ← distance between the j-th centroid and the i-th pixel
10:        end for
11:        assigend_cluster_i ← index of min centroid_distance
12:    end for
13:    previous_centroids ← cluster_centroids
14:    update cluster_centroids
15:    actual_error ← (Σ_{i=1}^{K} Σ_{j=1}^{L} |previous_centroids_{i,j} − cluster_centroids_{i,j}|) / (K·L)
16:    n_iter ← n_iter + 1
17: end while

Output: assigned_cluster, cluster_centroids
```

In Algorithm 1, lines 1 and 2 contain the initialization of the variables. In particular, cluster_centroids is initialized with K different hyperspectral pixels pseudo-randomly chosen from the input image Y. The variable actual_error is initialized with a huge value in order to ensure that the main loop of the algorithm (from line 5 to 17) is performed at least one time. Inside this main loop there are two *for* loops that iterate over the number of pixels N and the number of clusters K (lines from 6 to 12). For each pixel, a temporary array centroid_distances is set to 0, used for storing the distances between the considered hyperspectral pixel and the centroids. The distance metric used for hyperspectral pixels is usually the *Spectral Angle* (SA) which is defined as:

$$SA = \theta(x,y) = \cos^{-1}\left(\frac{\sum_{h=1}^{L} x_h y_h}{\left(\sum_{h=1}^{L} x_h^2\right)^{1/2}\left(\sum_{h=1}^{L} y_h^2\right)^{1/2}}\right) \tag{1}$$

where x and y are the spectral vectors and x_h and y_h represent the response of the h-th band of x and y respectively, being L the number of bands.

The label assigned to the i-th pixel corresponds to the group represented by the centroid with the minimum SA value, as shown in line 11. This phase is repeated for each pixel.

After these steps, the centroids used for the SAs computation are stored in the previous_centroids array. Successively, the centroids are updated by computing the barycenter of each group that is computing the mean value, for each band, of the pixels belonging to the group. Using the updated centroids and the previous ones, it is possible to evaluate the variation from the previous iteration. It represents how much the centroids have changed and it can be used as a stopping criterion when these variations become small (line 15). The last step of the *while* loop is the increment of the n_iter variable, used for controlling the maximum number of iterations performed by the algorithm.

The next section describes the serial and the parallel versions of this algorithm that we developed using different parallel approaches, together with a code profiling carried out in order to identify the heaviest code parts from the computational point of view.

3. Parallel K-Means Implementations

First, we developed a serial version of the K-mean algorithm written in C code. It serves both as reference for validating the results of the parallel implementations and for performing a careful code profiling needed to identify the most complex code parts. The numerical representation used is the IEEE-754 floating-point single precision.

3.1. Serial Code Profiling

The code profiling was performed using a dataset formed by real HS images and assuming $K = 24$, min_error $= 10^{-3}$ and max_iter $= 50$. This K value was stablished during the development of the HS brain cancer algorithm presented in [7]. Using this configuration, the execution of the algorithm never reached the maximum number of iterations. The characteristics of the dataset are shown in Table 1, while Figure 2 shows the RGB representation of the images.

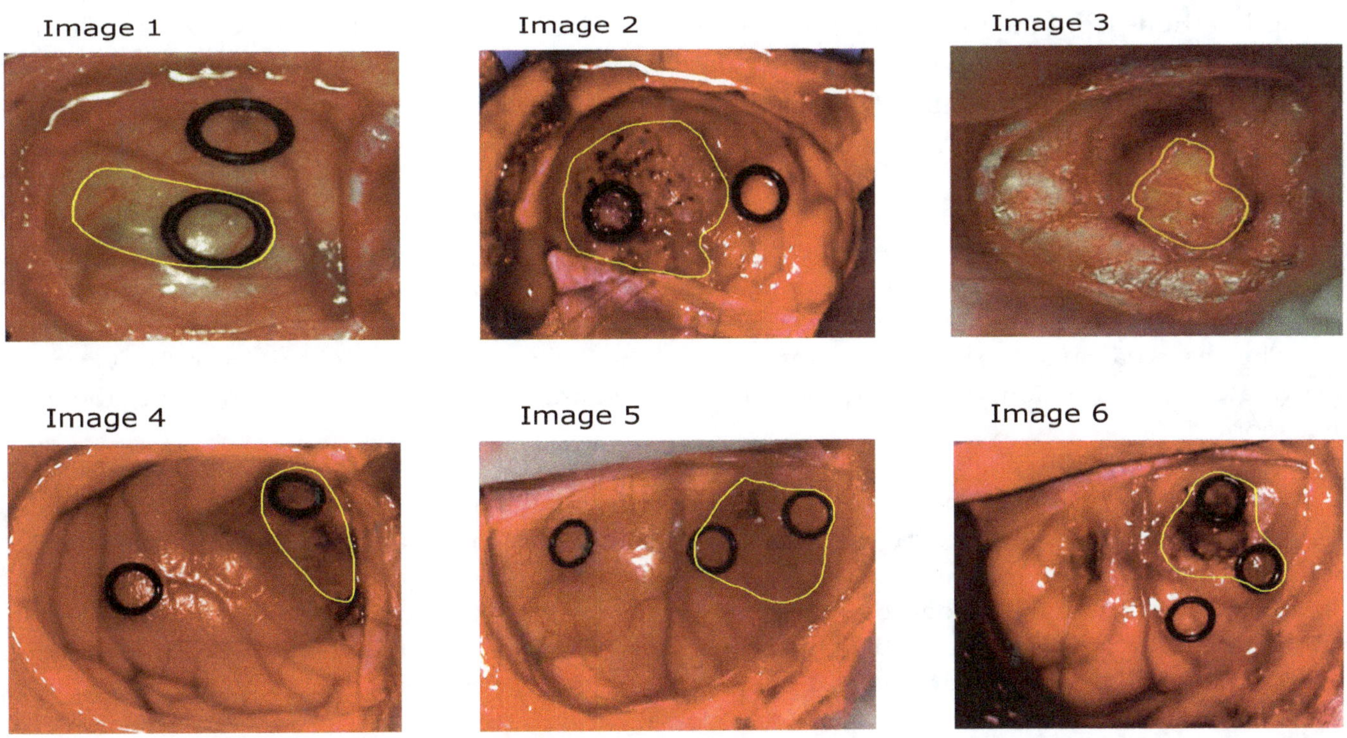

Figure 2. RGB representations of each hyperspectral cube of the brain cancer dataset. The yellow line represents the tumor location identified by the neurosurgeon.

Table 1. Dataset characteristics.

Image ID	# of Rows	# of Columns	Total # of Pixels	# of Bands	Size (MB)
Image 1	329	379	124,691	128	60.88
Image 2	493	376	185,368	128	90.51
Image 3	402	472	189,744	128	92.65
Image 4	496	442	219,232	128	107.05
Image 5	548	459	251,532	128	122.82
Image 6	552	479	264,408	128	129.11

The profiling highlighted that the heaviest code parts are the computation of distances, which are evaluated between each hyperspectral pixel and each centroid. In the considered cases, the *for* loops of lines 6–12 (Algorithm 1) take from 94 to 98% of the time for the smallest and the biggest image, respectively. Notice that these computations can be performed in parallel, since there is no dependency between the evaluations needed by a single pixel and the others.

3.2. OpenMP Algorithms

OpenMP (https://www.openmp.org/) is a parallel programming framework capable of exploiting multi-core architectures. It is based on a set of simple *#pragma* statements used for code annotations that indicates to the compiler which parts should be parallelized. An example is the *#pragma omp parallel for* statement, which generates a set of parallel threads and assigns to each one a group of iterations. It is also possible to indicate to the compiler which variables should be shared among the threads and which ones are private through the *shared* and *private* clauses, respectively. Finally, it is possible to choose the scheduling algorithm to use through the *schedule* option. The supported scheduling algorithms are *static*, *dynamic* and *guided*. In the first case, the number of iterations are equally or as equal as possible subdivided among the threads. Thus, each thread performs the same number of iterations. The *dynamic* scheduling uses the internal work queue to give a chunk-sized block of loop iterations to each thread. When a thread finishes, it retrieves the next block of loop iterations from the top of the work queue. The default value of the chunk size is 1, but it is possible to change it by a proper command. Finally, the *guided* scheduling is similar to the *dynamic* one, but the chunk size starts from a big value and then decreases in order to manage load imbalance between different iterations.

We developed two different OpenMP versions of the K-means algorithm. The first one parallelizes the *for* loop which iterates over the hyperspectral pixels (line 6, Algorithm 1). In this way, at each iteration of the main *while* loop, a set of parallel threads are generated and each one computes the SA between a certain group of pixels and the centroids. All the other operations are performed in a serial way. The shared arrays are the `cluster_centroids` and the input image Y, while all the other variables are private. In this version, the parallel region is created and destroyed at each iteration of the main *while* loop.

Concerning the second implementation, the majority of the operations are performed in parallel. The operations that continue to be performed sequentially are the `actual_error` computation and the increment of `n_iter`, at lines 15 and 16 of Algorithm 1, respectively. A barrier must be placed after the `actual_error` computation, in order to prevent the other threads to evaluate the *while* condition with an inconsistent old value. In this case, also the `centroid_distance` is declared as shared. Notice that, in this version, the parallel region is created and destroyed only once, at the beginning and at the end of the main *while* loop. However, in this case, it is necessary to introduce a barrier in order to ensure the correct execution of the program.

3.3. CUDA Algorithms

CUDA (https://developer.nvidia.com/cuda-zone) is a parallel programming framework developed by NVIDIA to exploit GPU computing power. In this framework, the GPU, also called *device*, is seen as a parallel co-processor, with separated address space with respect to the CPU, also called *host*. The execution of a CUDA program always begins from the host, using a serial thread. When it is necessary to perform a parallel operation, the host allocates memory on the GPU and transfers the data to that memory. Those two operations are performed through the *cudaFree* and *cudaMemcpy* routines. At this point, the GPU generates thousands of parallel threads, which cooperate in order to perform the desired computation. The function performed by the GPU is called *kernel*. When the kernel execution ends, the CPU retrieves the results from the GPU memory through memory transfer (*cudaMemcpy* routine). The GPU memory is then deallocated by the *cudaFree* routine. The execution proceeds then in a serial way.

The threads generated by the GPU are grouped into *blocks*, which form the *grid*. The blocks can be mono-dimensional, bi-dimensional, or three-dimensional and the number of threads within a block can be chosen by the programmer.

The typical bottleneck of GPU applications is represented by memory transfers. Therefore, it is necessary to properly manage them in order to achieve the best performance.

In this work, we present three different parallel versions of the K-means algorithm. The first one is based on the parallelization of the distance computation. In this case, the thread performs the computation of the distance between the assigned pixel and the K centroids. This kernel takes as inputs the hyperspectral image Y and the K centroids stored in the cluster_centroids variable. It produces as output a $N \times K$ array which contains the distances between each pixel and each centroid. In particular, the i-th row and the j-th column of this array store the distance between the i-th pixel and the j-th centroid. Therefore, it is necessary to add a supplementary temporary array ($N \times K$) with respect to the serial implementation. The schematization of this implementation is shown in Figure 3.

The hyperspectral image Y is copied to the GPU memory only once, before the beginning of the main *while* loop. This has been done since the image is not modified by the algorithm. At every iteration, the only data transferred to the GPU is the matrix containing the centroids, that is used, together with the image, to compute the distances, stored in a temporary matrix (distances_array in Figure 3). Data are sent back to the host, which computes the minimum distance for each pixel (i.e., each row of this matrix) and then updates the centroids and computes the error in order to evaluate convergence.

The second CUDA version has been developed in order to avoid the limit of the amount of data transferred during each iteration of the main *while* loop. Therefore, the minimum distance computations, the centroids update, and the error evaluation have been performed on the GPU side. Since the distances are stored in an $N \times K$ array, the kernel used to find the index of the minimum distance is executed by N threads. The i-th thread performs a *for* loop in order to evaluate the minimum distance of the i-th centroid. In other words, this task has been parallelized by assigning to each thread the computation of the minimum distance for one pixel. The index of the minimum distance is stored in the *assigned_cluster* array, which contains the classification obtained at the current iteration of the main loop. The update of the centroids has been performed by a simple kernel where the i-th thread computes the update of the i-th centroid. Concerning the error evaluation, it is possible to use the highly optimized routines offered by the CUBLAS library. In particular, it is possible to use the *cublasSasum* routine, which calculates the sum of the absolute values stored in the input array. Before activating this kernel the element-wise difference between the values stored in the *actual_centroids* and *previous_centroids* arrays must be computed. This is done by a kernel in which a single thread computes the difference between two elements. The sum computed by the *cublasSasum* routine is returned to the host, which performs the final division needed for error evaluation and increments the number of iterations. The schematization of this CUDA version is shown in Figure 4.

It is important to notice that, in this version, only a single precision floating-point value is transferred at each iteration of the main loop. However, an additional data transfer at the end of the main loop must be performed, since it is necessary to retrieve the *assigned_cluster* that contains the hyperspectral pixel classification.

The last CUDA version developed in this work exploits the *dynamic parallelism* introduced by CUDA 6.0. This allows to use a thread inside a kernel in order to generate a grid which executes another kernel. In the proposed case, it is possible to take advantage of dynamic parallelism by moving the main *while* loop inside the kernel. In other words, this version is made up of a single kernel executed on the GPU by a single thread, which manages the activation of the kernels already described for the second CUDA version. In this case, the only memory transfers are performed before (the hyperspectral image Y) and after the main loop (the classified pixels *assigned_cluster*). However, it is worth noting that the activation of a kernel from another kernel requires a launching overhead, which will be discussed in Section 4.

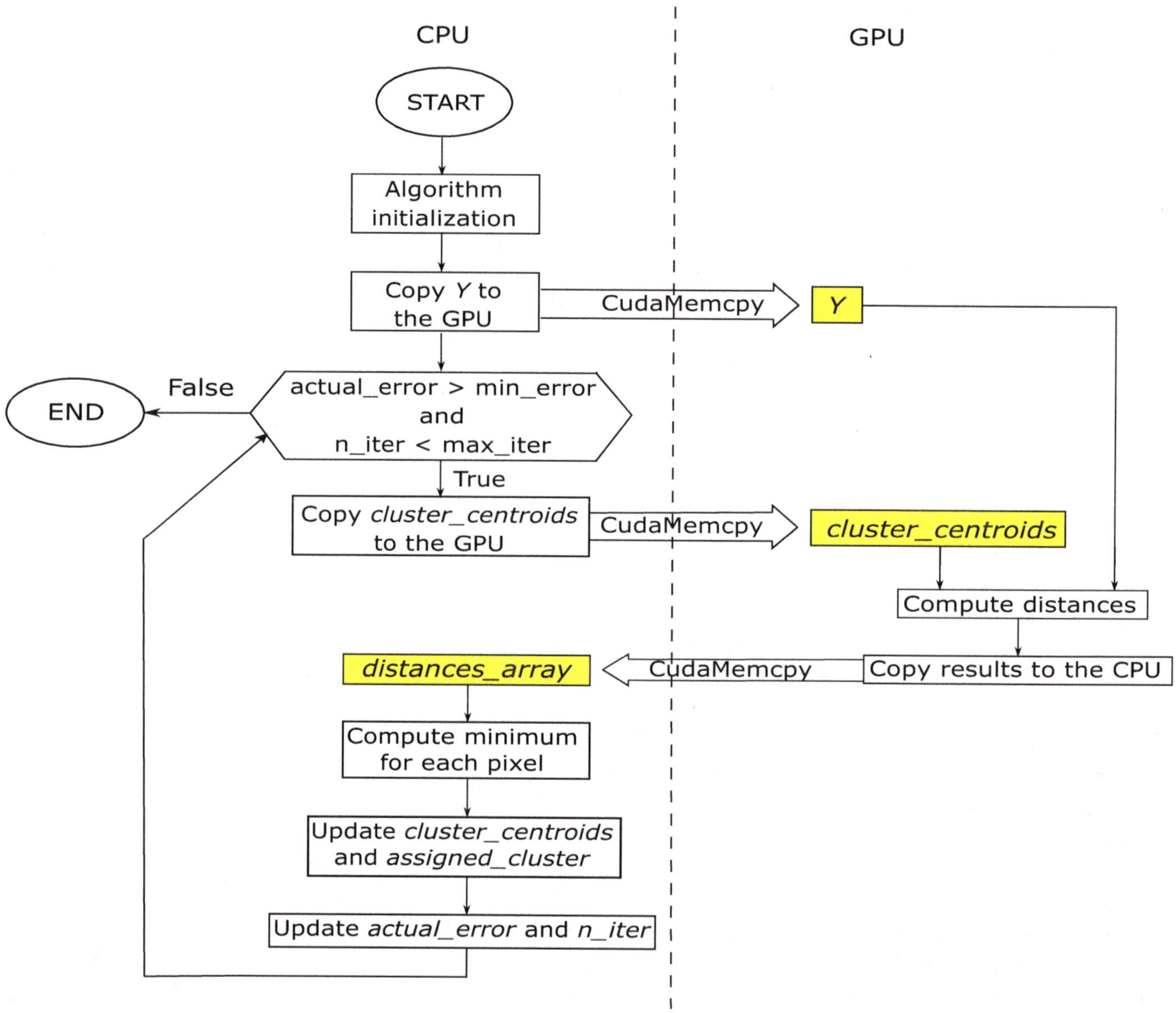

Figure 3. Schematization of the first GPU implementation. The operations are in white boxes, while data are in yellow boxes.

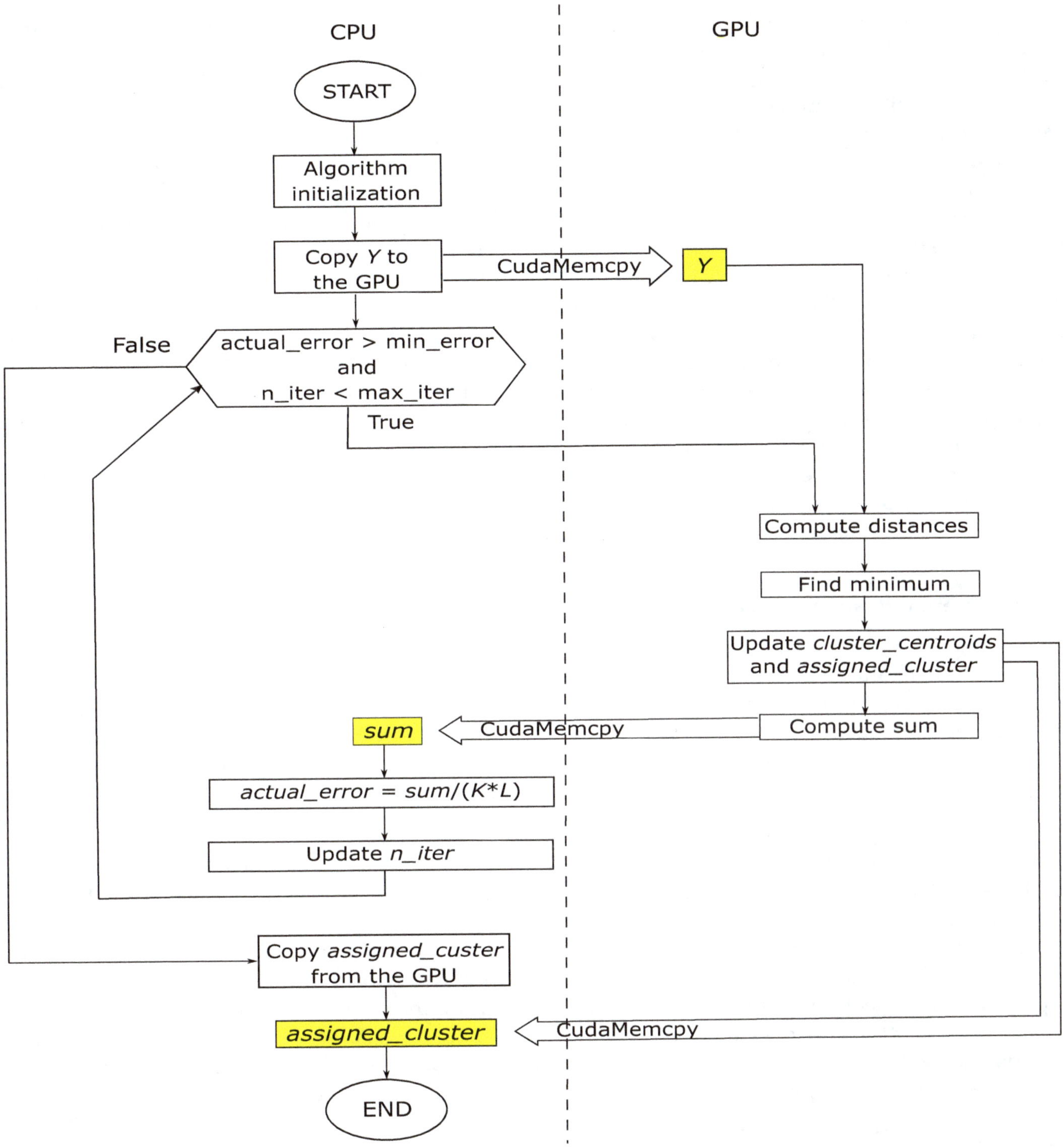

Figure 4. Schematization of the second GPU implementation. The operations are in white boxes, while data are in yellow boxes.

3.4. OpenCL Algorithms

OpenCL (https://www.khronos.org/opencl/) is a parallel programming framework maintained by the Khronos Group which addresses the issue of portability between devices from different vendors. It assumes a model similar to CUDA, with the difference that the blocks are called *working groups* and the threads are called *working items*. The computing platforms that can be programmed using OpenCL range from multi-core CPUs to manycore GPU and finally to Field Programmable Gate Arrays (FPGAs). Similarly to CUDA, this paradigm assumes that the computing platform is made up of a serial processor, called *host*, and one or more parallel *devices*. At the beginning of an OpenCL application, it is important to correctly initialize the execution context. This has the effect of pointing out to the OpenCL environment which devices will be used in the case that there are more than one OpenCL compatible boards installed on the same machine. Data that must be processed by the devices are stored into *buffers*, which can be of different types, depending on the targeting devices of the implementation. In particular, considering a generic GPU as a device, a buffer is a portion of the device memory where data are copied from the host memory. On the other hand, if we consider as a device a multi-core CPU or an integrated GPU which shared the RAM memory with the host, the buffer is only a reference to the RAM portion where data are stored. Notice that, in this last case, there will be no data transfers between host and device since the RAM address space is shared. An important difference when compared with CUDA is the absence of dynamic parallelism, thus, it is not possible to activate a kernel from another one. Therefore, we only developed two versions based on OpenCL. The first one performs the parallel computation of the distances on the device while the other operations are performed on the host. The second version performs all the operations inside the main *while* loop on the device, as we implemented in the second CUDA version already described. However, it is not possible to exploit the CUBLAS library, since it is strictly correlated with the adoption of NVIDIA devices. Therefore, we exploit the *clBLAS* library which is very similar to CUBLAS. In particular, we use the *clblasSasum* routine which performs the summation of all the elements stored in a given array. All the other operations have been performed as described for the second CUDA version.

4. Experimental Results and Discussion

All the parallel implementations have been tested with the hyperspectral dataset already used for serial code profiling and shown in Table 1. The images have been employed both to evaluate the processing times of the different versions and to validate the results. All the parallel versions have obtained the same results than the serial one when removing the random initialization. In other words, if the serial and the parallel versions have the same initialization, they perform the same number of iterations and produce the same outputs.

To graphically analyze the classification results, Figure 5A–F shows the RGB images where the tumor is highlighted. Moreover, Figure 5G–L depicts the supervised classification maps where the tumor is indicated with the red color, the healthy tissue in green, the hypervascularized in blue and the background in black. Images in Figure 5M–R are the segmentation maps produced by the K-means algorithm. As can be seen from the images, this algorithm is capable of distinguishing blood vessels, different tissue regions and the ring markers (used by neurosurgeons to label the image for the supervised classification). As said before, the algorithm defines with high accuracy the boundaries of each area, but the clusters do not correspond to specific classes. Moreover, colors are randomly assigned to each cluster. For this reason, it is crucial to combine this segmentation map with the supervised classification result in obtain the final output, shown in Figure 5S–X.

4.1. OpenMP Performance Evaluation

First, for each OpenMP implementation, several tests have been conducted in order to establish the optimal number of threads to be generated, using the biggest image (Image 6). These tests have been performed on an Intel i7 6700 processor working at 3.40 GHz equipped with 32 GB of RAM. The codes have been compiled with the *vc140* compiler, using compilation options to indicate the target architecture (i.e., x64 processor) and to maximize the processing speed. The processing times have been measured through the *omp_get_wtime* routine. The obtained results are shown in Figure 6.

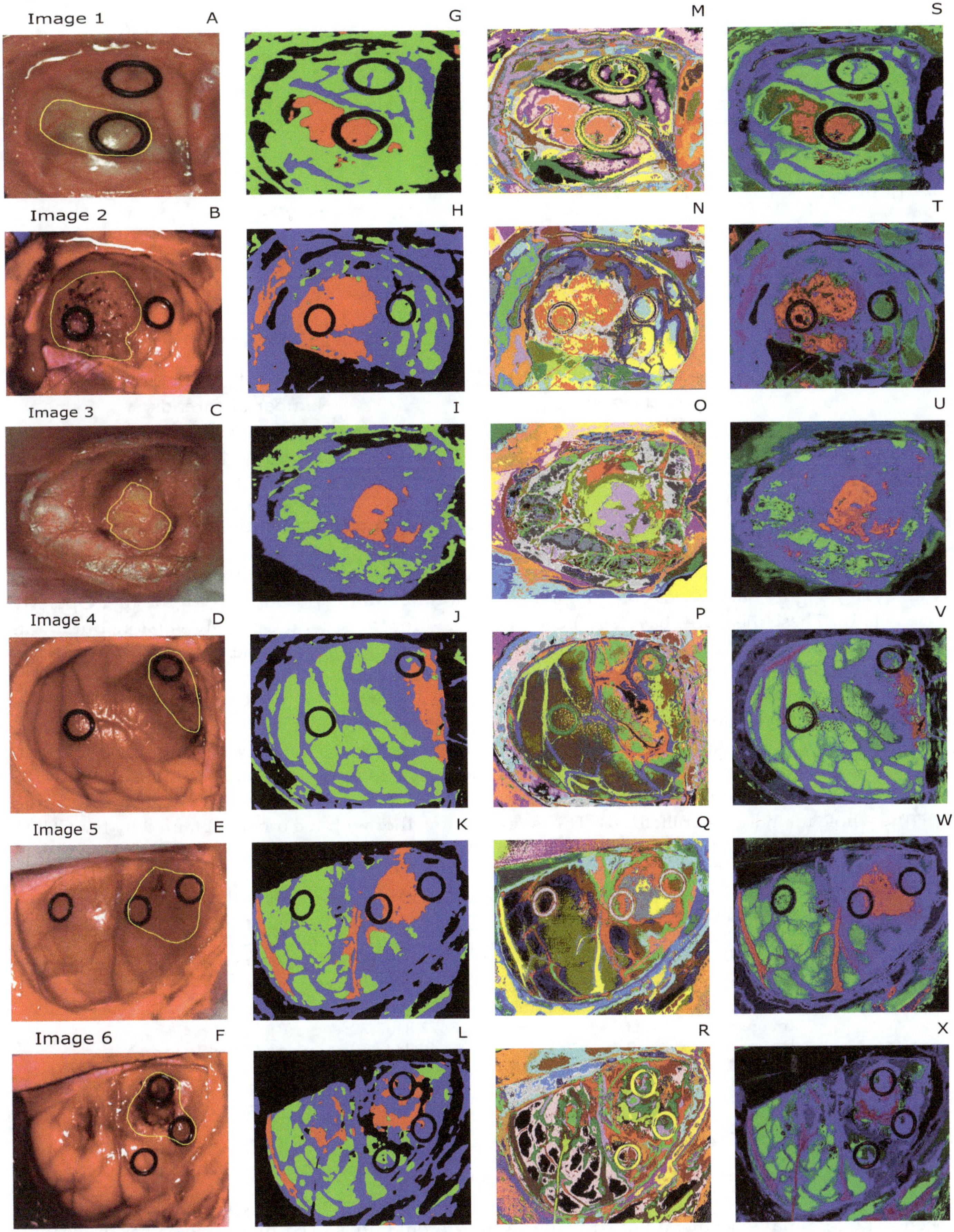

Figure 5. RGB representations of the dataset (**A–F**), supervised classification maps (**G–L**), segmentation maps (**M–R**), final output (**S–X**).

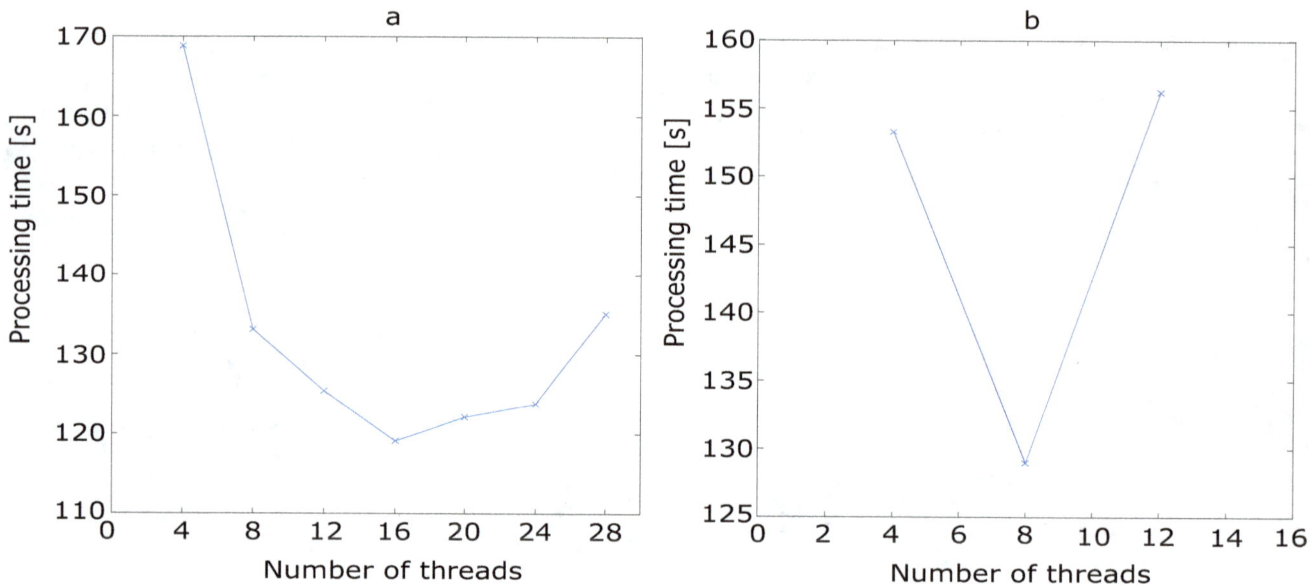

Figure 6. Processing time for Image 6 with respect to the number of threads for the first (**a**) and for the second (**b**) OpenMP version.

It is important to highlight that the experiments have been conducted with the same initialization, and they provide the same number of iterations and the same classification results. For the first OpenMP implementation, we measured the processing time from 4 to 28 threads. We did not test the application with more threads since the processing time begins to significantly grow after 28 threads. By analyzing Figure 6a, it is possible to see that the optimal number of threads for the first OpenMP version is 16. These measures have also been performed for the second OpenMP version, but in this case the maximum number of threads tested was 12 since the processing times begins to grow. In this case, as highlighted by Figure 6b, the optimal number of threads is 8.

After establishing the optimal number of threads, we tested the two OpenMP versions on the entire dataset presented in Table 1. In order to allow a direct comparison between the serial and the parallel versions, we initialized the algorithm with the same values for a given image. The obtained results, together with the speed-up values, are reported in Table 2, where OpenMPv1 indicates the first version (the parallelization of the distance metric computation), while OpenMPv2 indicates the second one (the whole main loop parallelized). Those results, together with the others obtained by the CUDA and OpenCL versions, will be discussed in Section 4.4.

Table 2. Comparison between the serial and the OpenMP versions of the algorithm. The speed-up is reported between brackets.

Image ID	# of Iterations	Serial [s]	OpenMPv1 [s]	OpenMPv2 [s]
Image 1	32	272.20	73.18 (3.72×)	75.88 (3.59×)
Image 2	13	162.37	44.42 (3.65×)	45.80 (3.55×)
Image 3	23	289.64	77.81 (3.72×)	81.35 (3.56×)
Image 4	10	151.50	40.98 (3.70×)	43.42 (3.49×)
Image 5	13	214.52	59.00 (3.64×)	63.09 (3.40×)
Image 6	25	465.51	118.31 (3.93×)	136.99 (3.40×)

4.2. CUDA Performance Evaluation

The three CUDA versions have been compiled using the NVIDIA *nvcc* compiler, which is part of the CUDA 9.0 environment. Compilation options have been chosen in order to maximize the execution speed. The tests have been conducted using two different GPUs. The first one is a NVIDIA Tesla K40 GPU equipped with 2880 CUDA cores working at 750 MHz and with 12 GB of DDR5 RAM.

It is based on the Kepler architecture that does not have a graphical output port since it is optimized for scientific computations. The second GPU is a NVIDIA GTX 1060 equipped with 1152 CUDA cores working at 1.75 GHz and with 3 GB of DDR5 RAM. This GPU is more recent than the first one and it is based on the Pascal architecture, having a graphical output port. In order to take full advantage of the specific architecture of each GPU, we indicate to the compiler which is the target micro-architecture. Specifically, we used the options *sm_35* and *compute_35* for the Tesla K40 GPU and the options *sm_60* and *compute_60* for the GTX 1060, where the values 35 and 60 represent the Kepler and the Pascal architecture, respectively. The results obtained using the Tesla K40 GPU are reported in Table 3, while the results obtained by the GTX 1060 GPU are reported in Table 4.

Table 3. Comparison between the serial and the CUDA versions of the algorithm on a Tesla K40 GPU. The speed-up is reported between brackets.

Image ID	# of Iterations	Serial [s]	CUDAv1 [s]	CUDAv2 [s]	CUDAv3 [s]
Image 1	32	272.20	87.48 (3.11×)	4.52 (60.22×)	4.87 (55.89×)
Image 2	13	162.37	54.51 (2.98×)	2.97 (54.67×)	3.34 (48.61×)
Image 3	23	289.64	100.67 (2.88×)	4.99 (58.04×)	5.12 (56.57×)
Image 4	10	151.50	56.41 (2.69×)	2.96 (51.18×)	3.47 (43.66×)
Image 5	13	214.52	79.74 (2.69×)	3.99 (53.76×)	4.14 (51.82×)
Image 6	25	465.51	159.77 (2.91×)	7.45 (62.48×)	7.83 (59.45×)

Table 4. Comparison between the serial and the CUDA versions of the algorithm on a GTX 1060 GPU. The speed-up is reported between brackets.

Image ID	# of Iterations	Serial [s]	CUDAv1 [s]	CUDAv2 [s]	CUDAv3 [s]
Image 1	32	272.20	80.84 (3.37×)	2.37 (114.85×)	4.21 (64.66×)
Image 2	13	162.37	44.54 (3.65×)	1.94 (83.70×)	2.93 (55.42×)
Image 3	23	289.64	98.61 (2.94×)	2.66 (108.89×)	2.96 (97.85×)
Image 4	10	151.50	52.47 (2.89×)	2.02 (75.00×)	3.25 (46.62×)
Image 5	13	214.52	75.00 (2.86×)	2.41 (89.01×)	3.48 (61.64×)
Image 6	25	465.61	147.50 (3.16×)	3.16 (147.34×)	3.69 (126.18×)

In both tables, CUDAv1 indicates the version where only the distance computation is computed on the GPU, CUDAv2 indicates the version where all the operations are performed in parallel and, finally, CUDAv3 indicates the version exploiting dynamic parallelism.

Concerning the GPU implementation, we also conducted a profiling using the NVIDIA Visual Profiler. This tool allows to profile the code execution on GPU together with memory transfers, in order to evaluate the efficiency of the implementation. Figure 7 shows the results obtained by profiling the Image 1 (the most demanding one) processing on the GTX 1060 with the CUDAv1 (a) and CUDAv2 (b) codes. Concerning the CUDAv2, in Figure 7b the different kernels executions percentage on the GPU are detailed. Profiling of CUDAv3 is not shown since it is very similar to CUDAv2 as well as the code profiling on the NVIDIA Tesla K40 GPU.

4.3. OpenCL Performance Evaluation

OpenCL codes have been compiled using vendor-specific compilers. In particular, the OpenCL version without memory transfers have been tested on an Intel i7 6700 processor working at 3.40 GHz, equipped with 32 GB of RAM and on an Intel HD Graphics 530 integrated GPU with 16 cores working at 350 MHz. The integrated board shares the RAM with the CPU. Concerning the OpenCL version which performs memory transfers, it has been tested on the NVIDIA GTX 1060 GPU. Results obtained by the OpenCL versions are reported in Table 5.

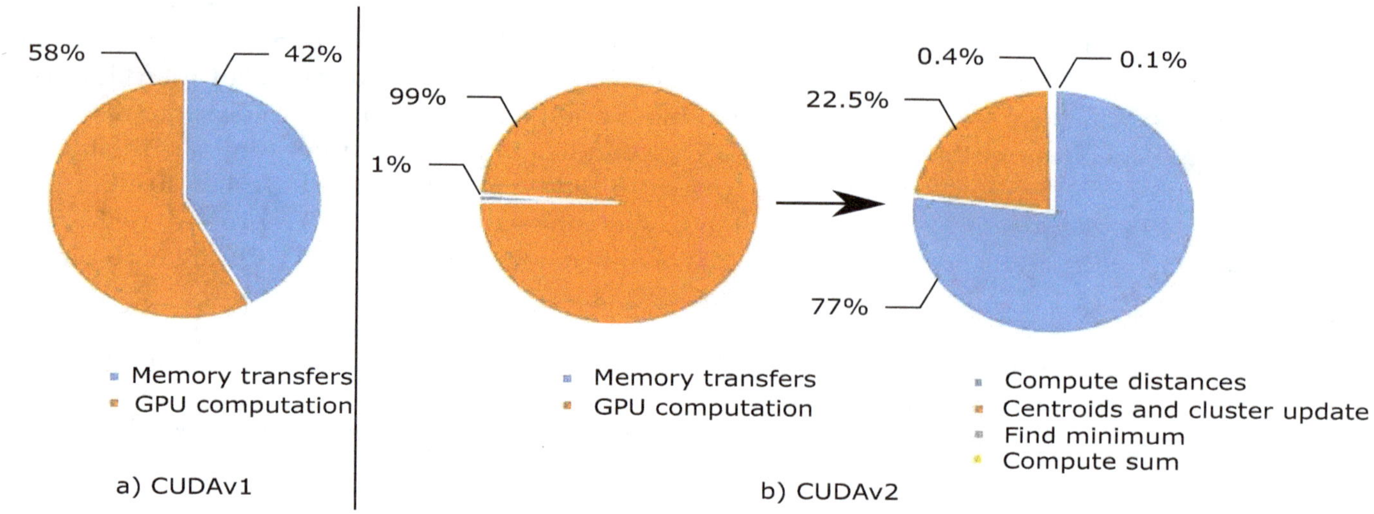

Figure 7. Profiling of GPU versions on the NVIDIA GTX 1060 board for the CUDA v1 (**a**) and CUDA v2 (**b**) versions.

Table 5. Comparison between the serial and the OpenCL versions of the algorithm. The speed-up is reported between brackets.

Image ID	# of Iterations	Serial [s]	Intel i7 [s]	Intel HD 530 [s]	GTX 1060 [s]
Image 1	32	272.20	74.13 (3.67×)	183.96 (1.48×)	57.61 (4.72×)
Image 2	13	162.37	44.32 (3.66×)	114.24 (1.42×)	35.61 (4.56×)
Image 3	23	289.64	79.52 (3.64×)	203.62 (1.42×)	63.75 (4.54×)
Image 4	10	151.50	40.52 (3.74×)	113.82 (1.33×)	35.36 (4.28×)
Image 5	13	214.52	59.92 (3.58×)	156.56 (1.37×)	47.03 (4.56×)
Image 6	25	465.51	121.59 (3.83×)	312.68 (1.49×)	93.65 (4.97×)

4.4. Comparisons and Discussion

The OpenMP version that offers the better results is the one where only the distance evaluations are processed in parallel. In this version, a parallel region is created and then destroyed at every iteration of the main loop, while in the second version the parallel region is created only once before the beginning of the main loop and is destroyed after the end of the main loop. However, the second version requires synchronization barriers between the threads, since there are operations that should be performed sequentially to obtain correct results. As an example, the increment of the number of iterations and the check of the conditions for repeating or not the main loop should be performed by a single thread. This is a critical issue since the advantage of creating and destroying the parallel region only once is thwarted by the synchronization bottleneck. The result analysis shows that the processing times are very similar, but the processor manages better the first version (OpenMPv1). Moreover, the speed-up values of the two versions are similar. Finally, it is important to highlight that the considered processor is equipped with 4 physical cores and the obtained speed-up is always greater than 3.5×. This means that the parallelization efficiency is close to the theoretical value.

Concerning the CUDA versions, by analyzing Tables 3 and 4, it is possible to observe that, for both GPU boards, the first CUDA version (CUDAv1) performs worse than the OpenMP ones. The reason is highlighted in Figure 7a, where the profiling results show that the memory transfers take about 42% of the time and only the remaining 58% is used for the computation. This is the typical bottleneck of GPU computing since the memory transfers are performed by the PCI-express external bus. The second CUDA version (CUDAv2) is not affected by this issue since the amount of data transferred at each main iteration is significantly lower than in the previous case. It is possible to parameterize the amount of transferred data at each iteration for these two versions. In the first case (CUDAv1), the data transferred is the distance_array matrix, which is made up of $N \times K$ elements represented in single precision floating-point arithmetic, while in the second case (CUDAv2) only one single precision floating-point value is copied back to the host. In the third case (CUDAv3), when dynamic parallelism is used, there are no data transfers inside the main loop. Therefore the third CUDA version is the one which transfers the minimum possible amount of data, but it does not perform better than the second version. This is because the dynamic parallelism produces an overhead due to the GPU switch between the main kernel and the subroutine kernel. This overhead affects every sub-kernel activation. In this specific case, four different sub-kernels are activated at every iteration. This overhead is not negligible and, as it can be seen form the results of Tables 3 and 4, it takes longer than the copy of a single float value from device to host. In other words, the time needed by the GPU to manage the generation of four sub-kernels (CUDAv3) is comparable with the time taken by a single value copy from the host to the device memory (CUDAv2). Finally, for all the CUDA versions, the GTX 1060 board performs better than the Tesla K40, even if the last board is optimized for scientific computations. This is because the first board is equipped with a more recent architecture which has better CUDA cores working at a higher frequency than the Tesla GPU.

The analysis of the OpenCL versions highlight that, considering the Intel i7, the processing times are close to the OpenMP ones. For what concerns the Intel HD 530 integrated GPU, the performance is very poor, and the speed-ups are negligible. This is probably due to the low-end integrated GPU with a working frequency of 350 MHz and only 16 parallel processing elements. Therefore, it is not possible to obtain a significant speed-up compared to the serial version. Comparing the OpenCL version and the CUDA versions running on the GTX 1060 GPU, it is possible to notice that the OpenCL version performs better than the CUDAv1, but is significantly slower than the other two CUDA versions. These CUDA versions (CUDAv2 and CUDAv3) employ highly optimized routines, which exploits all the hardware features of a GPU. Moreover, the CUDA versions have been compiled using compilation options in order to produce an executable code which fully exploits the specific target architecture. This is not possible in OpenCL since it targets portability between different devices as main feature.

We also performed a comparative study between the three best performing versions of the three considered technologies in order to characterize how the speed-up varies with respect to the number of clusters. In particular, we performed experiments using Image 6 and K values varying from 2 to 50. The speed-ups of the OpenMP, CUDA and OpenCL best versions with respect to the serial implementation are shown in Figure 8 using a semi-logarithmic scale. It is possible to see that the CUDA version has a speed-up that ranges from $10\times$ to $\sim 150\times$ and from 12 clusters on it becomes nearly constant. On the other hand, the solutions based on a multi-core processor have speed-ups that are close to $4\times$.

In the literature, there are different works about parallel K-means.

Baramkar et al. [18] performed a review of different parallel GPU-based K-means, but the considered works where focused only on general classification, without considering high data dimensionality, which is the case explored in our work. Therefore it is hard to perform direct comparisons with these works, which achieve very different speed-ups ranging from $11\times$ to $220\times$.

Zechner et al. [19] proposed a parallel implementation of this algorithm using both CPU and GPU. In particular, the GPU was only employed for distance computation, while centroids update was left to the CPU. They classified an artificial dataset with two-dimensional elements ranging from 500 to $500,000$. The maximum speed-up achieved was $14\times$, lower than the one obtained in our work. This is because the optimization proposed in [19] is only valid for low-dimensional data and cannot be employed for classifying high-dimensional data such as hyperspectral images.

A similar approach is shown in [20,21], with the difference that also the clusters update has been performed on the GPU. However, between the distance computation and centroids update they performed host computation for updating each pixel label. This choice leads to a maximum speed-up of 60 in both works, lower than our one, since we moved all the computation on the device side.

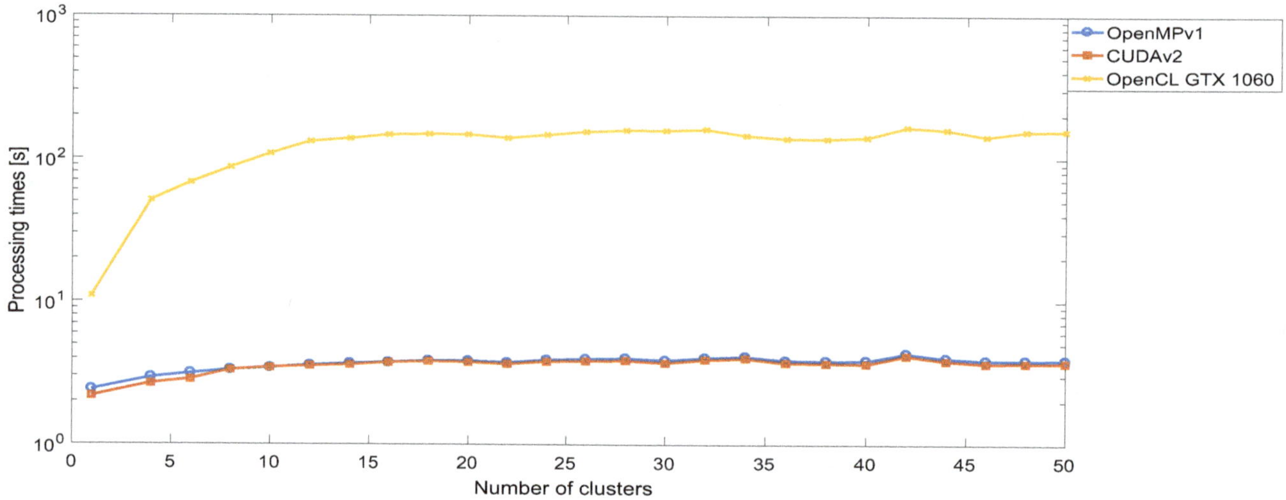

Figure 8. Speed-ups achieved by the three best parallel implementations (one for each evaluated parallel technology) with respect to the number of clusters.

In [22], a GPU-based K-means algorithm is proposed, with a distance computation that is evaluated through a simple Cartesian distance. Under this assumption, they classify 1,000,000 pixels with 32 features in 1.15 s. In our case, the bigger image has 264,408 pixels, the features (i.e., the bands) are 128 and it is processed in ~3.56 s. Moreover, the distance metric that we adopt (the spectral angle) is more complex than the one proposed in [22].

Baydoun et al. [23] developed a parallel K-means for RGB images classification. They adopted as metric a simple Cartesian distance and they parallelize only this computation, achieving a maximum speed-up of ~25×. In this case, the metric and the data dimensionality are very different compared to this work.

In [24], the K-means algorithm was modified to further reduce the distance computation. The speed-up varies from 4× to 386×, but also, in this case, it is not possible to perform a direct comparison since there are not enough details about the dataset composition. Finally, in [25], the K-means algorithm was developed on GPU with the Cartesian distance. They adopt a modern GPU with 1536 CUDA cores obtaining a maximum speed-up of 88×, which is very similar to our results.

Lutz et al. [26] proposed a parallel K-means implementation using an NVIDIA GTX 1080 GPU. They perfomed only experiments producing four groups and no further details are given in the paper about the dataset. They achieved a maximum speed-up of 18.5× which is nearly an order of magnitude smaller than one of our implementations.

A comparative analysis similar to the one we conducted is reported in [27]. Authors exploited GPUs, OpenMP, Message Passing Interface (MPI) and FPGAs. However, also in this case, they considered only a dataset made up of 10-dimensional points, therefore the computational complexity of the distance computation is lower than our one. On the other hand, the results were not as good as our ones, since the maximum GPU speed-up achieved is ~60×. They also demonstrated that the speed-up could reach a value up to 200× if the number of clusters to produce was significantly increased (i.e., more than 2000 clusters), but a study of how this speed-up varied also with respect to the data dimensionality were not carried out. Concerning OpenMP, the classification of 20,000 10-dimensionality points took ~3 s. Our smallest image is 6 times bigger than this one and with a dimensionality 18 times greater than the one considered. Keeping this in mind, the performance of our best OpenMP version is quite similar to this one. Finally, concerning the FPGA implementation, experiments were reported only with a 17,692 9-dimensionality dataset. Classification time is ~100 ms, but, as stated in [27], the FPGA resources, especially memory banks, were not enough to process bigger datasets. The authors of this work do not use external DDR memory, therefore, the FPGA performance is limited due to this design choice.

The comparison between our work and the literature is summarized in Table 6.

Table 6. Comparison between the proposed work and the literature.

Paper	Maximum Image Size	Data Dimensionality	Technology	Speed-Up
[18]	2,000,000	8	GPU NVIDIA GTX 280	220
[19]	500,000	2	GPU NVIDIA 9600 GT	14
[20]	1,000,000	2	GPU NVIDIA 8800 GTX	60
[21]	15,052,800	3	4 × GPU NVIDIA GTX 750Ti	60
[22]	1,000,000	32	GPU NVIDIA GTX 280	N. A.
[23]	16,777,216	3	GPU NVIDIA Tesla C2050	25
[24]	245,057	4	GPU NVIDIA GeForce 210	386
[25]	500,000	16	GPU NVIDIA Quadro K5000	88
[26]	N. A.	N. A.	GPU NVIDIA GTX 1080	18.5
[27]	20,000	10	2 × AMD Opteron quad-core	8
[27]	65,536	10	GPU NVIDIA Tesla 2050	60
[27]	17,692	9	Mitrion MVP FPGA Simulator	N. A.
Our work	264,408	128	GPU NVIDIA GTX 1060	126

5. Conclusions

In this paper, we presented different parallel implementations of the K-means algorithm for hyperspectral medical image clustering. In particular, we evaluated multi-core CPUs and manycore GPUs through the OpenMP and CUDA frameworks, respectively. Moreover, we also addressed the problem of code portability by developing OpenCL-based versions. We performed experiments with a dataset made up of *in-vivo* hyperspectral human brain images. Those experiments validated the results of all the proposed parallel implementations. Among them, CUDA achieved the better performance, outperforming OpenMP implementations. The cost of the better performance is the parallelization effort, which is significantly greater when working with CUDA. In fact, the development of the CUDA versions required the development of custom kernels and ad-hoc memory transfer management, while OpenMP only required code annotations with suitable pragmas. Code portability has also been addressed with OpenCL. However, this technology is not yet competitive with OpenMP or CUDA, achieving the worst results among the developed parallel applications. Moreover, OpenCL guarantees portability among different devices, but, for obtaining the best performance from a given device, it is necessary to tune the code with respect to specific hardware features. The comparison of the proposed implementations shows that the best one is based on CUDA and executed on the GTX 1060 board, achieving a maximum speed-up of ~125×. In particular, the best CUDA version performs all the computations on the GPU without exploiting dynamic parallelism.

We also made comparisons with other recent works in the literature, that only in one case achieved results comparable but not better than ours, except for the FPGA solution proposed in [27]. However, FPGA memory constraint does not allow to process images with more than 17,692 pixels. This limits the use of this technology and, in particular, it makes FPGAs not suitable for our target application.

Summarizing, the proposed work confirms that the GPU technology is the best solution for these class of problems, even when considering a data dimensionality bigger than the ones considered before. It also highlights that the GPU algorithm has a good scalability with respect to the number of clusters (K). Moreover, when considering high data dimensionality, the parallelization of the distance computation is not enough, since also the centroids update, and the error computation can be parallelized. This ensures a supplementary speed-up. Finally, the technological evolution of GPUs offers increasing computing power at relatively low cost. In our case, a consumer GPU sold at about $200 outperforms a more expensive Tesla K40 GPU (~$5000) of a previous generation, but optimized for scientific computations.

In conclusion, this work provides an efficient GPU implementation of the K-means algorithm, that will be included in the parallel version of the complete system already shown in Figure 1. Since the K-means is one of the most computational demanding algorithms in the system, this remarkable result is essential to satisfy the real-time constraint.

Future research will be focused on integrating this parallel algorithm in more complicated classification frameworks, such as the one proposed in [5,7].

Author Contributions: E.T. performed the GPU implementations, the algorithms optimizations, designed and performed experiments and wrote the manuscript. G.F. designed experiments and edited the manuscript. F.C. performed the GPU implementations and experiments. S.O., H.F. performed the serial algorithm implementation and edited the manuscript. G.M.C., M.M.-M., F.L. supervised the project and edited the manuscript.

Acknowledgments: The authors would like to thank NVIDIA Corporation for the donation of the NVIDIA Tesla K40 GPU used for this research.

References

1. Ferlay, J.; Soerjomataram, I.; Ervik, M.; Dikshit, R.; Eser, S.; Mathers, C.; Rebelo, M.; Parkin, D.M.; Forman, D.; Bray, F. *Cancer Incidence and Mortality Worldwide: IARC CancerBase No. 11*; International Agency for Research on Cancer: Lyon, France, 2013.
2. Louis, D.N.; Perry, A.; Reifenberger, G.; von Deimling, A.; Figarella-Branger, D.C.; Webster, K.; Ohgaki, H.; Wiestler, O.D.; Kleihues, P.; Ellison, D.W. The 2016 World Health Organization Classification of Tumors of the Central Nervous System: A summary. *Acta Neuropathol.* **2016**, *131*, 803–820. [CrossRef] [PubMed]
3. Sanai, M.; Berger, M.S. Operative techniques for gliomas and the value of extent of resection. *Neurotherapeutics* **2009**, *6*, 478–486. [CrossRef] [PubMed]
4. Fabelo, H.; Ortega, S.; Kabwama, S.; Callicó, G.M.; Bulters, D.; Szolna, A.; Pineiro, J.F.; Sarmiento, R. HELICoiD project: A new use of hyperspectral imaging for brain cancer detection in real-time during neurosurgical operations. *Proc. SPIE Int. Soc. Opt. Eng.* **2016**, *12*, 9860. [CrossRef]
5. Fabelo, H.; Ortega, S.; Lazcano, R.; Madronal, D.; Callicó, G.M.; Juárez, E.; Salvador, R.; Bulters, D.; Bulstrode, H.; Szolna, A.; et al. An intraoperative visualization system using hyperspectral imaging to aid in brain tumor delineation. *Sensors* **2018**, *18*, 430. [CrossRef] [PubMed]
6. Chang, C.-I. *Hyperspectral Data Processing: Algorithm Design and Analysis*; John Wiley & Sons: Hoboken, NJ, USA, 2013; ISBN 978-0-471-69056-6.
7. Fabelo, H.; Ortega, S.; Ravi, D.; Kiran, B.R.; Sosa, C.; Bulters, D.; Callicó, G.M.; Bulstrode, H.; Szolna, A.; Pineiro, J.F.; Kabwama, S.; et al. Spatio-spectral classification of hyperspectral images for brain cancer detection during surgical operations. *PLoS ONE* **2018**, *13*, e0193721. [CrossRef] [PubMed]
8. Torti, E.; Fontanella, A.; Florimbi, G.; Leporati, F.; Fabelo, H.; Ortega, S.; Callicó, G.M. Acceleration of brain cancer detection algorithms during surgery procedures using GPUs. *Microprocess. Microsyst.* **2018**, *61*, 171–178. [CrossRef]
9. Florimbi, G.; Fabelo, H.; Torti, E.; Lazcano, R.; Madronal, D.; Ortega, S.; Salvador, R.; Leporati, F.; Danese, G.; Báez-Quevedo, A.; et al. Accelerating the K-Nearest Neighbors Filtering Algorithm to Optimize the Real-Time Classification of Human Brain Tumor in Hyperspectral Images. *Sensors* **2018**, *18*, 2314. [CrossRef] [PubMed]
10. Lazcano, R.; Madronal, D.; Salvador, R.; Desnos, K.; Pelcat, M.; Guerra, R.; Fabelo, H.; Ortega, S.; Lopez, S.; Callico, G.M.; et al. Porting a PCA-based hyperspectral image dimensionality reduction algorithm for brain cancer detection on a manycore architecture. *J. Syst. Archit.* **2017**, *77*, 101–111. [CrossRef]
11. Madronal, D.; Lazcano, R.; Salvador, R.; Fabelo, H.; Ortega, S.; Callico, G.M.; Juarez, E.; Sanz, C. SVM-based real-time hyperspectral image classifier on a manycore architecture. *J. Syst. Archit.* **2017**, *80*, 30–40. [CrossRef]
12. Domingo, R.; Salvador, R.; Fabelo, H.; Madronal, D.; Ortega, S.; Lazcano, R.; Juarez, E.; Callico, G.M.; Sanz, C. High-level design using Intel FPGA OpenCL: A hyperspectral imaging spatial-spectral classifier. In Proceedings of the 2017 12th International Symposium on Reconfigurable Communication-centric Systems-on-Chip (ReCoSoC), Madrid, Spain, 12–14 July 2017; pp. 1–8. [CrossRef]
13. Fontanella, A.; Marenzi, E.; Torti, E.; Danese, G.; Plaza, A.; Leporati, F. A suite of parallel algorithms for efficient band selection from hyperspectral images. *J. Real-Time Image Process.* **2018**, 1–17. [CrossRef]
14. Marenzi, E.; Carrus, A.; Danese, G.; Leporati, F.; Callicó, G.M. Efficient Parallelization of Motion Estimation for Super-Resolution. In Proceedings of the 2017 25th Euromicro International Conference on Parallel, Distributed and Network-based Processing (PDP), St. Petersburg, Russia, 6–8 March 2017; pp. 274–277. [CrossRef]

15. Lopez-Fandino, J.; Heras, D.B.; Arguello, F.; Dalla Mura, M. GPU Framework for Change Detection in Multitemporal Hyperspectral Images. *Int. J. Parallel Program.* **2017**, 1–21. [CrossRef]
16. Florimbi, G.; Torti, E.; Danese, G.; Leporati, F. High Performant Simulations of Cerebellar Golgi Cells Activity. In Proceedings of the 2017 25th Euromicro International Conference on Parallel, Distributed and Network-based Processing (PDP), St. Petersburg, Russia, 6–8 March 2017; pp. 527–534. [CrossRef]
17. Feng, X.; Jin, H.; Zheng, R.; Zhu, L.; Dai, W. Accelerating Smith-Waterman Alignment of Species-Based Protein Sequences on GPU. *Int. J. Parallel Program.* **2015**, *43*, 359–380. [CrossRef]
18. Baramkar, P.P.; Kulkarni, D.B. Review for K-Means On Graphics Processing Units (GPU). *Int. J. Eng. Res. Technol.* **2014**, *3*, 1911–1914.
19. Zechner, M.; Granitzer, M. K-Means on the Graphics Processor: Design and Experimental Analysis. *Int. J. Adv. Syst. Meas.* **2009**, *2*, 224–235. [CrossRef]
20. Hong-tao, B.; Li-li, H.; Dan-tong, O.; Zhan-shan, L.; He, L. K-Means on Commodity GPUs with CUDA. In Proceedings of the WRI World Congress on Computer Science and Information Engineering, Los Angeles, CA, USA, 31 March–2 April 2009; pp. 651–655. [CrossRef]
21. Fakhi, H.; Bouattane, O.; Youssfi, M.; Hassan, O. New optimized GPU version of the k-means algorithm for large-sized image segmentation. In Proceedings of the Intelligent Systems and Computer Vision, Fez, Morocco, 17–19 April 2017; pp. 1–6. [CrossRef]
22. Li, Y.; Zhao, K.; Chu, X.; Liu, J. Speeding up k-Means algorithm by GPUs. *J. Comput. Syst. Sci.* **2013**, *79*, 216–229. [CrossRef]
23. Baydoun, M.; Dawi, M.; Ghaziri, H. Enhanced parallel implementation of the K-Means clustering algorithm. In Proceedings of the 3rd International Conference on Advances in Computational Tools for Engineering Applications (ACTEA), Beirut, Lebanon, 13–15 July 2016; pp. 7–11. [CrossRef]
24. Saveetha, V.; Sophia, S. Optimal Tabu K-Means Clustering Using Massively Parallel Architecture. *J. Circuits Syst. Comput.* **2018**, In press. [CrossRef]
25. Cuomo, S.; De Angelis, V.; Farina, G.; Marcellino, L.; Toraldo, G. A GPU-accelerated parallel K-means algorithm. *Comput. Electr. Eng.* **2017**, 1–13. [CrossRef]
26. Lutz, C.; Bress, S.; Rabl, T.; Zeuch, S.; Markl, V. Efficient k-means on GPUs. In Proceedings of the 14th International Workshop on Data Management on New Hardware, Huston, ID, USA, 11 June 2018. [CrossRef]
27. Yang, L.; Chiu, S.C.; Liao, W.K.; Thomas, M.A. High Performance Data Clustering: A Comparative Analysis of Performance for GPU, RASC, MPI, and OpenMP Implementations. *J. Supercomput.* **2014**, *70*, 284–300. [CrossRef] [PubMed]

9

Application of a Glucose Dehydrogenase-Fused with Zinc Finger Protein to Label DNA Aptamers for the Electrochemical Detection of VEGF

Jinhee Lee [1,†], Atsuro Tatsumi [2,†], Kaori Tsukakoshi [2,†], Ellie D. Wilson [1], Koichi Abe [2], Koji Sode [1] and Kazunori Ikebukuro [2,*]

[1] Joint Department of Biomedical Engineering, The University of North Carolina at Chapel Hill and North Carolina State University, Chapel Hill, NC 27599, USA; jh.lee@unc.edu (J.L.); elliedw@email.unc.edu (E.D.W.); ksode@email.unc.edu (K.S.)

[2] Department of Biotechnology and Life Science, Graduate School of Engineering, Tokyo University of Agriculture and Technology, 2-24-16 Naka-cho, Koganei, Tokyo 184-8588, Japan; atsuro0916tatsumi@gmail.com (A.T.); k-tsuka@cc.tuat.ac.jp (K.T.); abe79kou@gmail.com (K.A.)

* Correspondence: ikebu@cc.tuat.ac.jp

† These authors contributed equally to this work.

Abstract: Aptamer-based electrochemical sensors have gained attention in the context of developing a diagnostic biomarker detection method because of their rapid response, miniaturization ability, stability, and design flexibility. In such detection systems, enzymes are often used as labels to amplify the electrochemical signal. We have focused on glucose dehydrogenase (GDH) as a labeling enzyme for electrochemical detection owing to its high enzymatic activity, availability, and well-established electrochemical principle and platform. However, it is difficult and laborious to obtain one to one labeling of a GDH-aptamer complex with conventional chemical conjugation methods. In this study, we used GDH that was genetically fused to a DNA binding protein, i.e., zinc finger protein (ZF). Fused GDH can be attached to an aptamer spontaneously and site specifically in a buffer by exploiting the sequence-specific binding ability of ZF. Using such a fusion protein, we labeled a vascular endothelial growth factor (VEGF)-binding aptamer with GDH and detected the target electrochemically. As a result, upon the addition of glucose, the GDH labeled on the aptamer generated an amperometric signal, and the current response increased dependent on the VEGF concentration. Eventually, the developed electrochemical sensor proved to detect VEGF levels as low as 105 pM, thereby successfully demonstrating the concept of using ZF-fused GDH to enzymatically label aptamers.

Keywords: aptamer; labeling; enzyme; zinc finger protein; glucose dehydrogenase; electrochemical sensor; vascular endothelial growth factor

---

1. Introduction

Aptamers are DNA or RNA ligands that recognize a specific target molecule with comparable affinity and specificity to antibodies [1,2]. The utilization of aptamers in biosensing has several advantages over antibodies owing to their small size, high thermal stability, and ease of chemical modification. Accordingly, aptamers have become a major target recognition element in a variety of biosensing principles, including fluorescence, electrochemical, and colorimetric methods. In particular, since our first report on aptamer-based electrochemical sensors [3], many electrochemical aptamer sensors have been described for point of care testing purposes, taking advantage of rapid response times, ease of miniaturization, and cost-effectiveness owing to their established platform over other electrochemical detection principles.

To construct such electrochemical sensors, enzymes are attractive and often used as labeling molecules for high-sensitivity detection owing to their signal amplification ability. In reported electrochemical aptamer sensors, alkaline phosphatase and horse radish peroxidase are the most common enzymatic labels [4]. To label aptamers, avidin is typically conjugated to these enzymes, and this avidin-enzyme conjugate interacts with a biotinylated aptamer to form a chimeric aptamer-enzyme molecule. Historically, alkaline phosphatase and horse radish peroxidase are both difficult enzymes to produce recombinantly via prokaryotic host cells, such as *Escherichia coli*. Therefore, the preparation of avidin-enzyme complexes synthesized via chemical conjugation is favorable. However, the procedure to chemically conjugate and purify avidin and enzymes of interest before their use is not only laborious, but it can result in heterogenous molecules due to random conjugation [5] as well as the loss of protein function [6].

Alternatively, we have focused on glucose dehydrogenase (GDH) as a labeling enzyme for electrochemical aptamer sensors [3,7,8]. As GDH is the enzyme employed in the representative miniaturized electrochemical biosensor, the glucose sensor for the self-monitoring of blood glucose, well-established electrochemical principles and platforms are available. Importantly, GDH can be produced via prokaryotes while retaining a high specific activity, allowing for easy engineering of the enzyme [9]. Therefore, GDH would serve as an attractive labeling enzyme to engineer and perform simple and site-specific labeling for electrochemical aptamer sensors.

With regard to site-specific modifications, several methods are reported utilizing unnatural amino acids [6], intein [10], enzyme-catalyzed tags [11], self-labeling enzymes [12], or DNA-templated conjugation [13,14]. However, additional materials other than the DNA and protein are required to perform these conjugation methods. Kobatake and Gordon's group have developed a unique strategy for DNA–protein crosslinking through a DNA-binding enzyme-mediated covalent bond formation [15–17]. However, the method still suffered from low bioactivity of the conjugated enzyme. Inspired by our previous study [18], we have focused on the zinc finger protein (ZF), a monomeric double-stranded DNA-binding protein, to create a GDH-labelled aptamer. ZF is a DNA-binding protein which is capable of recognizing and binding to a specific sequence of double-stranded DNA [19,20]. On account of its small molecular weight, various molecules, including enzymes and fluorescent proteins, have been genetically fused to ZF for the purpose of gene editing and DNA detection, and are efficiently produced using prokaryotic cells without compromising its original function [21–25]. Previously, we have reported the use of ZF-fused GDH for the detection of PCR products, and successfully detected target DNA quantitatively [25]. This study demonstrated that the binding of ZF toward DNA happens spontaneously in a neutral buffer solution in a site-specific manner in vitro. Therefore, we assumed the aptamer labeling of GDH would occur by simply mixing the aptamer with ZF-fused GDH.

To this end, we present a novel GDH labeling method using ZF-fused GDH for aptamers. As a proof of concept, we have utilized vascular endothelial growth factor (VEGF) as a model target. VEGF plays an important role in the formation of new blood vessels of tissues [26]. As anti-VEGF pharmaceuticals are being used in tumor and age-related macular degeneration therapies, the detection of VEGF is important to predict the effectiveness of these treatments [27–29]. Moreover, VEGF is suggested as a biomarker for the early diagnosis of several diseases, such as lymphangioleiomyomatosis [30], major depressive disorder [31], and diabetic nephropathy [32]. Therefore, the rapid and sensitive detection of VEGF levels is crucial for clinical purposes. Here, we present the construction and results of an electrochemical sensor based on a GDH-labeled aptamer for VEGF detection with a lower detection limit of 105 pM.

2. Materials and Methods

2.1. Chemicals and Materials

All oligonucleotides were purchased from Eurofins Genomics (Luxembourg, Luxembourg). The sequences are indicated in the Supplementary Materials Table S1.

Phenazine methosulfate (PMS), 2,6-dichlorophenolindophenol (DCIP), D(+)-glucose, sodium chloride, 2-amino-2-hydroxymethyl-propane-1,3-diol (Tris), glycerol, and Tween-20 were purchased from Kanto Chemical Co. Inc. (Tokyo, Japan). Kanamycin sulfate and d-desthiobiotin were purchased from Sigma-Aldrich Co. LLC (St. Louis, MO, USA). A self-assembled monolayer (SAM) forming thiol reagent (dithiobis(succinimidyl undecanoate)) was purchased from Dojindo Laboratories Co., Ltd. (Kumamoto, Japan). LB broth, the bacterial host strain *Escherichia coli* BL21(DE3), and the expression vector pET30c(+) were purchased form Merck KGaA (Darmstadt, Germany). Anti-VEGF antibodies (MAB293 and BAF293) were purchased from R&D Systems, Inc. (Minneapolis, MN, USA). Gold and platinum wires were purchased from TANAKA Kikinzoku (Tokyo, Japan). A silver/silver chloride (3M NaCl) reference electrode RE-1B (Ag/AgCl) was purchased from BAS Inc. (Tokyo, Japan).

2.2. Investigation of Aptamer and Antibody Combination for the Sandwich Assay

Either biotinylated VEGF aptamers (30 pmol/well) or anti-VEGF antibody; BAF293 (20 pg/well) was diluted by TBS (10 mM Tris-HCl and 100 mM NaCl; pH 7.0) and immobilized on a streptavidin-coated micro-titer plate (Nunc, Rochester, NY, USA) by incubating for 1 h at 25 °C. Subsequently, the wells were washed with TBS-T (10 mM Tris-HCl, 100 mM NaCl and 0.05% Tween-20; pH 7.0) and blocked by blocking buffer (TBS-T containing 4% skim milk). After blocking, 0 or 100 nM VEGF was added, incubated for 1 h, and washed again by TBS-T. Next, the 300 nM of the labeling VEGF aptamer harboring the Zif268 binding site was added and incubated. Finally, 100 nM ZF-GDH was added to each well and incubated. After a final washing by TBS-T, the residual GDH activity was measured using PMS and DCIP. For this measurement, 100 μL of assay buffer (TBS containing 0.06 mM DCIP, 0.6 mM PMS, and 100 mM glucose) was added to each well and the absorbance change at 595 nm was measured using a plate reader (Wallac 1420 ARVO MX, Perkin-Elmer, Waltham, MA, USA).

2.3. Investigation of Binding Specificity of ZF-GDH Towards Its Target Sequence

Biotinylated VEGF-binding aptamer (2G19) or Zif268 recognition sequence-inserted 2G19 (2G19-Z) was first heat-treated at 95 °C for 10 min then gradually cooled down to 25 °C in TBS to let them fold into a stable structure. Then, 100 μL of the folded oligonucleotide solution was added onto a streptavidin coated micro-titer plate (Nunc, Rochester, NY, USA) at a concentration of 1 μM. After immobilization, each well was washed with TBS-T three times and blocked with a blocking buffer. Finally, 100 μL of 100 nM ZF–GDH solution was added and incubated for 1 h at 25 °C. After washing with TBS-T, the binding of ZF–GDH to each oligonucleotide was detected by measuring the residual GDH activity using PMS and DCIP using a plate reader (Wallac 1420 ARVO MX, Perkin-Elmer).

2.4. Investigation of VEGF Concentration Dependency on Plate Using Antibody and Aptamer

To select the pair of ligands for the sandwich binding assay, either biotinylated aptamer (30 pmol/well) or the anti-VEGF antibody BAF293 (20 pg/well) was immobilized on a streptavidin coated clear micro-titer plate by incubating for 1 h at 25 °C. Subsequently, the wells were washed with TBS-T and blocked using a blocking buffer. After blocking, 0 or 100 nM VEGF was added and incubated for 1 h, followed again by washing with TBS-T. Next, 100 μL of 300 nM 2G19-Z or V7t1 aptamer was added and incubated. Finally, 100 nM ZF–GDH was added to each well and incubated. After a final wash by TBS-T, the residual GDH activity was measured as described in Section 2.2. For the investigation of VEGF concentration dependency, 0–100 nM VEGF solution was added on the antibody-immobilized micro-titer plate and incubated for 1 h at room temperature. After washing, the captured VEGF was detected by GDH labeled 2G19-Z.

2.5. *Preparation of Antibody-Immobilized Gold Electrode*

For the formation of the self-assembled monolayer (SAM) on a gold wire electrode, the wire was cleaned by piranha solution and immersed in ethanol containing 1 mM thiol reagent (dithiobis(succinimidy undecanoate)) overnight at 25 °C. Next, the SAM-modified electrode was immersed into HEPES buffer (pH 7.0) containing 0.15 mg/mL streptavidin and incubated overnight at 4 °C. Followingly, the electrode was incubated for 30 min in HEPES buffer containing 5 μg/mL biotinylated anti-VEGF antibody (BAF293). Finally, the *N*-hydroxysuccinimide (NHS) ester was blocked through incubation of 1 M Tris-HCl (pH 8.0) for 15 min.

2.6. *Investigation of the Non-Specific Adsorption on a Gold Electrode*

A bare gold wire electrode, SAM-modified electrode, or antibody immobilized electrode was incubated with 100 nM ZF-GDH in TBS for 30 min. After washing, the residual GDH activity was electrochemically measured using chronoamperometry. The prepared gold electrode (working electrode) was immersed in 10 mL TBS containing 1 mM electron mediator (m-PMS: 1-methoxy-5-methylphenazinium methylsulfate) with Ag/AgCl and Pt wire as reference and counter electrodes, respectively. After applying a potential of 0.1 V (vs. Ag/AgCl) in a VersaSTAT4 potentiostat (Princeton Applied Research, Princeton, NJ, USA), the background response current was measured as the background in the absence of glucose. The applied potential was determined by considering the standard redox potential of mPMS (+0.063 V) [33], and we confirmed the potential was able to effectively oxidize mPMS in our previously reported GDH-based amperometric aptamer sensor [3,7,8]. Then, 25 s after application of the potential, glucose was added at a final concentration of 100 mM and the response current was measured for 100 s. The delta current was determined by subtracting the background current before the addition of glucose from the plateau signals after the addition of glucose.

2.7. *Electrochemical Detection of VEGF Using GDH-Labeled Aptamer*

The BAF293-immobilized gold wire electrode was blocked with 4% skim milk in TBS-T and incubated in TBS containing 0.25–25 nM of VEGF for 30 min at room temperature. Following washing with TBS-T, the electrode was incubated with 300 nM of 2G10-Z for 30 min and was subsequently incubated with 100 nM of ZF–GDH for 30 min again. After a final wash, residual GDH activity was detected via the same amperometric method described in the Section 2.6 with 1 mM m-PMS and 100 mM glucose utilizing VersaSTAT4 potentiostat (Princeton Applied Research, Princeton, NJ, USA). The calibration of VEGF was obtained by plotting the delta current against VEGF concentration. As a negative control, bovine serum albumin (BSA) was incubated with the electrode instead of VEGF, and after incubation of the aptamer and ZF-GDH, the residual GDH activity was measured by the chronoamperometry with an applied potential of 0.1 V (vs. Ag/AgCl).

3. Results

3.1. *GDH Labeling of VEGF-Binding Aptamer Using ZF-GDH and Characterization of the Labeled Aptamer*

To construct the fusion of GDH and ZF, we chose GDH derived from *Aspergillus flavus* (AfGDH) [34] and a mouse-derived ZF (Zif268) [35]. AfGDH is a monomeric flavin adenine dinucleotide-dependent GDH which has high catalytic activity of several hundred Unit/mg protein. Zif268 is a very well-characterized C_2H_2-type ZF which binds to its target double-stranded DNA (forward strand: 5′-GCGTGGGCG-3′ and reverse strand: 5′-CGCCCACGC-3′) in a one-to-one manner with high sequence specificity and binding affinity [35]. We confirmed the fusion protein maintained both the target double-stranded DNA binding ability of Zif268 [25] and the enzymatic activity of AfGDH. Remarkably, the enzymatic activity was the almost same level as that of original AfGDH (Supplementary Materials Figure S1). This is due to the small molecular weight of ZF (<10 kDa), one of the advantages of ZF as a fusion partner.

For electrochemical detection of VEGF, we selected a sandwich manner of detection. Therefore, first, the best combination of ligands was investigated on a sandwich plate assay. For this comparison, we chose two types of VEGF binding aptamers (Supplementary Materials Table S1). Both aptamers have a single binding region against VEGF with a nano-molar order K_d value, but fold into different unique structures. Moreover, 2G19 aptamer is predicted to form a stem loop structure [36], whereas V7t1 aptamer was revealed to form a G-quadruplex (G4) structure [37,38]. To label them by ZF-GDH, 2G19 and V7t1 were fused to a ZF recognition site and referred to as 2G19-Z and V7t1-Z, respectively (Supplementary Materials Figure S2). As the capture ligand, we immobilized either biotinylated VEGF aptamer or anti-VEGF antibody on a streptavidin-coated micro-titer plate. After the addition of 100 nM VEGF, GDH-labeled 2G19-Z or V7t1-Z was further added and washed. Eventually, the residual GDH activity was detected with a colorimetric redox dye.

When we used the anti-VEGF antibody as the capture ligand, the GDH-labeled aptamers showed a signal increase in the presence of VEGF (Figure 1). This indicated that both aptamers were correctly labeled by ZF-GDH and can be used to detect VEGF regardless of folding structure. Whereas, all of the aptamer-aptamer pairings showed a higher background signal without the addition of VEGF compared to that of antibody-aptamer pairs (Figure 1). Considering the low background signal with the antibody–aptamer pairs, this higher background signal would be due to the direct interaction between the capture and labeling aptamers rather than the non-specific adsorption of ZF-GDH. Therefore, we chose the anti-VEGF antibody and 2G19 aptamer pair to construct the VEGF sensor, as this combination provided the highest signal with the lowest background noise.

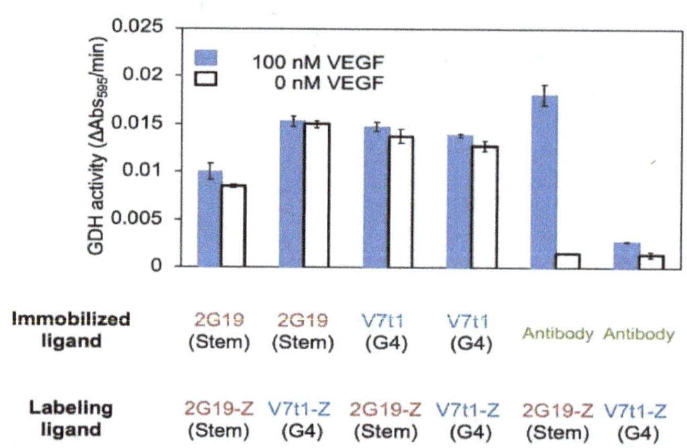

Figure 1. Investigation of aptamer and antibody combinations for the sandwich assay. To capture VEGF, aptamers (2G19 or V7t1) or anti-VEGF antibody (BAF293) was immobilized on a streptavidin-coated microtiter plate. As the detection ligand, ZF-GDH-labeled aptamers (2G19-Z or V7t1-Z) were used. Residual GDH activity on the plate was detected with colorimetric redox dye. Error bars indicate the standard deviation ($n = 3$).

The specific binding of ZF-GDH to the inserted Zif268-binding site in 2G19 was further investigated on a micro-titer plate. Here, we immobilized either the original 2G19 or Zif268 binding site inserted 2G19 (2G19-Z) using biotin-avidin interaction and allowed ZF-GDH to bind to the DNA. After washing, the residual GDH activity was measured with a colorimetric redox dye. We observed a significantly higher signal from the wells immobilized with 2G19-Z (Supplementary Materials Figure S3). This confirmed that ZF-GDH bound to the specific sequence inserted in the 2G19-Z aptamer. In other words, ZF-GDH labeled the aptamer with GDH.

Finally, we investigated VEGF concentration dependency using anti-VEGF antibody and GDH-labeled 2G19-Z on a micro-titer plate. Various concentrations of VEGF solution were added to the plate, and the VEGF captured by the antibody was detected using the GDH-labeled aptamer. When GDH activity was measured, signal increase was dependent on VEGF concentration, while there was no signal increase with the negative control protein, bovine serum albumin (BSA) (Supplementary

Materials Figure S4). Therefore, as we expected, ZF-GDH functioned to label the aptamer, which showed a specific binding against VEGF.

3.2. Construction of Electrochemical Detection System Using GDH-Labeled 2G19-Z to Detect VEGF

To construct the electrochemical VEGF detection system using the GDH-labeled aptamer, we modified the SAM on the gold wire electrode (approximate working surface area: 16 mm^2) using a decyl alkyl chain harboring a thiol group and *N*-hydroxysuccinimide (NHS) group to immobilize anti-VEGF antibody and to reduce the non-specific adsorption of ZF-GDH. The non-specific adsorption of ZF-GDH on the SAM-modified electrode was investigated by measuring the residual GDH activity after the electrode was immersed in the ZF-GDH solution. GDH activity was measured using the chronoamperometry in the presence of 1 mM m-PMS and 100 mM glucose with an applied potential of 0.1 V (vs. Ag/AgCl). When the bare gold electrode was incubated in the ZF-GDH solution, a high response current was observed even after washing with a buffer; however, the current was reduced with the SAM- and antibody-modified electrode (Supplementary Materials Figure S5). Therefore, the immobilization of this SAM on the electrode efficiently reduced non-specific adsorption.

To immobilize the antibody on the SAM-modified electrode, we used biotin-avidin interactions to control the orientation of the anti-VEGF antibody. First, streptavidin was immobilized on the SAM-modified electrode via amine coupling, and then biotinylated anti-VEGF antibody was immobilized on a streptavidin-modified electrode. After antibody immobilization, the surface was blocked by skim milk and used to detect VEGF. For this detection, we incubated the electrode with 0.25–25 nM of VEGF and after washing, the captured VEGF was labeled by 2G19-Z and ZF-GDH (Figure 2A). In this principle, the amount of GDH on the electrode would be dependent on the amount of the captured VEGF. Upon addition of glucose, GDH obtains an electron and the cofactor (flavin adenine dinucleotide) is reduced. Subsequently, the cofactor is then re-oxidized by the free electron mediator existing in solution, mPMS. Eventually, the reduced mPMS is oxidized by the electrode to generate the response current for the chronoamperometry measurement. Therefore, as the VEGF concentration increases, more reduced mediator is generated, and a higher response current is observed.

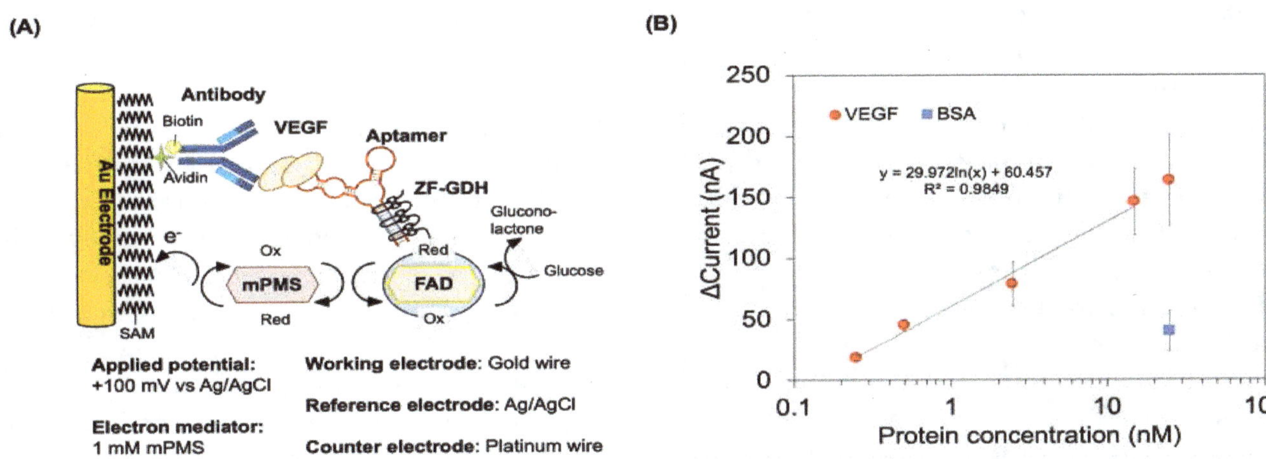

Figure 2. Electrochemical detection of VEGF. (**A**) Schematic diagram of the electrochemical detection of VEGF. (**B**) Electrochemical detection of VEGF by using ZF-GDH-labelled aptamer. The GDH activity was measured by chronoamperometry in the presence of 1 mM mPMS and 100 mM glucose with an applied potential of 0.1 V (vs. Ag/AgCl). The delta current is defined as the subtraction of background current before addition of glucose from the plateau signals after the addition of glucose. Error bars indicate standard deviations ($n = 3$).

As a result of detection, we observed a concentration-dependent signal increase with a linear relationship between the current responses and the logarithmic values of VEGF concentration ranging from 0.25–15 nM (Figure 2B). The limit of detection was calculated to be 105 pM according to the method of M_b + 3 SD (where M_b and SD are the mean value and standard deviation of the blank, respectively). However, the addition of the negative control, BSA instead of VEGF, gave a higher current value than the blank and was comparable to the current value obtained with 0.5 nM VEGF. This indicated that further optimization of the electrode surface modification is necessary.

Although the sensitivity can be improved as the estimated VEGF concentration in a sample would be sub-pico molar, these results showed that the aptamer was correctly labeled with GDH and generated an electrochemical signal. Most importantly, the spontaneous binding of the ZF to the binding sequence inserted into the aptamer enabled GDH labeling of the aptamer by merely mixing the solution.

4. Discussion

For the simple fabrication and construction of an enzyme-based amperometric aptamer sensor, we focused on GDH in terms of its facile recombinant production and engineering. Specifically, we circumvented GDH labeling via chemical conjugation by using ZF-fused GDH. As we expected, the ZF-GDH fusion protein was expressed as soluble protein in *E. coli*-based recombinant production system. In contrast to chemical conjugation, the fusion of ZF had little effect on GDH function, as ZF-fused GDH maintained more than 90% of original GDH activity (Supplementary Materials Figure S1). With chemical modification, surface lysine residues are commonly targeted, and the random modification of these residues can decrease the solubility and stability of protein. As we fused ZF genetically to the N-terminus of GDH, the surface lysine residues remained intact. Additionally, considering the fused position of ZF, which is separate from the active site, and the small molecular weight (<10 kDa) of ZF, the fusion of ZF did not alter protein folding of the GDH nor block the substrate access.

When we labeled two different VEGF-binding aptamers using ZF-GDH and performed sandwich detection of VEGF, both aptamers showed higher GDH activity in the presence of VEGF. Although their folding structures are different, both aptamers were labeled by GDH and served as a detection ligand for VEGF. Therefore, this suggests that this GDH labeling method can be generalized for different aptamers than those used in this study. In the sandwich assay, the G-quadruplex forming V7t1 aptamer showed lower signal intensity than 2G19 aptamer in spite of its better K_d value (1.4 nM vs. 52 nM). Therefore, the sensitivity depends on the paring of antibody and aptamer, not just on the aptamer's affinity.

We successfully detected VEGF electrochemically utilizing the aptamer labeled by ZF-GDH with a lower detection limit of 105 pM and a detection range of 250 pM to 15 nM. To date, several electrochemical aptamer sensors are reported for VEGF detection (Supplementary Materials Table S2). Some of these sensors utilize labeling enzymes, such as alkaline phosphatase or GDH, however they also require chemical conjugation of avidin. We were able to bypass this laborious process by using ZF-GDH to label the aptamer. Besides the simplicity of labeling, another advantage of the present system in comparison to other reported sensors is its detection principle. Namely, the system is an amperometric sensor based on GDH activity, and this principle is adopted in the commercially available glucose sensors. Therefore, we can construct this sensing system with already established platforms. On the other hand, the sensor showed a signal increase with BSA, a non-target molecule. This current increase can be attributed to the direct interaction of ZF-GDH with the non-specifically adsorbed BSA on the electrode surface. As seen in the result of the sandwich plate assay (Supplementary Materials Figure S4), once the surface was sufficiently blocked, the GDH-labeled 2G19-Z did not show a signal increase with the addition of BSA. Therefore, further optimization of the SAM composition and its density, as well as the conditions of blocking and washing would prove this signal increase with BSA.

Compared to previously reported GDH activity-based VEGF sensors, our sensor demonstrated a tenfold improvement in (Supplementary Materials Table S2). However, our sensor sensitivity was moderate in comparison to those reported for electrochemical sensors, as some demonstrated femto-molar levels of sensitivity. Indeed, the constructed sensor requires improvement considering the sub-pico molar concentration of VEGF in a clinical sample. To increase the signal, we can first consider fusing multiple GDH enzymes to ZF to obtain higher GDH activity. Secondly, we can increase the affinity of ZF to DNA by increasing the number of ZF motifs, as well as alter these motifs to recognize longer sequences. In this study, we used Zif268 which recognizes 9 bp and has a K_d with nanomolar affinity, but by fusing an additional ZF motif, we can improve the K_d to a picomolar level [39].

5. Conclusions

In this study, we employed GDH as a labeling enzyme for an amperometric aptamer sensor and developed a GDH labeling method for a VEGF-binding aptamer using ZF-fused GDH. Since GDH can be recombinantly produced and easily engineered, the connecter, ZF was genetically fused to GDH, eliminating the need for chemical conjugation methods to prepare ZF-fused GDH. The small molecular size of ZF (<10 kDa) contributed to the maintenance of GDH activity even after the fusion of ZF. Furthermore, the fusion protein enabled simple and easy labeling of the aptamer without laborious steps, such as purification and dialysis, to obtain the aptamer–GDH complex. Eventually, we could detect 105 pM VEGF in the GDH activity-based electrochemical detection system. Since the target specificity of ZF is designable, this GDH labeling method has the potential to be a universal labeling method to construct electrochemical aptamer sensors.

Author Contributions: Conceptualization, J.L., A.T., K.A., K.S., and K.I.; methodology, J.L., and A.T.; data collection, J.L. and A.T.; data curation, J.L. and A.T.; writing—original draft preparation, J.L., A.T., and K.A.; writing—review and editing, K.T., E.D.W., and K.I.; supervision, K.I.; All authors have read and agreed to the published version of the manuscript.

Acknowledgments: This work was supported by The Murata Science Foundation.

References

1. Tuerk, C.; Gold, L. Systematic evolution of ligands by exponential enrichment: RNA ligands to bacteriophage T4 DNA polymerase. *Science* **1990**, *249*, 505–510. [CrossRef] [PubMed]
2. Ellington, A.D.; Szostak, J.W. In vitro selection of RNA molecules that bind specific ligands. *Nature* **1990**, *346*, 818–822. [CrossRef] [PubMed]
3. Ikebukuro, K.; Kiyohara, C.; Sode, K. Electrochemical detection of protein using a double aptamer sandwich. *Anal. Lett.* **2004**, *37*, 2901–2909. [CrossRef]
4. Villalonga, A.; Pérez-Calabuig, A.M.; Villalonga, R. Electrochemical biosensors based on nucleic acid aptamers. *Anal. Bioanal. Chem.* **2020**, *412*, 55–72. [CrossRef]
5. Wang, L.; Amphlett, G.; Blattler, W.A.; Lambert, J.M.; Zhang, W. Structural characterization of the maytansinoid–monoclonal antibody immunoconjugate, huN901–DM1, by mass spectrometry. *Protein Sci.* **2005**, *14*, 2436–2446. [CrossRef]
6. Kazane, S.A.; Sok, D.; Cho, E.H.; Uson, M.L.; Kuhn, P.; Schultz, P.G.; Smider, V.V. Site-specific DNA-antibody conjugates for specific and sensitive immuno-PCR. *Proc. Natl. Acad. Sci. USA* **2012**, *109*, 3731–3736. [CrossRef]
7. Ikebukuro, K.; Kiyohara, C.; Sode, K. Novel electrochemical sensor system for protein using the aptamers in sandwich manner. *Biosens. Bioelectron.* **2005**, *20*, 2168–2172. [CrossRef]
8. Fukasawa, M.; Yoshida, W.; Yamazaki, H.; Sode, K.; Ikebukuro, K. An aptamer-based bound/free separation system for protein detection. *Electroanalysis* **2009**, *21*, 1297–1302. [CrossRef]
9. Ferri, S.; Kojima, K.; Sode, K. Review of glucose oxidases and glucose dehydrogenases: A bird's eye view of glucose sensing enzymes. *J. Diabetes Sci. Technol.* **2011**, *5*, 1068–1076. [CrossRef]

10. Barbuto, S.; Idoyaga, J.; Vila-Perello, M.; Longhi, M.P.; Breton, G.; Steinman, R.M.; Muir, T.W. Induction of innate and adaptive immunity by delivery of poly dA:dT to dendritic cells. *Nat. Chem. Biol.* **2013**, *9*, 250–256. [CrossRef]
11. Liang, S.I.; McFarland, J.M.; Rabuka, D.; Gartner, Z.J. A Modular approach for assembling aldehyde-tagged proteins on DNA scaffolds. *J. Am. Chem. Soc.* **2014**, *136*, 10850–10853. [CrossRef] [PubMed]
12. Duckworth, B.P.; Chen, Y.; Wollack, J.W.; Sham, Y.; Mueller, J.D.; Taton, T.A.; Distefano, M.D. A universal method for the preparation of covalent protein-DNA conjugates for use in creating protein nanostructures. *Angew. Chem. Int. Ed.* **2007**, *46*, 8819–8822. [CrossRef] [PubMed]
13. Yan, X.; Zhang, H.; Wang, Z.; Peng, H.; Tao, J.; Li, X.F.; Chris Le, X. Quantitative synthesis of protein–DNA conjugates with 1:1 stoichiometry. *Chem. Commun.* **2018**, *54*, 7491–7494. [CrossRef] [PubMed]
14. Rosen, C.B.; Kodal, A.L.; Nielsen, J.S.; Schaffert, D.H.; Scavenius, C.; Okholm, A.H.; Voigt, N.V.; Enghild, J.J.; Kjems, J.; Torring, T.; et al. Template-directed covalent conjugation of DNA to native antibodies, transferrin and other metal-binding proteins. *Nat. Chem.* **2014**, *6*, 804–809. [CrossRef] [PubMed]
15. Akter, F.; Mie, M.; Grimm, S.; Nygren, P.-Å.; Kobatake, E. Detection of Antigens Using a Protein–DNA Chimera Developed by Enzymatic Covalent Bonding with phiX Gene A*. *Anal. Chem.* **2012**, *84*, 5040–5046. [CrossRef] [PubMed]
16. Lovendahl, K.N.; Hayward, A.N.; Gordon, W.R. Sequence-directed covalent protein-DNA linkages in a single step using HUH-Tags. *J. Am. Chem. Soc.* **2017**, *139*, 7030–7035. [CrossRef] [PubMed]
17. Mie, M.; Niimi, T.; Mashimo, Y.; Kobatake, E. Construction of DNA-NanoLuc luciferase conjugates for DNA aptamer-based sandwich assay using Rep protein. *Biotechnol. Lett.* **2019**, *41*, 357–362. [CrossRef]
18. Abe, K.; Murakami, Y.; Tatsumi, A.; Sumida, K.; Kezuka, A.; Fukaya, T.; Kumagai, T.; Osawa, Y.; Sode, K.; Ikebukuro, K. Enzyme linking to DNA aptamers via a zinc finger as a bridge. *Chem. Commun.* **2015**, *51*, 11467–11469. [CrossRef]
19. Wolfe, S.A.; Nekludova, L.; Pabo, C.O. DNA recognition by Cys_2His_2 zinc finger proteins. *Annu. Rev. Biophys. Biomol. Struct.* **2000**, *29*, 183–212. [CrossRef]
20. Gaj, T.; Gersbach, C.A.; Barbas, C.F. ZFN, TALEN, and CRISPR/Cas-based methods for genome engineering. *Trends Biotechnol.* **2013**, *31*, 397–405. [CrossRef]
21. Urnov, F.D.; Rebar, E.J.; Holmes, M.C.; Zhang, H.S.; Gregory, P.D. Genome editing with engineered zinc finger nucleases. *Nat. Rev. Genet.* **2010**, *11*, 636–646. [CrossRef] [PubMed]
22. Stains, C.I.; Porter, J.R.; Ooi, A.T.; Segal, D.J.; Ghosh, I. DNA Sequence-Enabled Reassembly of the Green Fluorescent Protein. *J. Am. Chem. Soc.* **2005**, *127*, 10782–10783. [CrossRef] [PubMed]
23. Ooi, A.T.; Stains, C.I.; Ghosh, I.; Segal, D.J. Sequence-Enabled Reassembly of β-Lactamase (SEER-LAC): A Sensitive Method for the Detection of Double-Stranded DNA. *Biochemistry* **2006**, *45*, 3620–3625. [CrossRef] [PubMed]
24. Abe, K.; Kumagai, T.; Takahashi, C.; Kezuka, A.; Murakami, Y.; Osawa, Y.; Motoki, H.; Matsuo, T.; Horiuchi, M.; Sode, K.; et al. Detection of pathogenic bacteria by using zinc finger protein fused with firefly luciferase. *Anal. Chem.* **2012**, *84*, 8028–8032. [CrossRef]
25. Lee, J.; Tatsumi, A.; Abe, K.; Yoshida, W.; Sode, K.; Ikebukuro, K. Electrochemical detection of pathogenic bacteria by using a glucose dehydrogenase fused zinc finger protein. *Anal. Methods* **2014**, *6*, 4991–4994. [CrossRef]
26. Ferrara, N. Vascular endothelial growth factor: Basic science and clinical progress. *Endocr. Rev.* **2004**, *25*, 581–611. [CrossRef]
27. Burstein, H.J.; Chen, Y.-H.; Parker, L.M.; Savoie, J.; Younger, J.; Kuter, I.; Ryan, P.D.; Garber, J.E.; Chen, H.; Campos, S.M.; et al. VEGF as a marker for outcome among advanced breast cancer patients receiving anti-VEGF therapy with bevacizumab and vinorelbine chemotherapy. *Clin. Cancer Res.* **2008**, *14*, 7871–7877. [CrossRef]
28. Kim, K.J.; Li, B.; Winer, J.; Armanini, M.; Gillett, N.; Phillips, H.S.; Ferrara, N. Inhibition of vascular endothelial growth factor-induced angiogenesis suppresses tumour growth in vivo. *Nature* **1993**, *362*, 841–844. [CrossRef]
29. Girmens, J.-F.; Sahel, J.-A.; Marazova, K. Dry age-related macular degeneration: A currently unmet clinical need. *Intractable Rare Dis. Res.* **2012**, *1*, 103–114. [CrossRef]

30. Young, L.; Lee, H.-S.; Inoue, Y.; Moss, J.; Singer, L.G.; Strange, C.; Nakata, K.; Barker, A.F.; Chapman, J.T.; Brantly, M.L.; et al. MILES Trial Group Serum VEGF-D a concentration as a biomarker of lymphangioleiomyomatosis severity and treatment response: A prospective analysis of the Multicenter International Lymphangioleiomyomatosis Efficacy of Sirolimus (MILES) trial. *Lancet Respir. Med.* **2013**, *1*, 445–452. [CrossRef]
31. Lee, B.-H.; Kim, Y.-K. Increased plasma VEGF levels in major depressive or manic episodes in patients with mood disorders. *J. Affect. Disord.* **2012**, *136*, 181–184. [CrossRef] [PubMed]
32. Hanefeld, M.; Appelt, D.; Engelmann, K.; Sandner, D.; Bornstein, S.R.; Ganz, X.; Henkel, E.; Hasse, R.; Birkenfeld, A.L. Serum and plasma levels of vascular endothelial growth factors in relation to quality of glucose control, biomarkers of inflammation, and diabetic nephropathy. *Horm. Metab. Res.* **2016**, *48*, 529–534. [CrossRef] [PubMed]
33. Hisada, R.; Yagi, T. 1-Methoxy-5-methylphenazinium methyl Sulfate. A photochemically stable electron mediator between NADH and various electron acceptors. *J. Biochem.* **1977**, *82*, 1469–1473. [CrossRef] [PubMed]
34. Mori, K.; Nakajima, M.; Kojima, K.; Murakami, K.; Ferri, S.; Sode, K. Screening of *Aspergillus*-derived FAD-glucose dehydrogenases from fungal genome database. *Biotechnol. Lett.* **2011**, *33*, 2255–2263. [CrossRef]
35. Elrod-Erickson, M.; Rould, M.A.; Nekludova, L.; Pabo, C.O. Zif268 protein-DNA complex refined at 1.6 Å a model system for understanding zinc finger-DNA interactions. *Structure* **1996**, *4*, 1171–1180. [CrossRef]
36. Fukaya, T.; Abe, K.; Savory, N.; Tsukakoshi, K.; Yoshida, W.; Ferri, S.; Sode, K.; Ikebukuro, K. Improvement of the VEGF binding ability of DNA aptamers through *in silico* maturation and multimerization strategy. *J. Biotechnol.* **2015**, *212*, 99–105. [CrossRef]
37. Nonaka, Y.; Sode, K.; Ikebukuro, K. Screening and improvement of an anti-VEGF DNA aptamer. *Molecules* **2010**, *15*, 215–225. [CrossRef]
38. Marušič, M.; Veedu, R.; Wengel, J.; Plavec, J. G-rich VEGF aptamer with locked and unlocked nucleic acid modifications exhibits a unique G-quadruplex fold. *Nucleic Acids Res.* **2013**, *41*, 9524–9536. [CrossRef]
39. Moore, M.; Choo, Y.; Klug, A. Design of polyzinc finger peptides with structured linkers. *Proc. Natl. Acad. Sci. USA* **2001**, *98*, 1432–1436. [CrossRef]

10

A Self-Calibrating IoT Portable Electrochemical Immunosensor for Serum Human Epididymis Protein 4 as a Tumor Biomarker for Ovarian Cancer

Valentina Bianchi [1], Monica Mattarozzi [2,*], Marco Giannetto [2,*], Andrea Boni [1], Ilaria De Munari [1] and Maria Careri [2]

1 Department of Engineering and Architecture, University of Parma, 43124 Parma, Italy; valentina.bianchi@unipr.it (V.B.); andrea.boni@unipr.it (A.B.); ilaria.demunari@unipr.it (I.D.M.)

2 Department of Chemistry, Life Sciences and Environmental Sustainability, University of Parma, 43124 Parma, Italy; maria.careri@unipr.it

* Correspondence: monica.mattarozzi@unipr.it (M.M.); marco.giannetto@unipr.it (M.G.)

Abstract: Nowadays, analytical techniques are moving towards the development of smart biosensing strategies for the point-of-care accurate screening of disease biomarkers, such as human epididymis protein 4 (HE4), a recently discovered serum marker for early ovarian cancer diagnosis. In this context, the present work represents the first implementation of a competitive enzyme-labelled magneto-immunoassay exploiting a homemade IoT Wi-Fi cloud-based portable potentiostat for differential pulse voltammetry readout. The electrochemical device was specifically designed to be capable of autonomous calibration and data processing, switching between calibration, and measurement modes: in particular, firstly, a baseline estimation algorithm is applied for correct peak computation, then calibration function is built by interpolating data with a four-parameter logistic function. The calibration function parameters are stored on the cloud for inverse prediction to determine the concentration of unknown samples. Interpolation function calibration and concentration evaluation are performed directly on-board, thus reducing the power consumption. The analytical device was validated in human serum, demonstrating good sensing performance for analysis of HE4 with detection and quantitation limits in human serum of 3.5 and 29.2 pM, respectively, reaching the sensitivity that is required for diagnostic purposes, with high potential for applications as portable and smart diagnostic tool for point-of-care testing.

Keywords: human epididymis protein 4; competitive electrochemical immunosensor; WiFi portable potentiostat; on-board calibration; Internet of Things

---

1. Introduction

Ovarian carcinoma (OC) is the leading cause of death from gynecological malignancy worldwide: it is generally asymptomatic in the early stage, so the majority of women with OC are not diagnosed until the disease is in an advanced stage, with an overall five-year relative survival rate that is generally in the 30–40% range [1,2]. Therefore, it is crucial to detect OC as early as possible to correctly identify the cancer stage for effective treatment options and to early distinguish malignant from benign pelvic mass by means of annual routine gynecological and pelvic examinations, as well as dedicated screening programmes. In this context, noninvasive cancer detection at an early stage needs the identification of specific and sensitive biomarkers that are present at abnormal concentrations in body fluids, as well as the development of smart devices for analytical screening [3–6], in order to improve ovarian cancer survival rate [7]. Currently, carbohydrate antigen 125 (CA125) glycoprotein is the established biomarker for detecting OC occurrence and the monitoring therapeutic progress. However, the diagnostic potential of CA125 is mainly limited by its low specificity, since it can also be increased in a variety of other benign gynecological conditions affecting pre- and/or post-menopausal women, or in other malignant cancers [8]. In this context, over the last years, a number of alternative OC biomarkers, especially for the predominant OC subtype, i.e. epithelial ovarian cancer (EOC), have been identified and studied, either alone or combined, to improve the effectiveness of early diagnostic strategies. Among the recently proposed biomarkers, human epididymis protein 4 (HE4) resulted in being most promising in EOC differential diagnosis in detecting the disease at early stage, in monitoring the response to chemotherapy and in estimating the prognosis of ovarian cancer [1].

Electrochemical immunosensors are playing a growing role for improved clinical diagnosis and therapy monitoring by combining the specificity of antigen-antibody immunoreaction and the sensitivity of the electrochemical transduction [9]. As for HE4 determination, several sensing architectures that are based on "sandwich" approach have been recently exploited [10–13].

Electrochemical immunosensors can exploit enzyme labels for signal generation, such as the here presented study, but can also be designed according to label-free transduction and amplification mechanisms [14,15]. One of the main advantages associated to the enzyme-labelled electrochemical transduction is the possibility of method implementation on miniaturized electrodes as well as on portable and battery-operated devices [16]. Several instrumental approaches have been proposed in recent years and, some of these, such as 910 PSTAT and DropStat from Metrohm (Herisau, Switzerland), are already commercially available. DropStat, in particular, allows for making quantitative analyses and directly displaying the analyte concentration on the stand-alone device; the tool is custom configured with the electrochemical technique attending user's needs by simply inserting preprogrammed cards with calibration parameters available upon request from the producer. A PC connection is necessary to download acquired data for storage purposes. In addition, solutions by PalmSens (Houten, The Netherlands) and UNISCAN (Buxton, Derbyshire, UK) are battery-powered or USB-powered portable devices that are capable of performing voltammetric measurements, but they need to rely on external APP or software PC to determine the analyte concentration in a sample. Very recently, USB-based [17–19] and wireless [20–22] potentiostats were proposed, both involving data processing and visualization performed on an external device running a custom developed software. A Bluetooth communication for data collecting, processing, and sharing is exploited, even in the case of wireless potentiostats, thus requiring a PC that is close to the device. In 2015, Steinberg et al. proposed a device based on RFID or NFC data communication, where data are logged and then off-line analyzed in MS-Excel format [23]. However, all of the developed systems that allow for quantitative analyses to be performed involve off-line data processing based on a calibration function, even if using a Wi-Fi communication protocol. For example, Annamalai and coworkers recently described a Wi-Fi based solution for glucose determination, taking advantage from the Adafruit Cloud services to process and display data [24]. Chen et al. reported another recent example that involves Wi-Fi protocol that can locally visualize results on a TFT LCD display [25].

In this context, the possibility to perform data processing and calibration on-board, making the device completely autonomous, is very attractive. This approach allows, on the one hand, to reduce the device power consumption avoiding the raw data transmission and, on the other hand, to increase its portability, making it usable independently of connections or external devices at the time of measurement. However, the potentiostat portability must not affect the measurement accuracy in estimating the analyte concentration. Very recently, our research group proposed a new portable potentiostat having the Analog Front End (AFE) that was capable of very accurate analysis when compared to other portable solutions that are available in literature [26]. In this context, the present work represents a further improvement of that Wi-Fi portable potentiostat, proposing new additional functions through an enhanced firmware to introduce autonomous calibration and processing capabilities with the aim of applying it to the readout and processing of data from an innovative magneto-immunoassay for the determination of the ovarian cancer biomarker HE4 in human serum. This approach is consistent with the technological evolution of Analytics 4.0, representing the innovative integration of analytical chemistry into an Internet-of-Things (IoT) system, as recently defined by Mayer at al. [27].

2. Materials and Methods

2.1. Materials

Trizma® base, Tween-20, boric acid, sodium hydroxide, monosodium phosphate, disodium phosphate, magnesium chloride, human serum, albumin from bovine serum (BSA), Monoclonal Anti-WFDC2 clone 3F9 Antibody produced in mouse purified immunoglobulin (anti-HE4), PrEST Antigen WFDC2 (HE4) were purchased from Sigma Aldrich (Milan, Italy). Alkaline Phosphatase-conjugated secondary Rabbit Anti-Mouse IgG (RAM-AP), carcinoembryonic antigen (CEA), and Carbohydrate Antigen 125 (CA125) were purchased from Abcam (Cambridge, UK). DropSens® hydroquinone diphosphate (HQDP) was obtained from Metrohm Italiana (Origgio, Varese, Italy). The following buffers were prepared: 0.1 M borate buffer (BB) pH 9.5; 0.1 M Na-phosphate buffer (PB; 0.08 M Na_2HPO_4 and 0.02 M NaH_2PO_4) pH 7.4; 0.1 M TRIS Buffer (TB) containing 0.02 M of $MgCl_2$ pH 7.4; washing buffers PB-T and TB-T consisted, respectively, of PB and TB containing Tween-20 at 0.05 % (*v/v*). Reading buffer (RB) was prepared as TB, but adjusting the pH to 9.8.

Dynabeads®M-280 Tosylactivated (2.8 μm) MBs were purchased from Invitrogen (Thermo Fisher Scientific, Rodano, Milan, Italy). DropSens®Screen-Printed Carbon Electrodes (SPEs) for electrochemical readout were purchased from Metrohm Italiana; in particular, the working (WE; 4 mm diameter) and auxiliary (AE) electrodes are made of carbon, while pseudo-reference electrode (RE) is in silver.

2.2. Magnetic Immunoassay Set-Up

MBs were thoroughly suspended and a volume of 15 μL was transferred to a new tube, then, after triple-washing step with 200 μL of BB, the MBs were incubated with 400 μL of 10 μg mL^{-1} solution of HE4 antigen in BB (1 h; 37 °C; 1000 rpm). After the removal of unreacted HE4 solution by twice washing with BB, MBs were blocked with a 2% (*w/v*) solution of BSA dissolved in PB, and then washed with PB-T and PB. The HE4-modified MBs were used to carry out four independent competitive electrochemical immunoassays after their resuspension in 400 μL of TB and subdivision in four equivalent volume aliquots. After isolation, the MBs were resuspended with 100 μL of serum sample previously diluted ten-fold with TB and added with anti-HE4 monoclonal antibody to reach the final concentration of 1 μg mL^{-1}. The immunocompetition was left to undergo for 1 h at room temperature (RT) under agitation (1000 rpm), the reacted MBs was carefully washed with TB-T and TB and then incubated with 100 μL of 2 μgmL^{-1} RAM-AP secondary antibody (RT; 1 h; 1000 rpm). After washing with TB-T and TB, the beads were finally reacted with 100 μL of 1 mg mL^{-1} solution of HQDP enzyme substrate dissolved in RB for three minutes. Two 50 μL sub-aliquots of each sample were transferred on a SPE mounted on a DropSens®customized magnetic support that aimed at confining the MBs on the surface of WE and the electrochemical readout was carried out independently for each sub-aliquot of the sample suspension. Alkaline phosphatase (AP) dephosphorylates non-electroactive HQDP into hydroquinone (HQ), allowing for its electrochemical oxidation to quinone (Q) to achieve the signal related to the analyte.

Scheme 1 reports a schematic representation of the working principle of the electrochemical immunomagnetic assay.

The voltammetric readout of the assays were performed through our homemade IoT Wi-Fi portable potentiostat, while using the differential pulse voltammetry (DPV) scan. The potential was scanned between −0.4 and +0.2 V, setting on the IoT potentiostat a pulse amplitude of 0.05 V, a step potential of 0.005 V, and a pulse time of 100 ms. After the deposition of the MBs suspension on the SPE, a preconditioning step of 30 s at −0.4 V was applied to preconcentrate the reduced form of quinone.

The current responses observed for each concentration (S) were normalized with respect to the zero signal (S_0) obtained without HE4 in competition.

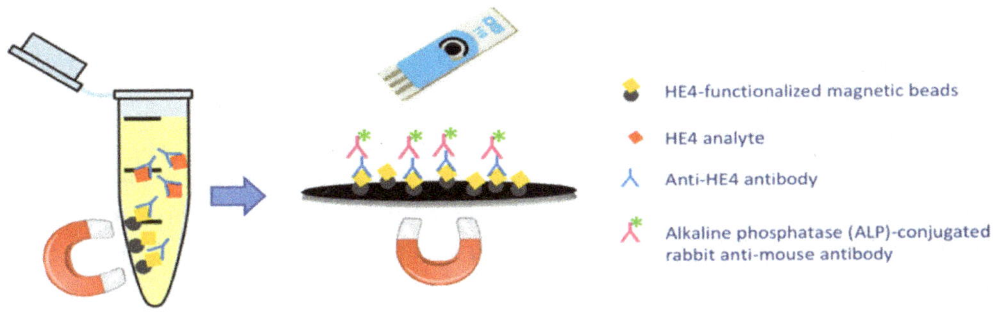

Scheme 1. Working principle of the electrochemical immunomagnetic assay on MBs supports.

2.3. *IoT Architecture*

The system architecture is depicted in the sketch that is shown in Scheme 2.

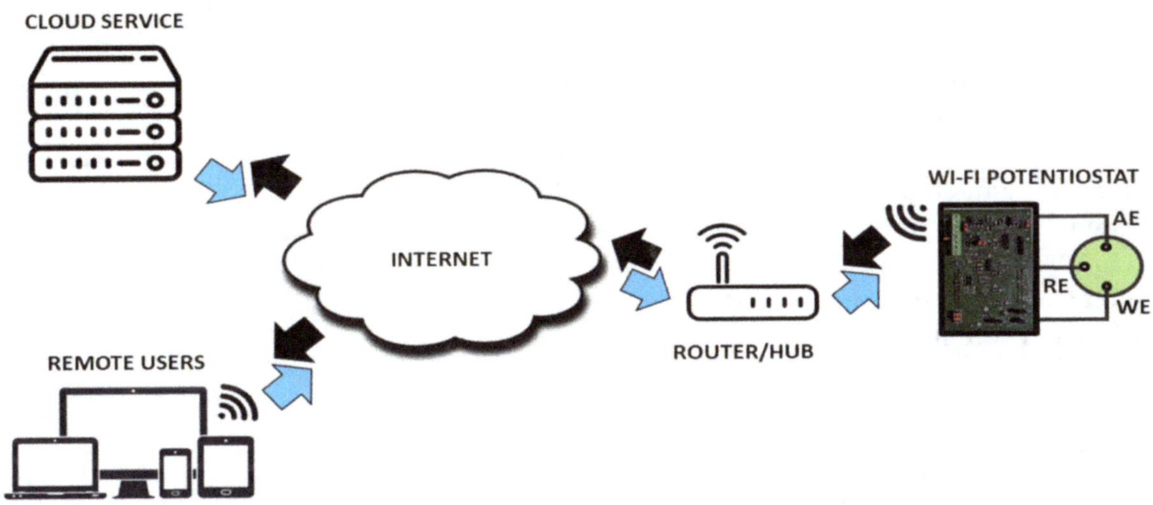

Scheme 2. Internet-of-Things (IoT) architecture for the proposed system.

The exploited AFE guarantees a sufficient measurement points to achieve higher accuracy with respect to other solutions presented in literature, as reported in our previous study [26]. In this work, the aforementioned AFE is connected to a CC3200 Microcontroller Unit (MCU) for signal processing with an improved firmware to develop a smart self-calibrating portable potentiostat, that was fully compliant with the IoT paradigm.

In particular, the proposed system takes a step forward with respect to current literature [17–25], since it is capable of on-board building a calibration function acquiring the signal from a given set of standards at known concentrations (*calibration mode*); this function is subsequently applied to calculate analyte concentration of unknown samples (*measurement mode*). Moreover, the proposed solution relies on a Wi-Fi connection to send the preprocessed data to a cloud service for storing and sharing exploiting the remote access feature. The on-board data elaboration allows for greatly reducing the device power consumption, enhancing battery lifetime. In fact, the main contribution to the device power consumption is the data transmission phase: sending preprocessed information allows to reduce the transmission task, with a benefit for the average absorbed current. In Bassoli et al. [28], a quantitative evaluation of this approach in the case of Wi-Fi protocol is reported. The data generated from the end device go directly, through the modem/router via Wi-Fi Protected Access (WPA) standard protocol, to the Internet cloud, where they are stored for subsequent sharing in a fast and efficient way. Thanks to the broad coverage guarantee by the Wi-Fi router, it is easy to ensure a stable sensor connection over a large area [29]. The scenario is fully compliant with an IoT paradigm, in which sensors "information flows rationally and orderly on the Internet, for being shared on a global scale" [30].

2.4. On-Board Data Management

The basedrift phenomenon has to be considered to correctly estimate the DPV peak current. In fact, the differential current baseline is often not parallel to the voltage axis, which prevents the computation of the peak by simply applying an algorithm for the search of the maximum. Hence, for each measurement point a baseline estimation algorithm is applied. Usually, for each curve, N minimum points have to be detected and the baseline is evaluated applying a polynomial fitting algorithm. Therefore, the baseline thus calculated is assumed as the reference for the correct evaluation of the peak current.

For calibration purposes, the peak current values have to be related to the HE4 concentration according to a suitable mathematical law. For this purpose, the normalized S/S_0 responses were plotted versus the HE4 concentration, so obtaining a dose-response inhibition curve, which was interpolated through a four-parameter logistic function (1) [31]:

$$S/S_0 = S_{min} + \frac{(S_{max} - S_{min})}{1 + ([C]/I_{50})^B}, \tag{1}$$

where S_{min} and S_{max} are the asymptotic minimum and maximum, I_{50} is the inflection point, namely the antigen concentration corresponding to 50% signal inhibition and B is the slope at I_{50}.

In the *calibration mode*, the device is able to compute on-board these four parameters when considering a set of measurements that were carried out on calibration standards. In particular, the parameters are computed, implementing the method of least squares according to the Levenberg–Marquardt algorithm [32,33]. When considering two vectors X and Y in Rn, containing, respectively, the n known concentration values and the n measurements of the corresponding peak current to be used for calibration, the vector of the residuals ε in Rn will be defined, as

$$\varepsilon = Y - F(X, \beta), \tag{2}$$

where F is the logistic function and β is the vector containing the four parameters to be computed. Hence, the aim of the proposed algorithm is to minimize the sum of the residual squares, SS, with an iterative approach. In doing so, the first step is to define the initial values for the parameters to be found, which are

$$S_{\text{max\_0}} = \max(Y), \tag{3}$$

$$S_{\text{min\_0}} = \min(Y), \tag{4}$$

$$B_0 = sign\left(\frac{y_n - y_1}{x_n - x_1}\right), \tag{5}$$

$$I_{50\_0} = X_k, \quad \text{k is the position where } \min\left(\left|Y - \frac{\max(Y) - \min(Y)}{2}\right|\right), \tag{6}$$

Subsequently, during a generic step i the β vector is updated as

$$\beta_i = \beta_{i-1} - \Delta_{\beta_{i-1}}, \tag{7}$$

where $\Delta_{\beta i}$ is defined as

$$\Delta_{\beta_i} = \left((J^T J)_{\beta_i} + \lambda (J^T J)_{\beta_i}\right)^{-1} J^T e_{\beta_i}, \tag{8}$$

λ is a parameter updated at each step and J is the Jacobian matrix defined as

$$J = \frac{\partial e}{\partial \beta}, \tag{9}$$

Finally, the sum of the residual square is computed as

$$SS_i = \sum_i (\varepsilon_i)^2 = \varepsilon_{\beta_i}^T \varepsilon_{\beta_i} \, , \tag{10}$$

If SS_i is equal to SS_{i-1} with a chosen tolerance of 1×10^{-6}, convergence is reached and the algorithm stops. Otherwise, the λ parameter is updated according the following law (11) and the algorithm continues.

$$\lambda_{i+1} = \begin{cases} 0.1\lambda_i \; if \; SS_i < SS_{i-1} \\ 10\lambda_i \; otherwise \end{cases} \, , \tag{11}$$

All of these operations were coded in C language for MCU programming and specific function to compute the derivative of residual with respect to each parameter in β vector was developed in order to compose the Jacobian matrix J.

Switching to the *measurement mode*, the inversion of the calibration function involves the computation of a B-th root. This type of calculation is trivial if it is performed on a platform with a high computing capacity, like the one made available by the main cloud services. However, processing the data in the cloud implies sending all of the collected raw data through the Wi-Fi energy-intensive connection, considerably increasing the power consumption and limiting the portability of the device. Processing data on board limits these issues, but, on the other hand, it entails fewer computational resources and the need to develop specific functions in C language. To implement the B-th root on the MCU platform, a generalization of the Heron's method was exploited [34]. Once the concentration has been computed, it can be made available on a cloud for remote monitoring or can be maintained in the device memory waiting a Wi-Fi connection.

2.5. *Immunosensor Validation*

The validation of sensing device was performed according to the Eurachem guidelines [35] on human serum as blank matrix. An assessment of the dose-response calibration curve was carried out using concentration values already corrected according to the serum dilution factor.

The detection (LOD) and quantitation (LOQ) limits were calculated from mean normalized signal (y_b) and standard deviation (s_b) recorded from ten independent replicates at HE4 level showing a not significant signal inhibition (35 fM, first point of dose-response curve, see 3.4 paragraph). More precisely, the corresponding signals were calculated, as $y_b - \left(3.3 \cdot \left(s_b / \sqrt{n}\right)\right)$ and $y_b - \left(10 \cdot \left(s_b / \sqrt{n}\right)\right)$, respectively, where n is the number of independent replicates for each concentration level. The linear dynamic range was determined as the concentration interval over which the slope (B parameter of the inhibition curve) varies within ±10%. Two concentration levels that were not explored for the calibration were used for the assessment of trueness.

3. Results and Discussion

3.1. *MBs Functionalization and Immunocompetition Study*

The competitive magneto-immunoassay was implemented on tosyl-activated magnetic microbeads as sensing substrate, involving the lysine residues of HE4 antigen for its covalent linking. The immobilization of the antigen is one of the most critical issues when developing immunoassays, as this procedure has to not compromise the immunoreactivity of the bioreceptor, i.e., not involving the antibody-binding regions.

Before carrying out the competition experiments, the maintenance of HE4 immunoreactivity was verified through direct binding titrations between the immobilized antigen and anti-HE4 antibody. These experiments were also aimed at investigating the dynamic range for the concentrations of (*i*) HE4 used for MBs functionalization and (*ii*) anti-HE4 used for the implementation of the immunocompetition. For this purpose, we fixed at 10 μg mL^{-1} the HE4 concentration for the MBs functionalization and, thus, we incubated the modified beads with anti-HE4 ranging from 0 to 2 μg mL^{-1}, and then with RAM-AP secondary antibody. Further experiments were carried out varying the antigen concentration from 0 to 20 μg mL^{-1}, keeping the anti-HE4 concentration at 2 μg mL^{-1} constant. The results of the immuno-titration experiments showed current responses increasing versus anti-HE4 and HE4 concentrations, with very low background signals recorded in the absence of antibody and antigen.

These findings can be rationalized as an evidence of the effective antigen immobilization, also being confirmed by the non-occurrence of unwanted non-specific binding on MBs surface.

On the basis of the above considerations, we performed a set of competition experiments keeping constant at 10 μg mL^{-1} the competing HE4 and varying the above discussed experimental parameters. The dataset of signal inhibition values, being calculated as 1-(S/S_0), was evaluated through a two-way Analysis of Variance (ANOVA), showing that the anti-HE4 factor and its interaction with HE4 factor significantly influence ($p < 0.01$) the immunosensor response, whereas the single HE4 factor resulted in being not significant ($p > 0.01$). Figure 1 reports the ANOVA interaction plot, showing the effect of the two studied factors. The observed trend clearly shows the higher signal inhibition rate being observed for the combination of the middle (1 μg mL^{-1}) anti-HE4 concentration level and the lowest (10 μg mL^{-1}) HE4 concentration explored for the functionalization of MBs. The best concentrations for the immunocompetition experiments were then chosen on the basis of these results.

As for functionalized MBs stability, intended as the maintenance of the reactivity of HE4 immobilized on the magnetic beads, it resulted in being good over at least two months stored in the dark at +4 °C.

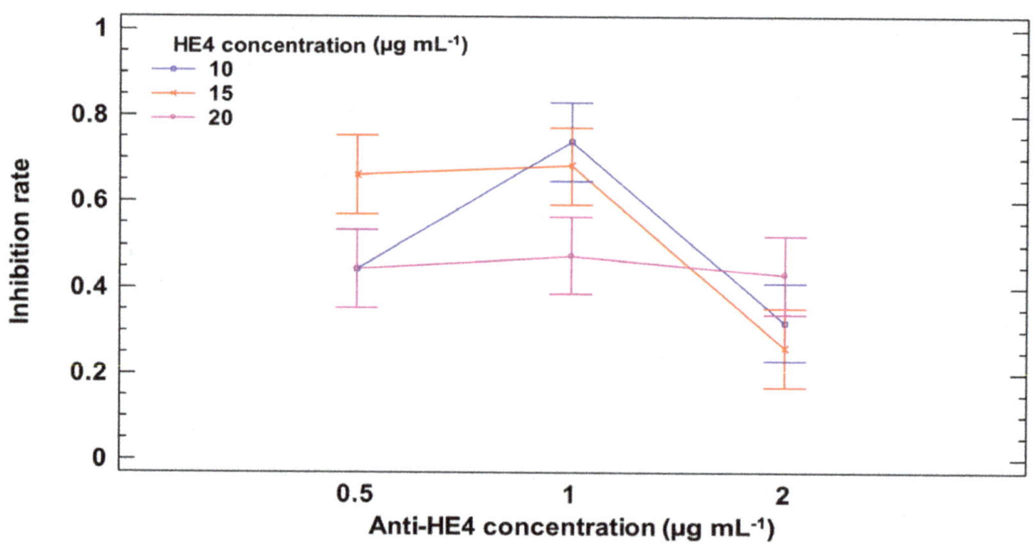

Figure 1. Interaction plot from two-way ANOVA. Factors: concentration of HE4 for functionalization and concentration of anti-HE4 antibody; Response: signal inhibition.

3.2. Data Acquisition and Processing

A *Vbias* ranging from −0.4 V to 0.2 V, which was suitable for acquisition of HQ oxidation current, was applied between WE and RE electrodes of the cell to measure the amperometric signal (i.e., the cell output current). Exploiting the high resolution of the AFE reported in our previous work [26], a total of 120 measurement points of differential output current were collected. Figure 2 shows the signals that were recorded over the 350 fM–350 nM HE4 concentration range.

In this application, a minimum number of point equal to 30 was set for baseline drift correction. Figure 3 illustrates an example of baseline estimation in the case of 350 fM HE4 concentration. The dots indicate the 30 minimum points that were exploited in the linear regression and the resulting baseline is shown. The actual peak value is calculated as the distance between the baseline and maximum current value.

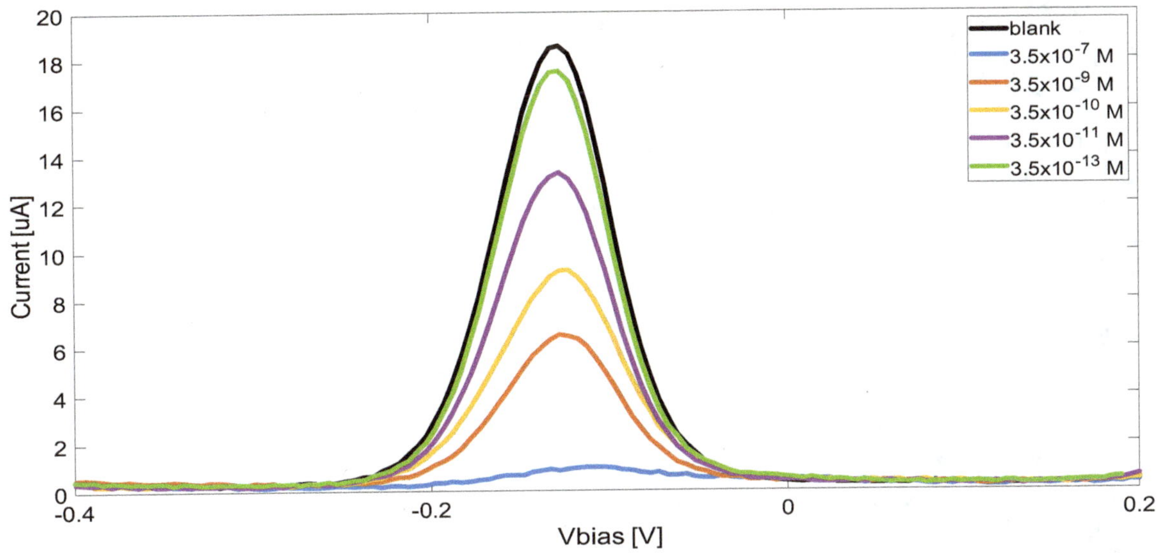

Figure 2. Differential pulse voltammetry (DPV) scans recorded carrying out immunocompetition assays over the 350 fM-350 nM HE4 concentration range in human serum samples.

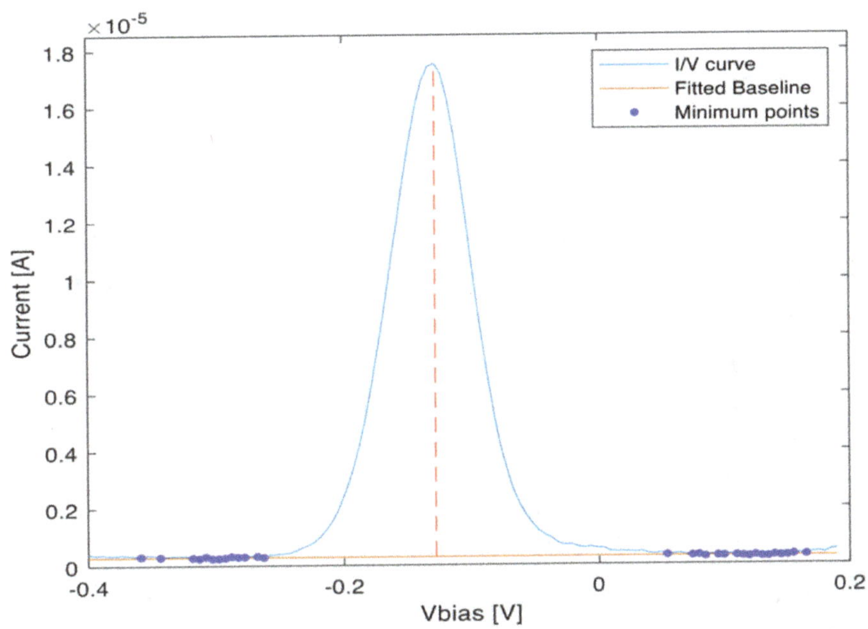

Figure 3. Example of baseline estimation from a voltammogram. Thirty minimum points were considered for the linear regression.

Figure 4 shows the dose-response inhibition curve that was obtained upon interpolation of the experimental dataset with the four-parameter logistic function (1). An increase of analyte concentration was found to reduce the amount of anti-HE4 that was bound to the antigen-modified MBs, thanks to the ability of HE4 to inhibit the antibody binding extent to the sensing surface that was functionalized with the antigen.

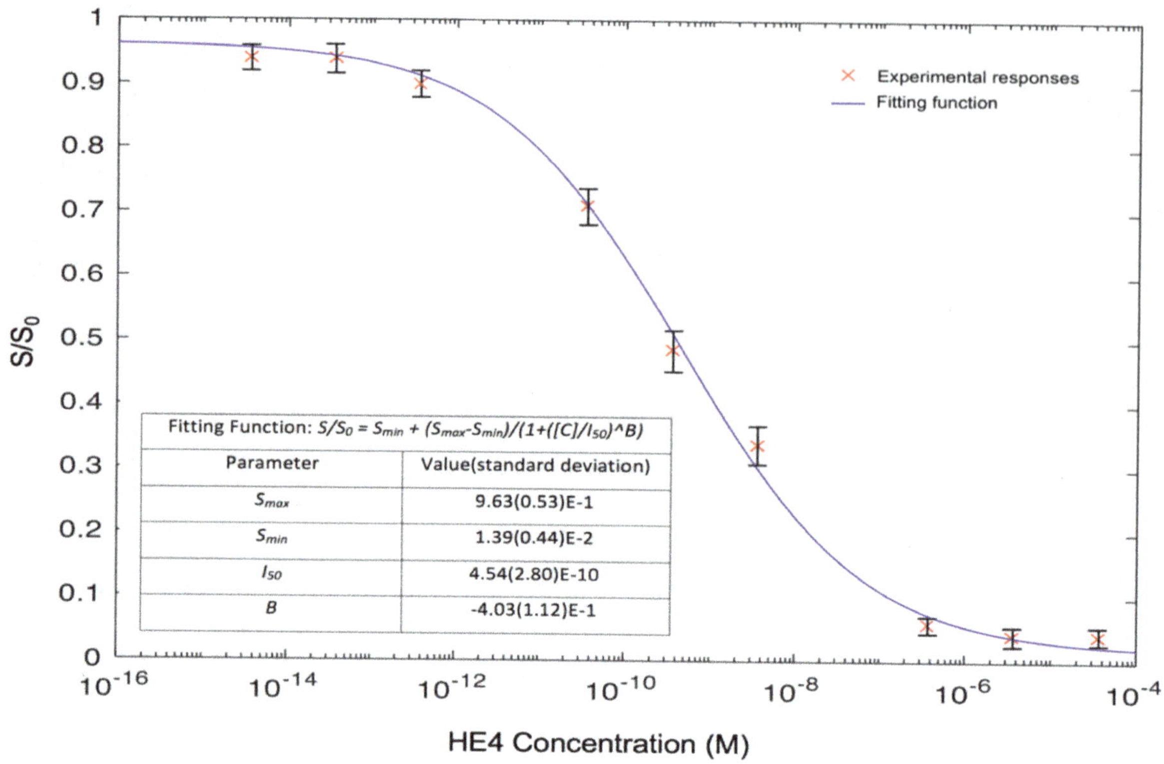

Figure 4. Dose-response inhibition curve for HE4-spiked human serum samples obtained interpolating the dataset from immunocompetition experiments carried out on HE4-modified MBs over the 3.5 fM–35 μM concentration range while using the four-parameter logistic function (1). Inset table: fitted curve parameters.

3.3. *Electrochemical Immunoassay Analytical Performance*

The developed IoT immunochemical device exhibited good analytical performance showing a linear dynamic range over three orders of magnitude. As for precision assessed on the basis of three independent assays, we observed relative standard deviations (RSD) always < 13%.

The analysis of HE4-spiked serum samples provided a LOD of 3.5 pM and a LOQ of 29.2 pM. A comparison of the calculated LOD with the threshold values set for premenopausal women (70 pM) and postmenopausal patients (140 pM) [36] highlights the suitability of the developed system in terms of quality criteria for routine analysis, while also considering the high automatization level in calibration and data processing and the assessment of all validation parameters in matrix, differently from previously published studies.

Trueness was assessed while using HE4-spiked serum samples with concentration levels that were not used for the calibration, i.e. LOQ and I_{50}, obtaining a mean recovery of 105 ± 12%. These values can be considered to be very satisfying while taking the developed on-board self-calibration innovative strategy, embedded in the portable automatized instrument, into account.

3.4. *Selectivity Assessment*

Protein markers potentially occurring in clinical samples of diagnostic interest for carcinomas of gynecologic concern were selected to assess the selectivity of the developed immunomagnetic assays. For this purpose, we evaluated the responses that were obtained with CA125 and CEA, both at I_{50} concentration levels, obtaining no significant signal inhibition ($p < 0.05$) with respect to blank reference samples only containing anti-HE4 antibody.

4. Conclusions

In the present work, we proposed an innovative approach to address disease diagnosis and management through the integration of IoT home-made portable potentiostat with electrochemical immunosensors for the determination of HE4 as ovarian cancer serological biomarker in the framework of the point-of-care (POC) testing. The choice of a mainstream protocol for the connection as Wi-Fi enhances the usability and portability of the system without requiring an additional device, such as PC or Smartphone. Thanks to the ability of the developed portable device to acquire a high number of measurement points (i.e. 350), an accurate quantitative evaluation of the analyte concentration can be carried out. The developed device is able to perform the interpolation of calibration function and the concentration evaluation directly on-board, enhancing the system portability, minimizing data transmission, and therefore the high power consumption that is generally required by the Wi-Fi connection. In the case of absence of connectivity, the device can store the data in a local memory waiting for an available wireless connection.

The analytical performance of the IoT-based competitive immunomagnetic electrochemical assay was assessed in human serum, obtaining LOD and LOQ values at the picomolar level, meeting the requirements for diagnostic applications in early diagnosis of OC. Finally, the sensing device was successfully applied in serum with adequate recovery values for the analysis of spiked samples as well as good selectivity toward potential protein interferents. This work shows great promise for the application of the developed self-calibrating IoT portable immunosensor for HE4 determination in serum samples, in accordance with Analytical 4.0 evolution towards smart platforms for decentralized POC testing.

Author Contributions: Conceptualization, V.B., M.M., I.D.M. and M.G.; methodology, V.B., M.M., M.G., A.B., I.D.M.; validation, M.M. and M.G.; investigation, V.B., M.M. and M.G.; writing—original draft preparation, V.B., M.M. and M.G.; writing—review and editing, V.B., M.M., M.G., A.B., I.D.M. and M.C.; funding acquisition, M.M., I.D.M. and M.C. All authors have read and agreed to the published version of the manuscript.

References

1. Granato, T.; Porpora, M.G.; Longo, F.; Angeloni, A.; Manganaro, L.; Anastasi, E. HE4 in the differential diagnosis of ovarian masses. *Clin. Chim. Acta* **2015**, *446*, 147–155. [CrossRef]
2. Reid, B.M.; Permuth, J.B.; Sellers, T.A. Epidemiology of ovarian cancer: A review. *Cancer Biol. Med.* **2017**, *14*, 9–32. [PubMed]
3. Bianchi, F.; Giannetto, M.; Careri, M. Advances in molecular analysis of biomarkers for autoimmune and carcinogenic diseases. *Anal. Bioanal. Chem.* **2014**, *406*, 15–20. [CrossRef] [PubMed]
4. Sharma, S.; Raghav, R.; O'Kennedy, R.; Srivastava, S. Advances in ovarian cancer diagnosis: A journey from immunoassays to immunosensors. *Enzyme Microb. Technol.* **2016**, *89*, 15–30. [CrossRef] [PubMed]
5. Ranjan, R.; Esimbekova, E.N.; Kratasyuk, V.A. Rapid biosensing tools for cancer biomarkers. *Biosens. Bioelectron.* **2017**, *87*, 918–930. [CrossRef]
6. Giannetto, M.; Bianchi, M.V.; Mattarozzi, M.; Careri, M. Competitive amperometric immunosensor for determination of p53 protein in urine with carbon nanotubes/gold nanoparticles screenprinted electrodes: A potential rapid and noninvasive screening tool for early diagnosis of urinary tract carcinoma. *Anal. Chim. Acta* **2017**, *991*, 133–141. [CrossRef]
7. De La Franier, B.; Thompson, M. Early stage detection and screening of ovarian cancer: A research opportunity and significant challenge for biosensor technology. *Biosens. Bioelectron.* **2019**, *135*, 71–81. [CrossRef]
8. Su, Z.; Graybill, W.S.; Zhu, Y. Detection and monitoring of ovarian cancer. *Clin. Chim. Acta* **2013**, *415*, 341–345. [CrossRef]

9. Sadighbayan, D.; Sadighbayan, K.; Tohid-kia, M.R.; Khosroushahi, A.Y.; Hasanzadeh, M. Development of electrochemical biosensors for tumor marker determination towards cancer diagnosis: Recent progress. *Trends Anal. Chem.* **2019**, *118*, 73–88. [CrossRef]
10. Wang, J.; Song, J.; Zheng, H.; Zheng, X.; Dai, H.; Hong, Z.; Lin, Y. Application of $NiFe_2O_4$ nanotubes as catalytically promoted sensing platform for ratiometric electrochemiluminescence analysis of ovarian cancer marker. *Sensor. Actuators B Chem.* **2019**, *288*, 80–87. [CrossRef]
11. Fan, L.; Yan, Y.; Guo, B.; Zhao, M.; Li, J.; Bian, X.; Wu, H.; Cheng, W.; Ding, S. Trimetallic hybrid nanodendrites and magnetic nanocomposites-based electrochemical immunosensor for ultrasensitive detection of serum human epididymis protein 4. *Sensor. Actuators B Chem.* **2019**, *296*, 126697. [CrossRef]
12. Yan, Q.; Cao, L.; Dong, H.; Tan, Z.; Liu, Q.; Zhang, W.; Zhao, P.; Li, Y.; Liu, Y.; Dong, Y. Sensitive amperometric immunosensor with improved electrocatalytic Au@Pd urchin-shaped nanostructures for human epididymis specific protein 4 antigen detection. *Anal. Chim. Acta* **2019**, *1069*, 117–125. [CrossRef] [PubMed]
13. Klein, T.; Wang, W.; Yu, L.; Wu, K.; Boylan, K.L.M.; Isaksson Vogel, R.; Skubitz, A.P.N.; Wang, J.-P. Development of a multiplexed giant magnetoresistive biosensor array prototype to quantify ovarian cancer biomarkers. *Biosens. Bioelectron.* **2019**, *126*, 301–307. [CrossRef]
14. Ramanavicius, A.; Oztekin, Y.; Ramanaviciene, A. Electrochemical formation of polypyrrole-based layerfor immunosensor design. *Sensor. Actuators B* **2014**, *197*, 237–243. [CrossRef]
15. Tan, Y.; Li, M.; Ye, X.; Wang, Z.; Wang, Y.; Li, C. Ionic liquid auxiliary exfoliation of WS2 nanosheets and the enhanced effect of hollow gold nanospheres on their photoelectrochemical sensing towards human epididymis protein 4. *Sensor. Actuators B* **2018**, *262*, 982–990. [CrossRef]
16. Giannetto, M.; Bianchi, V.; Gentili, S.; Fortunati, S.; De Munari, I.; Careri, M. An integrated IoT-Wi-Fi board for remote data acquisition and sharing from innovative immunosensors. Case of study: Diagnosis of celiac disease. *Sensor. Actuators B Chem.* **2018**, *273*, 1395–1403. [CrossRef]
17. Loncaric, C.; Tang, Y.; Ho, C.; Parameswaran, M.A.; Yu, H.-Z. A USB-based electrochemical biosensor prototype for point-of-care diagnosis. *Sensor. Actuators B Chem.* **2012**, *161*, 908–913. [CrossRef]
18. Adams, S.D.; Doeven, E.H.; Quayle, K.; Kouzani, A.Z. MiniStat: Development and evaluation of a mini-potentiostat for electrochemical measurements. *IEEE Access* **2019**, *7*, 31903–31912. [CrossRef]
19. Pruna, R.; Palacio, F.; Baraket, A.; Zine, N.; Streklas, A.; Bausells, J.; Errachid, A.; López, M. A low-cost and miniaturized potentiostat for sensing of biomolecular species such as TNF-α by electrochemical impedance spectroscopy. *Biosens. Bioelectron.* **2018**, *100*, 533–540. [CrossRef]
20. Hanitra, I.N.; Criscuolo, F.; Pankratova, N.; Carrara, S.; De Micheli, G. Multi-Channel Front-End for Electrochemical Sensing of Metabolites, Drugs, and Electrolytes. *IEEE Sens. J.* **2019**, *20*, 3636–3645. [CrossRef]
21. De Campos da Costa, J.P.; Bastos, W.B.; da Costa, P.I.; Zaghete, M.A.; Longo, E.; Carmo, J.P. Portable laboratory platform with electrochemical biosensors for immunodiagnostic of hepatitis C virus. *IEEE Sens. J.* **2019**, *19*, 10701–10709. [CrossRef]
22. Ma, L.; Ju, F.; Tao, C.; Shen, X. Portable, Low Cost Smartphone-Based Potentiostat System for the Salivary α-Amylase Detection in Stress Paradigm. In Proceedings of the 41st Annual International Conference of the IEEE Engineering in Medicine and Biology Society (EMBC), Berlin, Germany, 23–27 July 2019; pp. 1334–1337.
23. Steinberg, M.D.; Kassal, P.; Kereković, I.; Murković Steinberg, I. A wireless potentiostat for mobile chemical sensing and biosensing. *Talanta* **2015**, *143*, 178–183. [CrossRef] [PubMed]
24. Annamalai, P.; Slaughter, G. Wireless Bipotentiostat Circuit for Glucose and H_2O_2 Interrogation. In Proceedings of the 41st Annual International Conference of the IEEE Engineering in Medicine and Biology Society (EMBC), Berlin, Germany, 23–27 July 2019; pp. 1567–1570.
25. Chen, G.; Xie, J.; Zhang, Z.; Meng, W.; Zhang, C.; Kang, K.; Wu, Y.; Guo, Z. A portable digital-control electrochemical system with automatic ohmic drop compensation for fast scan voltammetry and its application to ultrasensitive detection of chromium(III). *Sensor. Actuators B Chem.* **2019**, *301*, 127135. [CrossRef]
26. Bianchi, V.; Boni, A.; Fortunati, S.; Giannetto, M.; Careri, M.; De Munari, I. A Wi-Fi cloud-based portable potentiostat for electrochemical biosensors. *IEEE Trans. Instrum. Meas.* **2019**, in press. [CrossRef]
27. Mayer, M.; Baeumner, A.J. ABC spotlight on analytics 4.0. *Anal. Bioanal. Chem.* **2018**, *410*, 5095–5097. [CrossRef]
28. Bassoli, M.; Bianchi, V.; De Munari, I.; Ciampolini, P. An IoT approach for an AAL Wi-Fi-based monitoring system. *IEEE Trans. Instrum. Meas.* **2017**, *66*, 3200–3209. [CrossRef]

29. Bassoli, M.; Bianchi, V.; De Munari, I. A plug and play IoT Wi-Fi smart home system for human monitoring. *Electronics* **2018**, *7*, 200. [CrossRef]
30. Huang, Y.; Li, G. Descriptive Models for Internet of Things. In Proceedings of the International Conference on Intelligent Control and Information Processing, Dalian, China, 12–15 August 2010; pp. 483–486.
31. Manfredi, A.; Giannetto, M.; Mattarozzi, M.; Costantini, M.; Mucchino, C.; Careri, M. Competitive immunosensor based on gliadin immobilization on disposable carbon-nanogold screen-printed electrodes for rapid determination of celiotoxic prolamins. *Anal. Bioanal. Chem.* **2016**, *408*, 7289–7298. [CrossRef]
32. Levenberg, K. A method for the solution of certain nonlinear problems in least squares. *Quart. Appl. Math.* **1944**, *2*, 164–168. [CrossRef]
33. Marquaradt, D.W. An algorithm for least-squares estimation of nonlinear parameters. *J. Soc. Ind. Appl. Math.* **1963**, *11*, 431–441. [CrossRef]
34. Taisbak, C.M. Cube roots of integers: A conjecture about Heron's method in Metrika III. 20. *Hist. Math.* **2014**, *41*, 103–106. [CrossRef]
35. Eurachem. The Fitness for Purpose of Analytical Methods: A Laboratory Guide to Method Validation and Related Topics. Available online: http://www.eurachem.org (accessed on 3 March 2020).
36. Dochez, V.; Caillon, H.; Vaucel, E.; Dimet, J.; Winer, N.; Ducarme, G. Biomarkers and algorithms for diagnosis of ovarian cancer: CA125, HE4, RMI and ROMA: A review. *J. Ovarian Res.* **2019**, *12*, 28. [CrossRef] [PubMed]

11

Secure Authentication and Prescription Safety Protocol for Telecare Health Services Using Ubiquitous IoT

Zahid Mahmood [1], Huansheng Ning [1,*], Ata Ullah [2] and Xuanxia Yao [1]

[1] School of Computer and Communication Engineering University of Science and Technology Beijing (USTB), Beijing 10008, China; b20140561@xs.ustb.edu.cn (Z.M.); kathy.yao@163.com (X.Y.)

[2] Department of Computer Science, National University of Modern Languages, Islamabad 44000, Pakistan; aullah@numl.edu.pk

[*] Correspondence: ninghuansheng@ustb.edu.cn

Abstract: Internet-of-Things (IoT) include a large number of devices that can communicate across different networks. Cyber-Physical Systems (CPS) also includes a number of devices connected to the internet where wearable devices are also included. Both systems enable researchers to develop healthcare systems with additional intelligence as well as prediction capabilities both for lifestyle and in hospitals. It offers as much persistence as a platform to ubiquitous healthcare by using wearable sensors to transfer the information over servers, smartphones, and other smart devices in the Telecare Medical Information System (TMIS). Security is a challenging issue in TMIS, and resourceful access to health care services requires user verification and confidentiality. Existing schemes lack in ensuring reliable prescription safety along with authentication. This research presents a Secure Authentication and Prescription Safety (SAPS) protocol to ensure secure communication between the patient, doctor/nurse, and the trusted server. The proposed procedure relies upon the efficient elliptic curve cryptosystem which can generate a symmetric secure key to ensure secure data exchange between patients and physicians after successful authentication of participants individually. A trusted server is involved for mutual authentication between parties and then generates a common key after completing the validation process. Moreover, the scheme is verified by doing formal modeling using Rubin Logic and validated using simulations in NS-2.35. We have analyzed the SAPS against security attacks, and then performance analysis is elucidated. Results prove the dominance of SAPS over preliminaries regarding mutual authentication, message integrity, freshness, and session key management and attack prevention.

Keywords: authentication; key agreement; telecare medical information system; anonymity; un-traceability

---

1. Introduction

With the development of computing technologies and the expansion of smart-devices and inter-network protocols, hospitals and healthcare organizations are adopting the Telecare Medical Information System (TMIS). The medical identification process has become more resourceful, trustworthy, and efficient by using TMIS. Some Telecare services have been projected in the modern age to ease the workload on the professionals, for example, by methods such as automated healthcare devices, distant health nursing, and patient's health monitoring for remote areas. It is considered as a time-saving, economical, and easy way to access health care facilities remotely. TMIS can lower societal and medical operating cost with improved quality and efficiency [1]. Patient authentication is mandatory to guard against data forgery, misuse, and falsifying the original information by unauthorized active or passive parties. In TMIS, a trusted medical server is responsible for registering all participants, including doctors, nursing staff, and patients, as illustrated in Figure 1. The remote healthcare server keeps the advanced clinical information of the register patients and gives different administrations like healthcare education, doctors, doctor's facilities, remote medical aid, general healthcare, private care benefit, and the most important is medical prescription. Registered TMIS users for medical services can utilize smart cards to access medical devices and transmit collected statistics to the medical server using a public channel. An intruder may likewise find access over the public open channel. The adversary can eavesdrop, block service, modify, delete records, and can also reply to a message broadcasted over an open channel. Therefore, authentication is mandatory for providing information security, records honesty, and confidentiality of data. It is necessary to overcome all existing threats that are major hurdles and make TMIS trustworthy. A session key must be established for a short-time secure communication between two parties where a new key is established for every new session. We have considered various advanced cryptographic calculations like non-revertible one-way hash function, Rivest-Shamir-Adelman (RSA), Elliptic Curve Cryptography (ECC), and chaotic maps cryptosystem. Despite the fact that both ECC and RSA cryptosystems offer an equal level of security, ECC is additionally advantageous as compared to RSA with respect to computational efficiency [2].

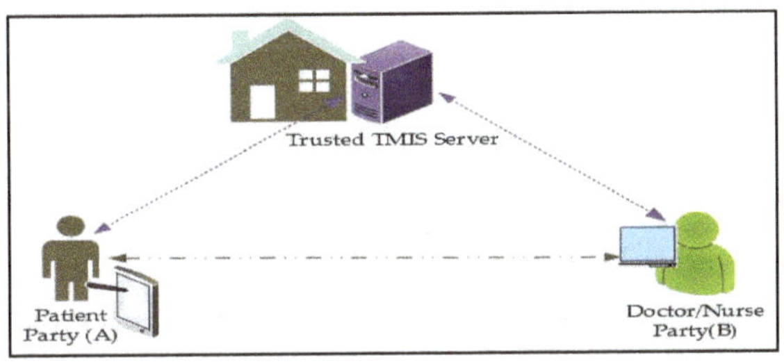

Figure 1. Telecare Medical Information System (TMIS) architecture.

An Internet of Things (IoT) is composed of a vast number of small and large devices that are using the internet for sharing data across the nodes of different networks. In an IoT environment, TMIS can serve patients to save time by remotely accessing consultants and doctors by using the new generation of internet. IoT supports a collection of objects, devices, and networks in surroundings to develop a large number of smart applications. It can undeniably improve the identification and dissemination of information regarding emergency situations where appropriate medical aid is mandatory to save precious lives. IoT can also support integration mechanisms for all physical objects with embedded systems or cyber physical systems for monitoring patients at distant locations. It improves diagnosis at the patient's home for better usefulness and effectiveness regarding medical services [3]. IoT promises an attractive future networking prototype.

Secure authentication and session key establishment schemes enable secure communication for health care services. A three-party password authentication key exchange (3-PAKE) scheme provides mutual authentication between doctor-patient-TS at the same time and hides identities from the adversary [4]. It helps in maintaining a secure link by using a common session key for specific communication. Schemes [5–7] discuss secure session key establishment between participants but later [8–10] identified that these plans are vulnerable to man-in-the-middle attack and undetectable online and offline dictionary attacks for guessing passwords. ECC-based schemes are also explored to evaluate the applicability of efficient solutions with desired security strengths using small key sizes as compared to preliminaries.

The main problem and common deficiency in these schemes are that user anonymity is not provided because the user's identity is sent without encryption on an open channel. The participants' credentials are insecure, causing a lack of anonymity and un-tractability [11]. The scheme is also vulnerable to identification-guessing attacks and tracking attacks. Specifically, a participant's identification might get exposed by an intruder when it gets disconnected from the internet. Furthermore, an adversary can tune into a selected user with the information the user provided within the login request message.

This paper presents a Secure Participant Authentication and Prescription Safety (SAPS) scheme for TMIS to accomplish participant's anonymity and un-traceability. The process begins when the patient registers with the trusted server that validates the communicating parties and then establishes the session key. We have used ECC in this study; results showed that an anonymous ECC-based presented technique has secure and well-organized authentication protocols with foolproof security along with user confidentiality protection which is practical for TMIS. Formal protocol secure analysis using Rubin Logic was used to evaluate their safety performance and reliability. Using the proposed protocol patient can get a medical prescription from physician securely and interacts with health service provider anonymously using TMIS keeping identities secret.

The rest of paper is organized as follows; Section 2 includes the previous work which has some related information regarding the present study and an overview of existing practices. The system model and problem statement are presented in Section 3. Section 4 explores the proposing anonymous SAPS scheme in details with formal steps. Formal analysis using Rubin Logic is presented along with security analysis in Section 5. The performance measures and results have been included in Section 6. Section 7 presents the conclusions of the work and a future roadmap.

2. Literature Review

This section explores some well-known existing schemes related to the security of TMIS and health care services. In this regard, different 3-PAKE and ECC-based schemes are reviewed to analyze the effectiveness, usefulness, and security strengths for providing reliable security solutions. Xie et al. have proposed an ECC-based efficient 3-PAKE scheme [12] that overcomes the flaws mentioned above but suffers from offline password guessing attacks. Che et al. have proposed modular exponentiation on an ECC-based 3-PAKE scheme [13] to make it more complicated for the attacker, but these operations require huge computational cost as compared to existing counterparts. Wu et al. have presented the concept of the secret password and smart card-based verification protocol [14] for TMIS by utilizing the discrete hard logarithm problem (DHLP). It pre-registers to stay away from the exponential mathematical computations during authentication stage. In three-party key exchanges (TPKE) [15], He et al. has found some flaws in [14] and presented an improved scheme that handles impersonation and insider attacks which made the existing scheme vulnerable. Later on, in scheme [16], Wei et al. explored both [14,15] schemes and identified the vulnerability of these schemes for offline password guessing attacks, dictionary attacks, and inability to maintain user un-traceability. To overcome these drawbacks, Wei et al. have improved protocols and presented a user authentication scheme for TMIS that can uphold different attacks. Moreover, Zhu et al. [17] also identified the offline password guessing attacks in these schemes. To overcome issues in [17], Pu et al. [18] has devised a new user authentication scheme applying smart care which is a user password-based identification that provides user anonymity. This scheme is based on an elliptic curve cryptosystem that provides the same security level as RSA with less key size.

Chen et al. [11] highlighted the client anonymity of Khan et al.'s technique [19] but it might be defenseless against insider attacks because all the lawful clients share the secret key. It presented an efficient and secret identity-based validation and secure protocol for TMIS that generates random identities for every exchange in a session to sustain a strategic distance bwetween individual data about the client and the danger of identity theft attack and ensured that their protocol accomplished client privacy. The scheme is a successor and much preferable to the previous responses for use on mobile devices. The scheme does not provide anonymity of the user and is vulnerable for identity guessing and tracking attacks.

In [20] Kumar et al. has presented a smart device authentication scheme in a WSN environment and found that these schemes are suitable for TMIS and fulfill all prerequisites for medical device networks. Later on, He et al. [21] found that some special insider attacks in medical device networks such as offline password guessing attacks occurred and the system was unable to handle anonymity in [20]. A user anonymous authentication scheme has been presented to handle remote medical services applying in WSN to resolve this issues. Nam et al. [22] pointed out some flaws in [21] for user anonymity and smart card theft. By exploiting symmetric encryption and secure key management for message integrity, Xue et al. [23] presented a temporary credential-based secure key using a one-way hash function and XOR operations. It enhances security fundaments without considerably expanding the memory requirements. In [24], Li et al. pointed out that scheme [23] is unable to protect against stolen-verifier attacks, denial of service attacks, smart card theft, and participant's signing attacks. Turkanovic et al. presented a secure hash function-based user prediction and secure key management protocol [25] that ensures security with low energy consumption. Amin et al. [26] identified that the scheme [25] is vulnerable to offline dictionary attacks, password guessing attacks, smart card theft, and has an inefficient authentication process.

IoT can be an appropriate approach to support health care systems by the technological advancements that enable the outlining of new advanced strategies for the treatment of many diseases, e.g., by the surveillance of chronic diseases to assist doctors to work out the best treatments, as projected by [27]. Due to the ubiquitous computational nature of IoT, all the TMIS entities may be monitored and managed continually. Mobile healthcare (m-Healthcare) is an associate economic model to give patients with the right of entry to resources, about past and present health records, blood pressure, and heart rate measurements. Additionally, hospitals and healthcare associations offer on-demand services hosted in the cloud, reducing the equipped costs and overcoming the constraints of standard medical treatment. On the contrary, the privacy of private healthcare information continues to be a challenge to be faced [28].

Rahimi et al. [29,30] introduced a more secure and powerful user authentication and key agreement technique for fitness-IoT structures which requires considerable processing power. It exploits the property of a sensible gateway in fog computing for critical and security services-associated organization. IoT technologies for healthcare achieve standardized medical care [31] that is frequently improved by further automating the tasks that can be performed without human interaction. In this experience, IoT-based healthcare permits remote monitoring and management of large amounts of medical data using cloud services. Yeh et al. [32] highlighted the idea of an ECC-based unique participant's verification protocol to get higher performance and security in a smart medical information system. ECC was first presented in [33,34] by utilizing a logarithm problem that can do a much better job with a smaller key length as compared to well-known existing schemes with larger key sizes [35]. By these assumptions, it is stated that ECC authentication schemes are very appropriate for resource-constrained and remotely accessible devices.

3. System Model and Problem Identification

TMIS requires strong security to provide a dependable user validation and secret key management system for an IoT-based medical environment as depicted in Figure 2. In TMIS, patients remotely present their healthcare services information to a trusted server using a medicinal gadget. Subsequently, accepting the medical records of patients in the network, the servers diagnose the issue and suggest medicines to the online patients. Such systems are rapidly growing in our society and hence require privacy of patient's data. Nonetheless, the private data transmitted over the internet using the public network are not ensured in many TMIS conditions. The system can be subject to a variety of attacks from external parties. Social insurance solutions linked with TMIS should fulfill critical security and protection necessities to ensure patient's medical records and prescriptions are secure, and that they are constantly provided validation, privacy, trustworthiness, and anonymity. Authentication restricts the medical data from being accessed by malicious and dangerous attackers. The secret key is used to encrypt the data packet to guarantee the confidentiality of medical information during data exchange.

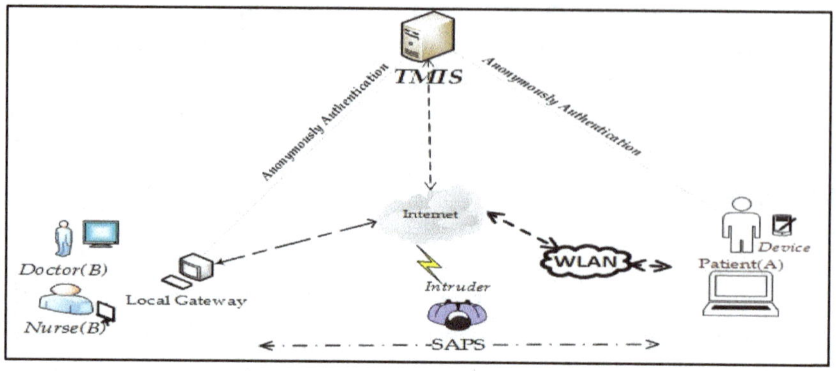

Figure 2. TMIS System Model.

In TMIS, when a patient wishes to become a new legitimate user, denoted as U_i, then the following steps are accomplished; validity of server-assigned timestamp and IDs. The user authenticated process is done after verifying smart card holding parameters to grant or reject authentication. Anonymity and un-traceability are two fundamental and attracting concerns during basic user privacy, where the former ensures secure user identity in transit, and no one else knows the exact IDs except the communication agents. The stronger property of privacy is un-traceability of the user, such that no one can find the sources of secret data during mutual authentication of the two parties by the trusted third party. Due to un-traceability, the outflow of client personal information in one session would be unusable for the adversary to recognize the user characteristics in another session [36].

Security Model

In this section, the identification of the possible threat scenarios that can be launched by exploiting user identity is discussed. An adversary can expose the user ID through exhaustive offline guessing because it is usually shorter and has a certain format which can be easily guessed [37]. To secure participants' medicinal prescription, the identity must not be disclosed at intermediate nodes when the information is being exchanged over the uncertain channel. An intruder can attempt to get the private information of the participant from the system, causing a potential risk for confidential data. There is no check of the rightness of a client's old secret key amid the secret password change stage, implying that an individual [38] who has other individual's smart card can change secret code and bio-metric without giving the original password. Other conceivable assaults are participant impersonation attacks, brute-force attacks, or dictionary assaults. Furthermore, an illegal participant may misuse the other participant's personal information to conduct various login sessions and follow participant's exercises by phishing techniques [30]. Also, the breaching of user privacy and their routine activities may likewise encourage an unapproved user to follow the participant's login history and even their current location. After obtaining the password by off-line password guessing, the user can easily guess or deduce common shared secret keys between end users like A and B after intercepting the transmitted messages R_A and R_B.

An intruder can attempt to retrieve the identity of the legitimate user from their login message. As the user's identity is short, the adversary (A) finds AId_i with polynomial time by executing exhaustive guessing. During multiple valid user sessions using the same unique password, forgery is possible [37]. The well-known threats that can be launched to breech the security of legitimate users are as follows.

(i) Applying reverse engineering by monitoring user activities, the adversary extracts the privately stored data in the participant's device [38].

(ii) During private information transmission over an open channel, there are possibilities of eavesdropping, intercepting, content modification, and reply attacking to influence overall communication.

(iii) A user registers with a true identity but acts as a malicious user in the TMIS.

(iv) To overcome low entropy issues, the password must be robust enough to defend against password guessing attacks.

Using two parameters, such as a secret password and unique identity, is more feasible and is cannot be guessed by an attacker in polynomial time. Considering this assumption, a malicious user can obtain private data from the location of data storage of the user and re-transmit all messages using the public channel. In case a security protocol is unable to handle these issues, then it cannot protect users from password guessing attacks (which is possible offline), replay attacks (by altering the original message), denial of services, man-in-the-middle attacks, and cannot provide seamless forward privacy.

By the above analysis, Chen's scheme [11] cannot survive tracking attacks and it has failed to uphold user un-traceability. It is defenseless against guessing attacks and tracking attacks. A smart card holds a secret number (r) and this can be determined from the fix value of $W = h(r||pw_i)$. An adversary (A) can eavesdrop on a legal user's login request message $R_m = h(Id_i, W)$ and get the value of W to subvert the privacy of the participant unless a new authentication session is established [37]. Moreover, tracking attacks are possible by monitoring different session of same user using W.

4. Secure Authentication and Prescription Safety Protocol

A novel protocol for TMIS is presented to protect patient's privacy and satisfy the security requirements. Mutual authentication enables the communicating parties to verify each other's identities. The proposed Secure Authentication and Prescription Safety (SAPS) protocol demonstrates that it is dynamic and overcomes the above-highlighted flaws in the existing schemes. In SAPS, user authentication and verification are performed by the trusted server (*TS*). The patient and doctor/nurse are the sender and receiver nodes, respectively, in the proposed scenario to establish the secret keys using SAPS. In this section, all the protocol steps are elaborated on, along with a description of the message contents of a SAPS scenario. It includes a trusted server (*TS*), patient (A), and a doctor/nurse (B). ASAP provides a secure link for the Patient (A) to communicate securely with a physician to obtain a medical opinion. We highlight that ECC-based mutual authentication is secure against numerous significant attacks and improves the communication and memory requirements of authentication. Considering the positive characteristics of ECC, such as the shorter secret key size and computational efficiency, it is attractive to establish an ECC-based anonymous 3-PAKE protocol to protect TMIS users. By exploring existing literature and studies, there is no such system based on ECC that gives anonymous 3-PAKE protocol to authenticate users without knowing their private information publicly. It achieves its security benefits due to the hardness property of the EC Discrete Logarithm Problem (ECDLP). A list of useful notation for SAPS is listed in Table 1.

In the SAPS protocol, we have assumed that during the registration phase, the TS provides masked identities for both the patient and doctors at the point of registration. Participants provide some secret credentials, such as biometrics, to verify their original identities and record the time of service request. The TS uses the parties' secret credentials for future verification, keeping their original identities and private information secret. Besides this, the authentication protocol satisfies the following functions and security requirements to achieve credible and secure authentication and data sharing in TMIS.

Table 1. Abbreviations and acronyms for Secure Authentication and Prescription Safety (SAPS).

Notations	Descriptions
$TMIS$	Telecare medical information system
E	A large-order finite field on elliptic curve
P	EC generator of a large order n
$H(.)$	Digestive Hash Function.
A	Patient that is participant A in TMIS
B	Doctor/nurse that is user B in TMIS
MAC	Message Authentication Code
$E_{K_{A-TS}}$	Pre-Shared key between TS and User A
$E_{K_{B-TS}}$	Pre-Shared key between TS and User B
TS	Trusted Server as a trusted third party in TMIS
Pw_P	TS shared password for Patient
$Pw_{D,N}$	Doctor/Nurse password shared with TS
ID_A, ID_B, ID_{TS}	Masked Identities of A, B and TS respectively
$E_{K_{TS-A/B}}$	Temporary Encryption key between TS & Ends
d	Private/Public key of TS
$E_k(.), D_k(.)$	Using key (k) perform Encryption/Decryption
T_1, T_2, T_3	User (A, B, TS) Time Stamp
N_1, N_2, N_3	User (A, B, TS) Nonce No
M_A, M_B	Message at User A (Patient) & B (Doctor/Nurse)
C_A, C_B	Cipher Text at A and B

1. Person anonymity: In an authentication mechanism, despite the fact that an attacker extracts some and can eavesdrop on the shared message within the communication network, the legal participant's identity is kept anonymous from the intruder.
2. Identity proof: the process in which both the user and authentication server prove their identities before accessing each other. Numerous steps are performed to achieve mutual authentication to check the integrity of all transmitted messages.
3. Session key management: When the verification method is consummated, the consumer and server must present the consultation key to each other.
4. Password verification manner: If a person has entered an incorrect password within the authentication section, the password has to be detected earlier than the check phase.
5. Person cordiality: An authentication mechanism system provides a password change method through which an individual may facilely change their password without communicating with the server.
6. Robustness: An authenticated key acquisition mechanism has been engendered, and has to be resistant to extraordinary types of assaults, insider attacks, off-line password conjecturing attacks, replay assaults, and consumer impersonation assaults. Besides this, in the proposed protocol, the TS partially establishes a session key between each party. Using the secret credentials generated by the TS, the ends parties establish a session key for the particular session which helps to protect participant identities and ensure un-traceability.

During authentication, a new patient (A) and doctor (B) submit their original identity to the TS using a secure channel. After receiving their network joining request, the TS generates shadow-IDs for each participant and stores them in its database. The shadow-IDs of each participant is to establish anonymous joining of the patient and doctor and to keep prescriptions and private data secret. SAPS is explored in a stepwise manner as follows.

A. Step-I: Initialization by Patient (A)

At the beginning, Patient (A) chooses a random number R_p from a finite field and computes secret parameters. After that, X_A is calculated by multiplying random number R_p by an ECC-based generator P of large order n. Similarly, Y_A is the resultant of R_p and the TS's public key F that is equal to dP, where d is random number a from finite field selected by TS. For level 1 encryption of security credentials, a hash of Y_A is taken to prepare key H_{Y_A}. Patient (A) prepares a message M_A that contains hash of IDs and PW_p as the patient's password and Message Authentication Code (MAC) is used for providing message integrity on the server side. Patient (A) calculates $H(PW_p||ID_A||ID_B)$ and includes PWp to keep it more secure. In our proposed scheme, an intruder is not able to get the IDs of A and B but if in any case these values are exposed, then the exact hash value cannot be calculated because of the missing PWp that is held by the Patient (A) and TS only. For transmission to the server, the patient computes cipher text P_A which is encrypted by the patient's generated secret key H_{Y_A} as shown in step (iv). After that, a cipher text C_A is generated using a pre-established key K_{A-TS}. In step (vi), a temporary ID as ID_{A_T} of the patient is obtained by taking the hash of the $H(X_A, P_A, N_1)$ and is used for the current session only. The new $ID_{A\sim T}$ is never transmitted and can be calculated at the TS using $H(X_A, P_A, N_1)$ where N_1 can be extracted after decryption. It encrypts the parameters $\{X_A, P_A, T_1\}$ using K_{A-TS} where, T_1 is timestamp. Patient (A) transmits $\{ID_{A\sim T}, C_A\}$ to trusted server $\{TS\}$ for authentication.

(i) $X_A = R_pP$
(ii) $Y_A = R_pF$
(iii) $M_A = H(PW_p||ID_A||ID_B)$
(iv) $P_A = E_{H_{Y_A}}(ID_A||M_A||N_1||\ \mathrm{MAC}(M_A)\ ||ID_B)$
(v) $C_A = E_{K_{A-TS}}(X_A||\ P_A||\ T_1)$
(vi) $ID_{A\sim T} = \{H(X_A, P_A\ , N_1)\}$

B. Step-II: Verification at Trusted Server

Upon receiving $\{ID_{A\sim T}, C_A\}$ form Patient (A), the TS decrypts the cipher text C_A to get $(X_A||\ P_A||\ T_1)$. It also checks the message freshness by taking the difference from T_1 to guard against replay attacks. After that, the TS computes the temporary key of the patient by multiplying the received X_A with d which was pre-generated by the TS as $Y'_A = dX_A$. To verify whether the message is original, the TS computes the Patient's (A) masked identity as $R_pF = R_pdP = dX_A$. It also decrypts P_A to obtain security credentials, including ID_A, M_A, N1, MAC (M_A), and ID_B. The hash of these values is calculated as $M'_A = H(PW_p||ID_A||ID_B)$ and is then compared to verify the equality of M_A and M'_A to ensure message integrity. Otherwise, the message is discarded. The (MAC(M_A)) provides data integrity for M_A. The trusted server computes the following steps.

(i) Decrypt C_A using K_{A-TS} to get $\{(X_A||\ P_A||\ T_1)\}$
(ii) Computer $Y'_A = dX_A$
(iii) Decrypts P_A using $K_{H(YA)}$ to get $\{ID_A, M_A, N_1, \mathrm{MAC}(M_A), ID_B\}$
(iv) Compute: $M'_A = H(PW_p||ID_A||ID_B)$
(v) If Verify $(MAC'(M_A) != \mathrm{MAC}(M_A))$ then discard
(vi) If M_A NOT equals M'_A then discard message

C. Step-III: TS-based Mutual Authentication of B&A

After verification, the TS picks a random number R_{Ts} and then computes $Z_{TS} = H(ID_{TS}||ID_B||R_{Ts})$ using identities of B and TS. It also generates a nonce number N_2 to get its hash with identities of communicating parties A and B. After that, TS calculates the XOR of hash value with Z_{TS} to get a new temporary ID for B. The value of C_{TS} is obtained by encrypting $(ID_A||Z_{TS}||\ T_2||\ N_2)$ using the pre-established key K_{TS-B}. The TS transmits the temporary identity ID_{B_T} and cipher text C_{TS} to B.

(i) $Z_{TS} = H(ID_{TS}||ID_B||R_{Ts})$
(ii) $ID_{B\sim T} = Z_{TS}\ XOR\ \{H(ID_B||ID_A||N_2)\}$

(iii) $C_{TS} = E_{K_{TS-B}}(ID_A||Z_{TS}||\ T_2||N_2||ID_{B\sim T})$

$TS \rightarrow B: \{ID_{TS},\ C_{TS}\}$

Doctor/Nurse (B) receives the message $\{ID_{TS},\ C_{TS}\}$ and decrypts it to get the other party's prescription details and TS validity by computing the set time stamp threshold value, nonce number, received masked-ID values, and decrypted message using the pre-share key from the TS. At each end, entity $E_{K_{TS}}$ is used as a key to encrypt secure credentials in addition to MAC and the hash function application to make them more secure.

(i) Decrypt using K_{TS-B} to get $\{(ID_A||Z_{TS}||\ T_2||\ N_2)\}$
(ii) If $\{Z_{TS}\ XOR\ \{H(ID_B||ID_A||N_2)\}\}$ NOT Equals $ID_{B\sim T}$ then discard
(iii) $X_B = R_B P, Y_B = R_B F$
(iv) $M_B = H(PW_B||ID_{TS}||ID_B)$
(v) $P_B = E_{H_{Y_B}}(ID_B||M_B||N_3||\ \mathrm{MAC}(M_B)||ID_{TS})$
(vi) $C_B = E_{K_{B-TS}}(X_B||\ P_B||\ T_3)$

$B \rightarrow TS: \{ID_{B\sim T},\ C_B\}$

TS receives the message $\{ID_{B\sim T},\ C_B\}$ and decrypts it to get $(X_B||\ P_B||\ T_3)$. After that, the TS computes $Y'_B = dX_B$ which is equal to $dR_B P = R_B dP = R_B F = Y_B$ calculated at Doctor/Nurse (B). It further decrypts the P_B to get $ID_B,\ M_B, N_3, \mathrm{MAC}(M_B)$ and ID_{TS}, as illustrated in steps below. After that, the TS verifies the message's integrity by computing and comparing the hash of the message. Finally, it computes the common parameters CP_A and CP_B for both parties and forwards them to the Patient (A) and doctor/nurse (B) for session key computation.

(i) Decrypt C_B to get $[(X_B||\ P_B||\ T_3)]$
(ii) Computes $Y'_B = dX_B$
(iii) Decrypt P_B to get $[(ID_B||M_B||N_3||\ \mathrm{MAC}(M_B)||ID_{TS})]$
(iv) Calculate $M'_B = H(PW_B||ID_{TS}||ID_B)$
(v) If M'_B *NOT equals* M_B then drop message
(vi) $CP_A = \{\ E_{H_{Y'_A}}(X_B||ID_A||ID_B||\ Y'_A||N_1\ )\}$
(vii) $CP_B = \{\ E_{H_{Y'_B}}(X_A||ID_A||ID_B||\ Y'_B||N_2\ )\}$

$TS \rightarrow A: \{ID_{A\sim T},\ CP_A\}$
$TS \rightarrow B: \{ID_{B\sim T},\ CP_B\}$

D. Step-IV: Participant Validation and Common Session Key Generation

Patient (A) decrypts CP_A, verified by its own nonce and MAC which provide integrity and validity of the TS and the message. The common parameters generated by the trusted server are transmitted securely on each end. Upon receiving the secret credentials, the participating parties first verify message integrity and authority by verifying Y'_A and Y'_B, respectively. After that, MAC, nonce, TS-ID, and the time stamp are also used for double-checking the source's integrity before processing secret credentials. After successful validation of both parties' identities and that of the TS, participants start to compute the common key. The proposed protocol along with stepwise execution is elaborated in Figure 3.

a. Party (A) gets: $\{X_B, ID_A,\ ID_B,\ Y'_A\}$
b. Patient (A): $S_{kA} = H(dX_B, ID_B,\ ID_A)$
a. Party (B) gets: $\{X_A\ , ID_A,\ ID_B,\ Y'_B\}$
b. Doctor/Nurse (B): $S_{kB} = H(dX_A, ID_B,\ ID_A)$

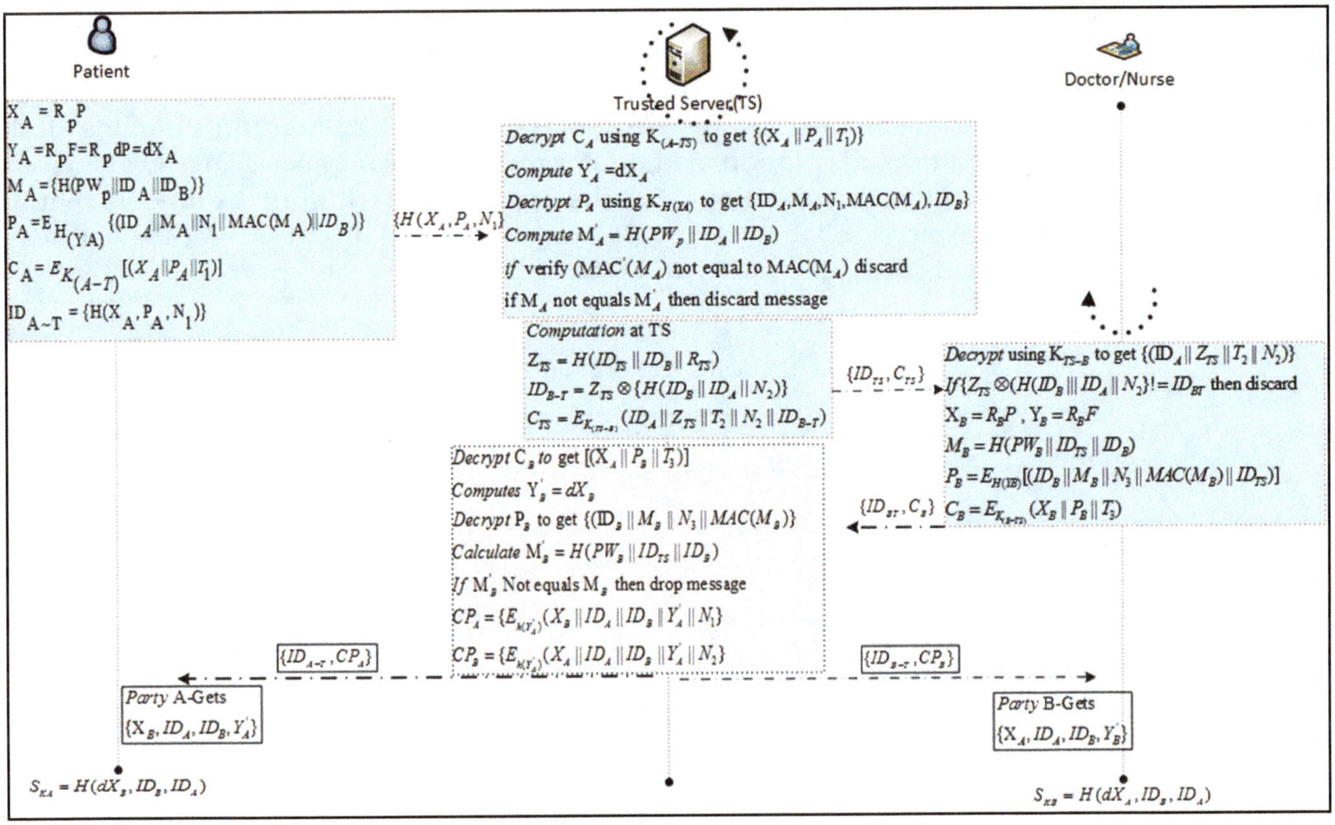

Figure 3. Secure authentication and prescription safety protocol steps.

The novelty of our study is relying upon the creation of secret credentials of the session key for multiparty computing using ECC and symmetric parameters which have less computation cost and are hard to compromise. Upon successful authentication of end parties and common session key generation, both ends share private data securely and efficiently. SAPS attains shared verification, better forward privacy, un-traceability, and participant anonymity. It can launch a secure data sharing connection between the end user and a trusted authority. It also ensures that various attacks, such as offline password guessing, untraceable online secret parameters guessing, confidential insider attacks, card theft attacks, and replay attacks. Intruders cannot enter the system, and the user remains protected at all times.

5. Formal Modeling and Analysis of SAPS

We have performed formal modeling using a method known as Nonmonotonic Cryptographic Protocol (NCP), also called Rubin Logic [39]. The analysis verification of the SAPS protocol is as per its previous terms and specification of NCP. NCP authenticates the proposed scheme as per the regular necessities of cryptographic procedures, considering parameters such as authenticity, data integrity, the freshness of received data, message encryption, and decryption, etc. This will also help identify the lack of certain properties in the presented scheme and for potential data compromising scenarios. This analysis is similar to the actual operation functionalities in a programming scenario. When we talk about Rubin Logic, the units are assigned specific roles, and a universal set of information is maintained. It also maintains current state of the parameters of users after each update operation. Global sets are accessible to all the member nodes and can be categorized into four types which are secret, observer, rule, and first sets. A detailed discussion of the formal specification for WSAN protocols is provided in [26,29], along with appropriate case studies. Entity or node contains a local set that can be categorized into ownership, represented as POSS (), a set of beliefs known as belief BEL (), and to represent the behavior, set BL (). Detailed specification of these sets can be explored in [14,30]. Table 2 represents the local set for the application scenario of Rubin logic on SAPS-AN. The details of SAPS, its verification, and analysis provide a detailed overview of all sets maintained under the category of the local set. All the participating entities, including sender, receiver, and Trusted Server are separately maintained locally. An ownership set, POSS (entity), contains all the parameters involved in encryption, decryption, and other processes accomplished in a local memory of each entity, as described in the section below. For the operations and input arguments that are performed in implementation steps, a Behavior List BL () is maintained. Local sets for the entities of the Trusted Server (TS), patient (A) as first party, and Doctor (B) as the second party are presented in Tables 2–4, respectively.

Table 2. Local set at (Patient) (A).

$POSS(A) = \{ID_A, P, R_p, K_{A\text{-}TS}, F, PW_p\}$
$BEL(A) = \{\#(ID_A), \#(P), \#(R_p), \#(K_{(A\text{-}TS)}), \#(F), \#(PW_p)\}$
$BL(A) =$
Mul $(R_p, P) \rightarrow X_A$, Mul $(R_p, F) \rightarrow Y_A$
Hash(h(.); Concat$(PW_p, ID_A, ID_B)) \rightarrow M_A$
Concat$(ID_A, M_A, N_1, MAC(M_A), ID_B) \rightarrow Q_A$
Hash(h(.); $Y_A) \rightarrow H_{YA}$
Encrypt$(\{Q_A, H_{YA}\}) \rightarrow P_A$
Encrypt(\{Concat$(X_A, P_A, T_1), K_{(A\text{-}TS)}\}) \rightarrow C_A$
Hash(h(.); Concat $(X_A, P_A, N_1)) \rightarrow ID_{A\sim T}$
Send$(\{ID_{A\sim T}, C_A\})$ to TS and Update $(ID_{A\sim T})$
Receive(TS, $(CP_A\})$
Decrypt$(\{ID_{TS}, CP_A\}\ H_{Y'A})$ and Split to get $[X_B, ID_A, ID_B, Y'_A, N_1]$
Hash(h(.); Concat $(dX_B, ID_B, ID_A)) \rightarrow S_{kA}$

Table 3. Local Set at Trusted Server (TS).

$POSS(T_S) = \{ID_{TS}, d, K_{(TS-A\}\}}, K_{(TS-B)}\}$
$BEL(T_S) = \{\#(ID_{TS}), \#(K_{(TS-A\}\}}, \#K_{(TS-B)})\}$
$BL(T_S) =$
Receive(A, $\{C_A\}$)
Decrypt$(\{ID_{A\sim T}, C_A\}K_{TS\text{-}A})$ and Split to get $[X_A, P_A, T_1]$
check$(T'_1 - T_1) \geq \Delta T$ then abort
Hash(h(.); Mul$(d, X_A)) \rightarrow H_{Y'A}$
Decrypt$(\{P_A\}H_{Y'A})$ and Split to get $[ID_A, M_A, N_1, MAC(M_A), ID_B]$
Hash(h(.); Concat$(PW_p, ID_A, ID_B)) \rightarrow M'_A$
if MAC(M'_A) equals MAC(M_A) else discard
if M'_A NOT equals M_A then discard
Hash(h(.); Concat$(ID_{TS}, ID_B, R_{TS})) \rightarrow Z_{TS}$
Hash(h(.); Concat$(ID_A, ID_B, N_2)) \rightarrow Q_{TS}$
XOR $(Z_{TS}, Q_{TS}) \rightarrow ID_{B\sim T}$
Encrypt(\{Concat$(ID_A, Z_{TS}, T_2, N_2, ID_{B\sim T}), K_{(TS\text{-}B)}\}) \rightarrow C_{TS}$
Send$(\{ID_{TS}, C_{TS}\})$ to B and Update $(\mathbf{ID_{B\sim T}})$
Receive(B, $\{C_B\}$)
Decrypt$(\{ID_{B\sim T}, C_B\}K_{TS\text{-}B})$ and Split to get $[X_B, P_B, T_3]$
check$(T'_3 - T_3) \geq \Delta T$ then abort
Hash(h(.); Mul $(d, X_B)) \rightarrow H_{Y'B}$
Decrypt$(\{P_B\}H_{Y'B})$ and Split to get $[ID_B, M_B, N_3, MAC(M_B), ID_{TS}]$
Hash(h(.); Concat$(PW_B, ID_{TS}, ID_B)) \rightarrow M'_B$
if MAC(M'_B) equals MAC(M_B) else discard
if M'_B NOT equals M_B then discard
Encrypt(\{Concat$(X_B, ID_A, ID_B, Y'_A, N_1), H_{Y'A}\}) \rightarrow CP_A$
Send$(\{ID_{A\sim T}, CP_A\})$ to A
Encrypt(\{Concat$(X_A, ID_A, ID_B, Y'_B, N_2), H_{Y'B}\}) \rightarrow CP_B$
Send$(\{ID_{B\sim T}, CP_B\})$ to B

Table 4. Local set at Patient/Doctor (B).

POSS(B) = $\{ID_B, P, R_B, K_{B\text{-}TS}, F, PW_B\}$
BEL(A) = $\{\#(ID_B), \#(P), \#(R_B), \#(K_{(B\text{-}TS)}), \#(F), \#(PW_B)\}$
BL(A) =
Receive(TS, $\{C_{TS}\}$)
Decrypt($\{ID_{B\sim T}, C_{TS}\}K_{B\text{-}TS}$) and Split to get $[ID_A, Z_{TS}, T_2, N_2]$
Hash(h(.); Concat(ID_A, ID_B, N_2)) $\rightarrow Q'_{TS}$
check(XOR($Z_{TS}, Q'_{\mathbf{TS}}$) ! equals $ID_{B\sim T}$) then abort
Mul (R_B, P) $\rightarrow X_B$, Mul (R_B, F) $\rightarrow Y_B$
Hash(h(.); Concat(PW_B, ID_{TS}, ID_B)) $\rightarrow M_B$
Concat(ID_B, M_B, N_3, MAC(M_B), ID_{TS}) $\rightarrow Q_B$
Hash(h(.); Y_B) $\rightarrow H_{YB}$
Encrypt($\{Q_B, H_{YB}\}$)$\rightarrow P_B$
Encrypt($\{$Concat(X_B, P_B, T_3),$K_{(B\text{-}TS)}\}$) $\rightarrow C_B$
Send($\{ID_{B\sim T}, C_B\}$) to TS and Update($ID_{B\sim T}$)
Receive(TS, ($CP_B\}$)
Decrypt($\{ID_{TS}, CP_B\}$ $H_{Y'B}$) and Split to get $[X_A, ID_A, ID_B, Y'_B, N_2]$
Hash(h(.); Concat(dX_A, ID_B, ID_A)) $\rightarrow S_{kB}$

5.1. SAPS Analysis and Verification

In this section, SAPS is analyzed for secure session key establishment for the patient to access their physicians anonymously for medical prescription, as discussed in section IV. In this scenario, the establishment request is initiated by the patient (A) by transmitting secret credentials generated using secure methodology established through the TS. After the sending operation, an update operation performed by the sender to refresh the security credentials for future sessions is as shown below.

- Concat(IDA, MA, N1, MAC(MA), IDB) $\rightarrow$ QA
- Encrypt($\{$QA,$H_{YA}\}$) $\rightarrow P_A$
- Encrypt($\{$Concat(X_A, P_A, T_1), $K_{(A\text{-}TS)}\}$) $\rightarrow C_A$
- Send($\{ID_{A\sim T}, C_A\}$) to TS and Update($ID_{A\sim T}$)
- Update()

To observe, a list of associated factors, messages, nonce numbers, actual key, ciphers, pseudo-dynamic, finite field, and one-way hash values, are kept in a possession set at the sender node, i.e., with the patient (A). In this case, during the authentication for key establishment phase, the following steps are performed.

- POSS(A) = $\{ID_A, P, R_p, K_{A\text{-}TS}, F, PW_p\}$
- BEL(A) = $\{\#(ID_A), \#(P), \#(R_p), \#(K_{(A\text{-}TS)}), \#(F), \#(PW_p)\}$
- BL(A) = Mul(Rp, P) $\rightarrow$ XA, Mul(Rp, F) $\rightarrow$ YA

After sending messages to the other party and the authentication request is sent to the trusted authority, the TS decrypts the received message to get the secret credentials necessary for verification and to explore the request message. The freshness of the message is checked by comparing the timestamp threshold value, nonce number, and masked IDs value with set values. If we fulfill the threshold parameter and verify the answer, then further process calculations are processed. Otherwise, the message is discarded. MAC is calculated for message integrity and compared to hash values to ensure integrity. The participant verification and message integrity steps performed at the TS are as follows.

- Receive(A, $\{C_A\}$)
- Decrypt($\{ID_{A\sim T}, C_A\}K_{TS\text{-}A}$) and Split to get $[X_A, P_A, T_1]$
- check($T'_1 - T_1$) $\geq \Delta T$ then abort
- Hash(h(.); Mul(d, X_A)) $\rightarrow H_{Y'A}$

- Decrypt({P_A}$H_{Y'A}$) and Split to get [ID_A, M_A, N_1, MAC(M_A), ID_B]
- Hash(h(.); Concat(PW_p, ID_A, ID_B)) $\rightarrow$ M'_A
- if MAC(M'_A) equals MAC(M_A) else discard
- if M'_A NOT equals M_A then discard

After Patient (A) verification, the TS calculates some parameters and generates a message for the other party that can provide medical services to the patient (A) as follows.

- Hash(h(.); Concat(IDTS, IDB, RTS)) $\rightarrow$ ZTS
- Hash(h(.); Concat(IDA, IDB, N2)) $\rightarrow$ QTS
- XOR(ZTS, QTS) $\rightarrow$ IDB~ T
- Encrypt({Concat (IDA, ZTS, T2, N2, IDB~T), K(TS-B)}) $\rightarrow$ CTS
- Send({IDTS, CTS}) to B and Update (IDB~ T)

Upon receiving the secret credentials sent by the TS, Doctor (B) verifies the message integrity and the TS as follows:

- Decrypt({$ID_{B\sim T}$, C_{TS}}$K_{B\text{-}TS}$) and Split to get [ID_A, Z_{TS}, T_2, N_2]
- Hash(h(.); Concat (ID_A, ID_B, N_2)) $\rightarrow$ Q'_{TS}
- check(XOR(Z_{TS},Q'_{TS}) ! equals $ID_{B\sim T}$) then abort

Following the authentication and verification of Party (B) by the TS, party (B) also computes some secret credentials and provides a reply message for the TS. The secret credentials are used by both parties to generate a secret key, and the transmission is secured using the shared key, as well as by calculating the hash, adding a nonce, and MAC. The steps performed at the physician's side for session key establishing are as follows:

- Mul(R_B, P) $\rightarrow$ X_B, Mul(R_B, F) $\rightarrow$ Y_B
- Hash(h(.); Concat (P_{WB}, ID_{TS}, ID_B)) $\rightarrow$ M_B
- Concat(ID_B,M_B, N_3, MAC(M_B), ID_{TS}) $\rightarrow$ Q_B
- Hash(h(.);Y_B) $\rightarrow$ H_{YB}
- Encrypt({QB, H_{YB}}) $\rightarrow$ P_B
- Encrypt({Concat(X_B, P_B,T_3), K(B-TS)}) $\rightarrow$ C_B
- Send({ID_B~T, C_B}) to TS and Update (ID_B~ T)

For verification and checking of message integrity of party (B), the TS performs the same steps as Party (A). The TS securely generates secret credentials based on the information gathered from both ends, and distributes a common key which is partially completed. Secure parameter distribution steps are shown as below, which are transmitted securely to the participants.

- Encrypt({Concat (X_B, ID_A,ID_B,Y'_A, N_1), $H_{Y'A}$}) $\rightarrow$ CP_A
- Send({$ID_{A\sim T}$, CP_A}) to A
- Encrypt({Concat (X_A, ID_A,ID_B, Y'_B, N_2), $H_{Y'B}$}) $\rightarrow$ CP_B
- Send({$ID_{B\sim T}$, CP_B}) to B

Although data/credentials transmission is performed using strong encryption techniques by the TS to increase security and un-traceability of participants, the proposed scheme has a novel approach in its partial session key mechanism. After successful authentication and session key establishment, a "Forget Operation" performed at each participating entity will result in removing temporary values like nonce value, time stamp, temporary encryption key H*, and MAC calculating parameters. These operations ensure security against forwarding secrecy and user traceability issues.

5.2. User Anonymity

The user's identity, ID, cannot be stored in plaintext at the user level, nor at the TS, and it can be transmitted via the login request. In our scheme, user identity is masked in both M_A and P_A, after the original identity registration, session request, and end-user joining request is sent to the TS in the encrypted form. The secret parameters are generated by party (A) and party (B) by choosing secret number d_A, d_B, respectively, from E with large order n as shown in steps I–III. It is not feasible for any third party to get these secret parameters and it is almost impossible to recover messages M_A, M_B to get identities without knowing the one-way hash function. It is not viable for an adversary to compute the original identities of the participant. The TS has private and public key pairs and the participants use their MAC for message integrity, masked-IDs, nonce number, and time stamp (T) for message freshness. At the trusted sever, a randomized symmetric encryption technique is used to conceal the random number $\{R_{TS}\}$ generated by the TS instead of using the XOR. Before communicating the session request of party(A) to party(B), the TS first verifies the original identity of the requested party and the message freshness by computing the inverse functions as shown in Protocols II and III. It generates a temporary public ID of each participant instead of using their original identities. The public identity, say IDV, can run the protocol. Therefore, on the basis of the above analysis, it is impossible for the adversary to get the user's identity from the proposed protocol during authentication, forwarding, the joining request, or the session key computing procedure. Therefore, we know that the proposed protocol is able to provide user anonymity.

5.3. User Un-Traceability

In our scheme, each session-based communication contains parameters $\{X_A,\ P_A,\ T_1\}$ based on X_A and P_A that are dynamic for each authentication/verification session of all participants and are different for each transmission. Moreover, a timestamp is appended to every session. The value of $(X_A,\ P_A)$, Z_{TS} and X_B, P_B, as shown in the proposed protocols to fulfill the requirements for common session key establishment, are executed in a distributed manner. Consequently, the adversary is unable to figure out that two procedures have the same users involved. It ensures that our proposal accomplishes user un-traceability. According to the pattern of the projected protocol, the participant generates a new random number $r \in Z^*_q$ to compute X_A , Z_{TS} and X_B in each session. Due to the randomness of the secret parameters, the adversary cannot find and link among messages sent by the end parties or the trusted server, and therefore is unable to follow their actions. Therefore, the proposed protocol is able to provide un-traceability during authentication, session key management, and the following data transmission procedures.

5.4. Offline Password Guessing Attacks

In offline password guessing, the adversary tries to capture the entire communication between party (A) and the TS or between the TS and party (B), but is unable to get the password. The next adversary attack may be possible.

i. $\{X_A,\ P_A,\ T_1\} \rightarrow$ {TS} from party(A) to TS, $\{ID_{TS},\ Z_{TS}\}$ are TS parameters, $(\{X_B,\ P_B\}, T_3)$ *Party(B) to TS* and $\{CP_A,\ CP_B\}$ are the communications between A, B, and the TS known by the adversary. To commence the offline secret password estimating attack, the adversary tries to regenerate PW_p', an inverse password of party (A) and computes $M_A{}'$. Still, if the adversary gets the IDs of both participants, it is not possible for the adversary to compute $E_{H(YA)}$ and they are unable to verify the P_A as used in the protocols which contains the message and the identities of the participants.

ii. Appropriate to the un-traceability of the Computational Diffie-Hellman assumption (CDH) a difficult adversary does not get $\{Y_A = R_pF := R_pdP \rightarrow Y_A = dX_A\ F\}$ and it is impossible for the adversary to get the password.

iii. If an adversary gets party B's password to compute the random R_{Ts} number generated by the TS, as shown in protocol-III, to compute the parameters after the received connection establishing request from party (A), it is not possible for the adversary to compute B's password without knowing YB because $Y_B = \{d_B F\}$ and has ECDLP, as shown in step-3 of protocol-III.

As a result, the proposed protocol can oppose offline password guessing attacks. To deal with online password guessing attack, the TS detects the encounter during the message validation process and the freshness procedure at the beginning of the communication.

5.5. Perfect Forward Secrecy

In our scheme, the un-traceability of CDH plays a vital role in resisting guessing previous session keys by the adversary. The session key is generated using $H(d_A, d_B P, ID_B, ID_A)$, where d_A, d_B are nonce numbers chosen by both participants specially for the specific session and are different from the nonce numbers used during the authentication process, such as N_1, N_2, N_3. In the proposed protocol, the end parties compute the session key, SK, as $H(dX_B, ID_B, ID_A)$ and $H(dX_A, ID_B, ID_A)$, where dX_A and dX_B are computed by randomly chosen numbers by both parties at their end with the help of the trusted server. Knowing the secret key of the server and the password does not help the adversary to compute a previously established session key, because the secret credentials used to compute the secure key are not based on the password and server's public key. If the adversary wants to know an old session key he /she must compute dX_A, dX_B. However, since the adversary does not know the R_p due to the hardness of ECDLP, the adversary cannot compute the secret credentials. Therefore, the proposed scheme provides perfect forward secrecy.

5.6. Replay Attack

Replay attacks can be launched while an attacker replays the original message parameters at some other time to impersonate any legal participant. In the proposed scheme, messages between the ID_A, TS, and ID_B are transmitted on the public channel. An attacker might try to use these conversations to launch a replay attack. However, in our protocol, replay attacks can be easily thwarted because an adversary cannot produce an updated timestamp. Both end parties and the TS verify message freshness with a threshold for timestamp and nonce number. If the difference exceeds this threshold, it will abort the session. It is not easy for an adversary to impersonate participants' reply messages because the nonce numbers N_1, N_2, N_3 during the authentication process, d_A, d_B for key session key generation and R_{Ts} used by the TS are newly chosen for every session. For this scenario, an adversary cannot compute the $\{X_A,\ P_A,\ T_1\}$, $S_K = H(d_A X'_B, ID_B,\ ID_A)$, and $(\{X_B,\ P_B\}, T_3\ )$ communication patterns of the entire network.

5.7. Forgery Attacks and Impersonation

In our scheme, TS has a pair of public-private secret keys (d, $F = dP$), and if an adversary attempts to impersonate the participants or the TS and sends a message to the TS acting as the participants or tries to establish a connection with any party, they will remain unable to verify themself. For the verification process, it is necessary for an adversary to know the password or private key of the TS, d.

5.8. Man in the Middle Attack

An adversary may intercept the messages sent between the parties and the TS and replace them with their own messages. These forged messages need to be verified by the TS before getting the session key. However, it is not feasible as the adversary does not know the TS secret key and secret passwords of the parties. So, our scheme resists a man in middle attack.

6. Results and Analysis

We have simulated the SAPS protocol by deploying nodes for the patient, doctor/nurse, and the trusted server using TCL script in NS 2.35.The simulation parameter and system setting defined in Table 5. We have separately configured the patient and doctor/nurse for low power devices. The server is configured for high residual and transmission power. In the TCL file, communication messages are initiated and traffic sources are also configured along with packet sizes. Moreover, C/C++ files are developed for providing device-level functionalities, including send, receive, hash, encrypt, and decrypt functions. Results are extracted from the trace file by executing the AWK scripts. We have used a 160-bit key along with $f(x) = x^{167} + x^9 + x^7 + x^5 + x^3 + 1$ where the tuple $T = (m, f, (x)a, b, G, n, h)$. The performance of SAPS is evaluated regarding storage, computation, and communication costs for the base scheme TPKE [15], A-TMIS [16], EAKA [40], and AAS [41]. A list of simulation parameters is shown in Table 4.

Table 5. Simulation Parameters.

Parameters	Values
Network Field	1300 × 1300 m
Initial Energy at Smart Device	1000 Joules
Tx Power at Smart Device	0.819 Joules
Receiving Power	0.049 Joules
Queue Type	Queue/DropTail/PriQue
Max Packet in Queue	55 Packets
Agent Trace	ON
Router Trace	ON
Number of Nodes	500 Nodes

6.1. Storage Overhead

In the proposed protocol, we outlined the storage overhead and memory requirement, including the public/private key of the TS and the communication parties, IDs, random number, timestamp, and resultant length of the session key, as shown in Figure 4. In the view of the used parameters between the patient (A), TS, and Doctor (B), we have analyzed and compared the storage cost of TPKE [15], the smart card keeps $\{ID, B, p\}$ and thus the storage overhead is $(160 + 1022 \times 2) = 2208$ bits. A-TMIS [16] stores $(1600 + 1024 \times 3) = 3232$ bits and an efficient authentication and key agreement EAKA protocol [40] requires $(160 \times 5) = 800$ bits in the smart card for basics parameters. The AAS [41] scheme improves the protocol for TMIS and consumes 960-bits storage to process authentication and authorization which contains $\{P, u, B, R, p, q\}$.

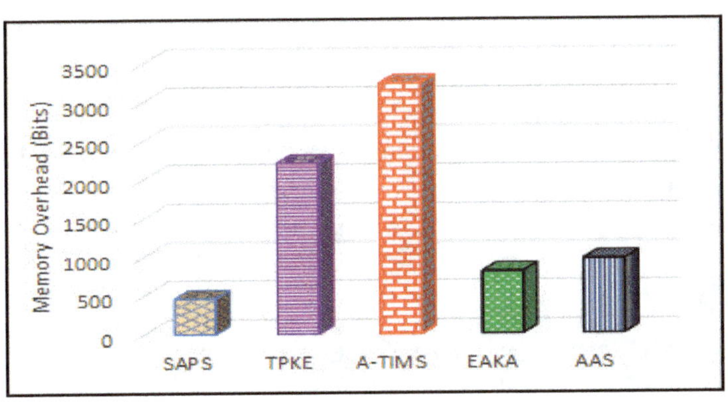

Figure 4. Storage cost for Secure Authentication and Prescription Safety (SAPS).

In our SAPS protocol, the end parties need to keep {P_W, ID, X_A, N_i, T_i, $E_{K_{A-TS}}$} for identification, authentication, and session key establishment. From an evaluation point of view, it has been supposed that secret identity, one-way hash operation, and timestamps are 160-bits in size, whereas the ECC recommended size by NIST for a key is 160-bits and 64-bit for the secret key for encrypting passwords generated using the TS's shared credentials. So, the total storage overheads of proposed scheme are $(160 + 160 \times 2) = 480$ bits, which is stored at both ends and the TS has more computation and storage capabilities. In our scenario, more parameters such as ID masking, public/private key and pseudorandom generation processes are accomplished at the TS.

6.2. Communication Overhead

To appraise the message exchanging overhead of the presented protocol, the data that is transmitted between the participating parties and the TS during the identification and session key generation phase need to be considered. It is identified that the secret key of size 160-bit using ECC can yield equal security to a 1024-bit RSA secret key. For the evaluation phase, we believe that the resultant one-way hash function, participant's identities, timestamp, and nonce number are 160 bits in length. The end party sends three parameters which are $\{XA,\ PA,\ T1\}$ to the TS for authentication, and their lengths are $(160 \times 3) = 480$ bits. On the other side, in the party verification phase, the TS sends an encrypted packet CP_A using a 160-bit ECC key to the end party for session key establishment and its length is $(160 \times 2) = 320$ bits. On the basis of these computations in the proposed SAPS protocol, Patient (A) and Doctor (B) have the same communication cost during their end user confirmation and secure key generation processes. On the other hand, existing ECC- and RSA-based schemes have greater communication overheads, as depicted in Figure 5.

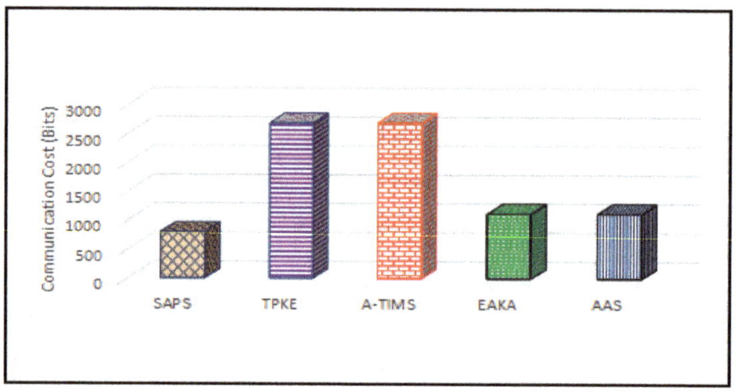

Figure 5. Communication overheads during authentication.

TPKE [15] is based on RSA which requires 1344 bits for the authentication method and 1344 bits for server to end party communication. Similarly, A-TMIS [16] consumes the same communication cost as TPKE for the whole procedure. In the login phase of Xu et al.'s protocol for EAKA [40], the server requires 640 bits of communication cost, and the server to the user requires 480-bits. AAS [41] requires 640 bits and 480 bits communication from the user to server and the server to user, respectively. By the above analysis, the proposed scheme has less communication cost by ensuring user anonymity.

6.3. Computation Complexity

Based on the simulation results and defined parameters, a 5 MHz frequency is required to compute the 160-bit elliptic curve, where 5 MHz is for one small data module in which multiple modules are included in the calculation of the elliptic curve and related mathematical operations. To elaborate in detail, we have defined some notations to describe the function of protocol like, T_E , T_{EPM} , T_{EDs} , T_H , T_X which are the time for performing an exponential operation, time for performing an elliptic curve point multiplication operation, time for computing EC point multiplication function, symmetric encryption/decryption operation time, the one way hash function computation time, and XOR operation, respectively.

According to [42,43], the computation time for an exponential operation is 0.522 ms, EC point multiplication process consumes 0.063075 ms, one-way hash operation implementation time is 0.0005 ms, and the encryption/decryption operation time is 0.0087 ms. On the user's side, the proposed scheme has lower computational overheads, as shown in Figures 6 and 7. Our SAPS protocol is more suitable for a mobile scenario when compared to existing schemes, because it has fewer rounds needed for authentication. Computing complexity for the adversary is high, whereas fewer communication rounds make it more efficient and secure.

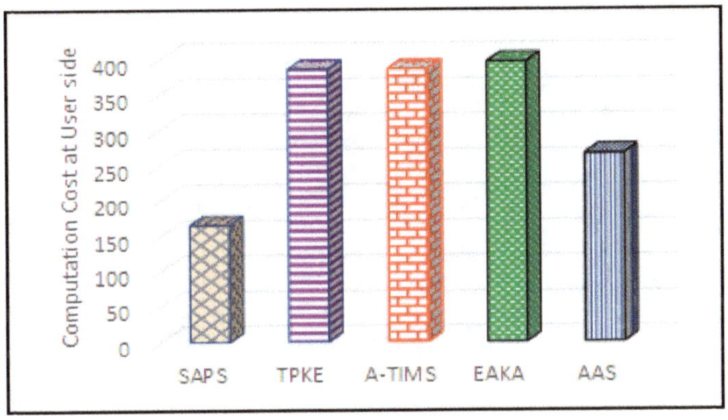

Figure 6. Computation cost at user side.

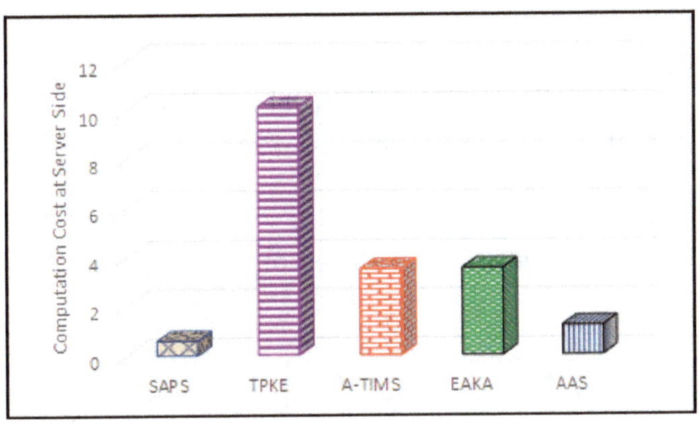

Figure 7. Computation cost at server side.

6.4. Resilience

During secure communication between the patient and doctor, devices from different regions communicate using intermediate devices. The chance of compromised devices in the path exists. The probability Pr_β that an intermediate node is compromised is given in Equation (1), where N is the number of devices in the network and β is number of devices compromised by adversary. The term $N-2$ represents that sender and receiver are considered uncompromised, whereas $N-3$ means to exclude one more intermediate device which is a direct neighbor of the sender.

$$Pr_\beta = 1 - \binom{N-3}{\beta} / \binom{N-2}{\beta} = \frac{\beta}{N-2} \tag{1}$$

Figure 8 elucidates the scenario for measuring the impact of compromising intermediate devices by calculating the probability Pr_β when the number of devices in the network varies from 100 to 500. In the case of 300 devices, the probability is 0.0167, 0.033, 0.050, and 0.067 for β = 5, 10, 15, and 20 compromised devices, respectively. If an intermediate device is compromised, then data and security credentials stored in that device are exposed. Moreover, the probability Pr_{ω} that a particular session key and its related credentials are compromised is given in Equation (2), where ω credentials are compromised out of a total of M devices in the network.

$$Pr_{\omega} = 1 - \binom{M-1}{\omega-1} / \binom{M}{\omega} = \frac{\omega}{M} \tag{2}$$

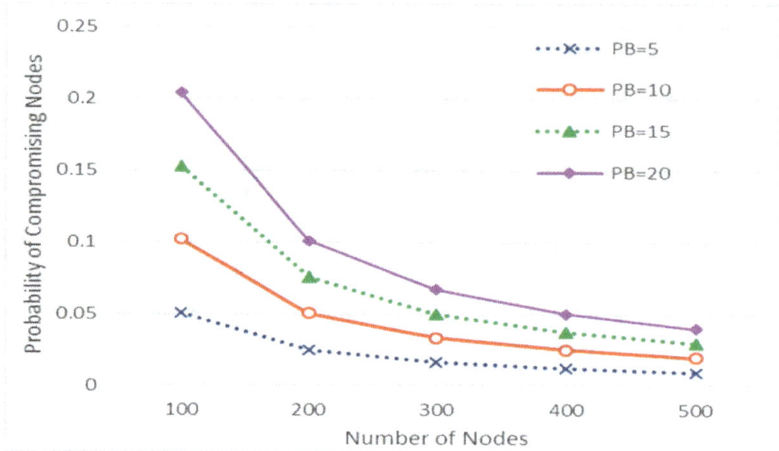

Figure 8. Probability of compromised intermediate device.

Figure 9 shows that different security credentials stored in devices can be revealed to intruders when the devices are compromised. We have considered the scenario where the number of devices is varied from 100 to 500, and the number of compromised nodes is varied from 5 to 25, respectively. In the case of 400 devices in the network where 20 of them are compromised, the number of compromised bytes are 15.62 KB, 18.75 KB, 43.12 KB, and 63.12 KB for EAKA, AAS, TPKE, and A-TIMS respectively. Our proposed SAPS method dominates and achieves better resilience against node capture attack by revealing only 8.98 KB.

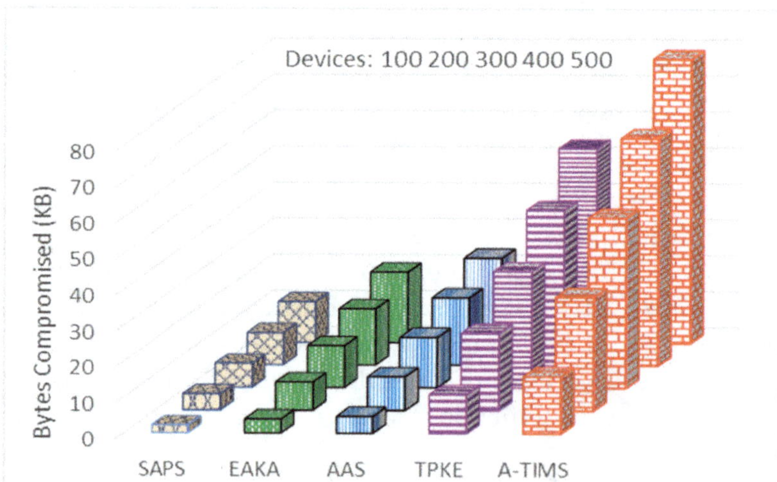

Figure 9. Bytes revealed upon device compromise.

7. Conclusions

A secure three-party key establishment technique for TMIS is presented to secure patients' medical prescriptions. It uses ECC for end-user anonymity, using the secure authentication and prescription safety (SAPS) protocol that can establish a secure connection between patients and a doctor/nurse without revealing their secret identities. The proposed scheme achieves anonymity and un-traceability of the participants. The SAPS protocol has been analyzed by applying Rubin Logic to verify security, user anonymity, and un-traceability of participants during session key generation for secure information sharing between the doctor and the patient in TMIS. Public attacks and their countermeasures are analyzed at each level. For validation of SAPS, we have performed simulation using NS-2.35 to compare the performance of SAPS for storage, communication, and computation overheads, as compared to other methods to prove its suitability for the ubiquitous TMIS network. The storage cost reduction of the proposed scheme at the user side and at the server side is approximately 38% and 41%, respectively, as compared with the mean of the four latest existing techniques. The average computation overhead reductions at both the user side and the server side are 37% and 49%, respectively, as compared with the mean average of existing four schemes. Our future work will aim to analyze the impact of chaotic map-based keying for multi-party authentication between doctors and patients to get a medical prescription for common diseases without revealing either identities on an open network.

Acknowledgments: This work was funded by the National Natural Science Foundation of China (61471035), and Fundamental Research Funds for the Central Universities (06105031, 06500010). In particular, it was supported by Cybermatics and Cyberspace International Science and Technology Cooperation Base.

Author Contributions: Zahid Mahmood and Ata Ullah conceived and designed the experiments; Zahid Mahmood performed the experiments; Huansheng Ning analyzed the data and overall proposed protocols, models, structure and flow of entire paper; Xuanxia Yao and Ata Ullah performed the formal modeling and verification of proposed scheme. Zahid Mahmood contributed reagents/materials/analysis tools and also wrote the paper along with literature.

References

1. Wu, Z.-Y.; Tseng, Y.-J.; Chung, Y.; Chen, Y.-C.; Lai, F. A reliable user authentication and key agreement scheme for web-based hospital-acquired infection surveillance information system. *J. Med. Syst.* **2012**, *36*, 2547–2555. [CrossRef] [PubMed]
2. Giri, D.; Maitra, T.; Amin, R.; Srivastava, P. An efficient and robust rsa-based remote user authentication for telecare medical information systems. *J. Med. Syst.* **2015**, *39*, 145. [CrossRef] [PubMed]
3. Xie, Q.; Zhang, J.; Dong, N. Robust anonymous authentication scheme for telecare medical information systems. *J. Med. Syst.* **2013**, *37*, 9911. [CrossRef] [PubMed]
4. Abdalla, M.; Fouque, P.-A.; Pointcheval, D. Password-based authenticated key exchange in the three-party setting. *IEEE Proc. Inf. Secur.* **2006**, *153*, 27–39. [CrossRef]
5. Chung, H.-R.; Ku, W.-C. Three weaknesses in a simple three-party key exchange protocol. *Inf. Sci.* **2008**, *178*, 220–229. [CrossRef]
6. Guo, H.; Li, Z.; Mu, Y.; Zhang, X. Cryptanalysis of simple three-party key exchange protocol. *Comput. Secur.* **2008**, *27*, 16–21. [CrossRef]
7. Lu, R.; Cao, Z. Simple three-party key exchange protocol. *Comput. Secur.* **2007**, *26*, 94–97. [CrossRef]
8. Huang, H.F. A simple three-party password-based key exchange protocol. *Int. J. Commun. Syst.* **2009**, *22*, 857–862. [CrossRef]
9. Nam, J.; Paik, J.; Kang, H.-K.; Kim, U.M.; Won, D. An off-line dictionary attack on a simple three-party key exchange protocol. *IEEE Commun. Lett.* **2009**, *13*, 205–207.
10. Phan, R.C.-W.; Yau, W.-C.; Goi, B.-M. Cryptanalysis of simple three-party key exchange protocol (S-3PAKE). *Inf. Sci.* **2008**, *178*, 2849–2856. [CrossRef]
11. Chen, H.-M.; Lo, J.-W.; Yeh, C.-K. An efficient and secure dynamic id-based authentication scheme for telecare medical information systems. *J. Med. Syst.* **2012**, *36*, 3907–3915. [CrossRef] [PubMed]

12. Xie, Q.; Dong, N.; Tan, X.; Wong, D.S.; Wang, G. Improvement of a three-party password-based key exchange protocol with formal verification. *Inf. Technol. Control* **2013**, *42*, 231–237. [CrossRef]
13. Wu, S.; Chen, K.; Pu, Q.; Zhu, Y. Cryptanalysis and enhancements of efficient three-party password-based key exchange scheme. *Int. J. Commun. Syst.* **2013**, *26*, 674–686. [CrossRef]
14. Wu, Z.-Y.; Lee, Y.-C.; Lai, F.; Lee, H.-C.; Chung, Y. A secure authentication scheme for telecare medicine information systems. *J. Med. Syst.* **2012**, *36*, 1529–1535. [CrossRef] [PubMed]
15. Debiao, H.; Jianhua, C.; Rui, Z. A more secure authentication scheme for telecare medicine information systems. *J. Med. Syst.* **2012**, *36*, 1989–1995. [CrossRef] [PubMed]
16. Wei, J.; Hu, X.; Liu, W. An improved authentication scheme for telecare medicine information systems. *J. Med. Syst.* **2012**, *36*, 3597–3604. [CrossRef] [PubMed]
17. Zhu, Z. An efficient authentication scheme for telecare medicine information systems. *J. Med. Syst.* **2012**, *36*, 3833–3838. [CrossRef] [PubMed]
18. Pu, Q.; Wang, J.; Zhao, R. Strong authentication scheme for telecare medicine information systems. *J. Med. Syst.* **2012**, *36*, 2609–2619. [CrossRef] [PubMed]
19. Khan, M.K.; Kim, S.-K.; Alghathbar, K. Cryptanalysis and security enhancement of a 'more efficient & secure dynamic ID-based remote user authentication scheme'. *Comput. Commun.* **2011**, *34*, 305–309.
20. Kumar, P.; Lee, S.-G.; Lee, H.-J. E-SAP: Efficient-strong authentication protocol for healthcare applications using wireless medical sensor networks. *Sensors* **2012**, *12*, 1625–1647. [CrossRef] [PubMed]
21. He, D.; Kumar, N.; Chen, J.; Lee, C.-C.; Chilamkurti, N.; Yeo, S.-S. Robust anonymous authentication protocol for health-care applications using wireless medical sensor networks. *Multimed. Syst.* **2015**, *21*, 49–60. [CrossRef]
22. Nam, J.; Choo, K.-K.R.; Han, S.; Kim, M.; Paik, J.; Won, D. Efficient and anonymous two-factor user authentication in wireless sensor networks: Achieving user anonymity with lightweight sensor computation. *PLoS ONE* **2015**, *10*, e0116709. [CrossRef] [PubMed]
23. Xue, K.; Ma, C.; Hong, P.; Ding, R. A temporal-credential-based mutual authentication and key agreement scheme for wireless sensor networks. *J. Netw. Comput. Appl.* **2013**, *36*, 316–323. [CrossRef]
24. Li, C.-T.; Weng, C.-Y.; Lee, C.-C. An advanced temporal credential-based security scheme with mutual authentication and key agreement for wireless sensor networks. *Sensors* **2013**, *13*, 9589–9603. [CrossRef] [PubMed]
25. Turkanović, M.; Brumen, B.; Hölbl, M. A novel user authentication and key agreement scheme for heterogeneous ad hoc wireless sensor networks, based on the Internet of Things notion. *Ad Hoc Netw.* **2014**, *20*, 96–112. [CrossRef]
26. Amin, R.; Islam, S.H.; Biswas, G.; Khan, M.K.; Li, X. Cryptanalysis and enhancement of anonymity preserving remote user mutual authentication and session key agreement scheme for e-health care systems. *J. Med. Syst.* **2015**, *39*, 140. [CrossRef] [PubMed]
27. Whitmore, A.; Agarwal, A.; Da Xu, L. The Internet of Things—A survey of topics and trends. *Inf. Syst. Front.* **2015**, *17*, 261–274. [CrossRef]
28. Dinh, H.T.; Lee, C.; Niyato, D.; Wang, P. A survey of mobile cloud computing: Architecture, applications, and approaches. *Wirel. Commun. Mob. Comput.* **2013**, *13*, 1587–1611. [CrossRef]
29. Moosavi, S.R.; Gia, T.N.; Nigussie, E.; Rahmani, A.-M.; Virtanen, S.; Tenhunen, H.; Isoaho, J. Session Resumption-Based End-to-End Security for Healthcare Internet-of-Things. In Proceedings of the 2015 IEEE International Conference on Computer and Information Technology; Ubiquitous Computing and Communications; Dependable, Autonomic and Secure Computing; Pervasive Intelligence and Computing (CIT/IUCC/DASC/PICOM), Liverpool, UK, 26–28 October 2015; pp. 581–588.
30. Moosavi, S.R.; Gia, T.N.; Rahmani, A.-M.; Nigussie, E.; Virtanen, S.; Isoaho, J.; Tenhunen, H. SEA: A secure and efficient authentication and authorization architecture for IoT-based healthcare using smart gateways. *Procedia Comput. Sci.* **2015**, *52*, 452–459. [CrossRef]
31. Rahmani, A.M.; Gia, T.N.; Negash, B.; Anzanpour, A.; Azimi, I.; Jiang, M.; Liljeberg, P. Exploiting smart e-health gateways at the edge of healthcare internet-of-things: A fog computing approach. *Futur. Gener. Comput. Syst.* **2017**, *78*, 641–658. [CrossRef]
32. Yeh, H.-L.; Chen, T.-H.; Liu, P.-C.; Kim, T.-H.; Wei, H.-W. A secured authentication protocol for wireless sensor networks using elliptic curves cryptography. *Sensors* **2011**, *11*, 4767–4779. [CrossRef] [PubMed]

33. Miller, V.S. Use of Elliptic Curves in Cryptography. In *Conference on the Theory and Application of Cryptographic Techniques*; Springer: Berlin/Heidelberg, Germany, 1985; pp. 417–426.
34. Koblitz, N. Elliptic curve cryptosystems. *Math. Comput.* **1987**, *48*, 203–209. [CrossRef]
35. Hankerson, D.; Menezes, A.J.; Vanstone, S. *Guide to Elliptic Curve Cryptography*; Springer Science & Business Media: New York, NY, USA, 2006.
36. Li, X.; Qiu, W.; Zheng, D.; Chen, K.; Li, J. Anonymity enhancement on robust and efficient password-authenticated key agreement using smart cards. *IEEE Trans. Ind. Electron.* **2010**, *57*, 793–800.
37. Ying, Z.; Chiou, S.-Y.; Liu, J. An Efficient Privacy Authentication Scheme Based on Cloud Models for Medical Environment. In Proceedings of the 2015 18th International Conference on Network-Based Information Systems (NBiS), Taipei, Taiwan, 2–4 September 2015; pp. 628–633.
38. Zhang, L.; Zhu, S.; Tang, S. Privacy protection for telecare medicine information systems using a chaotic map-based three-factor authenticated key agreement scheme. *IEEE J. Biomed. Health Inf.* **2017**, *21*, 465–475. [CrossRef] [PubMed]
39. Rubin, A.D.; Honeyman, P. Nonmonotonic Cryptographic Protocols. In Proceedings of the Computer Security Foundations Workshop VII (CSFW 7), Franconia, NH, USA, 14–16 June 1994; pp. 100–116.
40. Xu, X.; Jin, Z.P.; Zhang, H.; Zhu, P. A Dynamic ID-Based Authentication Scheme Based on ECC for Telecare Medicine Information Systems. In *Applied Mechanics and Materials*; Trans Tech Publ: Zürich, Switzerland, 2014; pp. 861–866.
41. Islam, S.H.; Khan, M.K. Cryptanalysis and improvement of authentication and key agreement protocols for telecare medicine information systems. *J. Med. Syst.* **2014**, *38*, 135. [CrossRef] [PubMed]
42. He, D.; Kumar, N.; Khan, M.; Lee, J.-H. Anonymous two-factor authentication for consumer roaming service in global mobility networks. *IEEE Trans. Consum. Electron.* **2013**, *59*, 811–817. [CrossRef]
43. Jiang, Q.; Ma, J.; Li, G.; Yang, L. An efficient ticket based authentication protocol with unlinkability for wireless access networks. *Wirel. Pers. Commun.* **2014**, *77*, 1489–1506. [CrossRef]

12

Unobtrusive Sleep Monitoring Using Movement Activity by Video Analysis

Yuan-Kai Wang [1,2,*], Hung-Yu Chen [1] and Jian-Ru Chen [1]

1 Graduate Institute of Applied Science and Engineering, Fu Jen Catholic University, New Taipei 24205, Taiwan
2 Electrical Engineering, Fu Jen Catholic University, New Taipei 24205, Taiwan
* Correspondence: ykwang@fju.edu.tw

Abstract: Sleep healthcare at home is a new research topic that needs to develop new sensors, hardware and algorithms with the consideration of convenience, portability and accuracy. Monitoring sleep behaviors by visual sensors represents one new unobtrusive approach to facilitating sleep monitoring and benefits sleep quality. The challenge of video surveillance for sleep behavior analysis is that we have to tackle bad image illumination issue and large pose variations during sleeping. This paper proposes a robust method for sleep pose analysis with human joints model. The method first tackles the illumination variation issue of infrared videos to improve the image quality and help better feature extraction. Image matching by keypoint features is proposed to detect and track the positions of human joints and build a human model robust to occlusion. Sleep poses are then inferred from joint positions by probabilistic reasoning in order to tolerate occluded joints. Experiments are conducted on the video polysomnography data recorded in sleep laboratory. Sleep pose experiments are given to examine the accuracy of joint detection and tacking, and the accuracy of sleep poses. High accuracy of the experiments demonstrates the validity of the proposed method.

Keywords: sleep pose recognition; keypoints feature matching; Bayesian inference; near-infrared images; scale invariant feature transform

---

1. Introduction

Sleep disorders induce irregular sleeping patterns and sleep deprivation that have serious impacts on health. Obstructive sleep apnea (OSA) [1] is one of the most well recognized sleep disorders. OSA is characterized by repetitive obstruction of the upper airways during sleep, resulting in oxygen de-saturation and frequent brain arousal. It is a symptom that not only decreases sleep quality by sleep disturbance, but also has severe influence which may be life-threatening. Reduction in cognitive function, cardiovascular diseases, stroke, driver fatigue and excessive day time sleepiness are common among OSA patients.

Sleep monitoring systems [2] are an important objective diagnosis method to assess sleep quality and identify sleep disorders. They provide quantitative data about irregularity of brain and body behaviors in sleeping periods and duration. This information helps the analysis of sleep-wake state, diagnosis of the severity of disorders, and prompt treatment of sleep-related diseases.

Polysomnography (PSG) is a standard diagnostic tool in sleep medicine [3] that measures a wide range of biosignals, including blood oxygen, airflow, electroencephalography (EEG), electrocardiography (ECG), electromyography (EMG) and electro-oculography during sleep time. The subject monitored by PSG has to sleep by carefully wearing a lot of sensors with numerous electrodes attached to his whole body, which increases sleep disturbance and discomfort. A sleep technician has to read these overnight data and mark sleep status manually according to the standardized scoring rule. It is a complex, costly and labor-intensive instrument that is absolutely not adequate for sleep care at home.

Alternative approach with minimized contact-based sensors has been developed [3,4]. Unconstrained portable biosensors, accelerometer, RFID (Radio Frequency IDentification), pressure sensors and smartphone are individually-applied or combined to detect sleep behaviors such as limb movement, body movement and sleep position. Detected sleep behaviors are further analyzed to inference sleep-wake pattern and assess sleep disorder. Actigraphy is a good representative that is commonly used with a watch-like accelerometer device attached typically to the wrist. These alternatives apply contact-based sensors and are disadvantageous to the data acquisition and sleep quality.

The noncontact approach usually employs imaging sensors such as microwave, thermal imaging and near-infrared (NIR) camera to non-intrusively detect sleep behaviors. Among these imaging modalities, NIR camera is more desired for home sleep analysis because it is low-cost, easily accessible and highly portable. Sivan et al. (in 1996) and Schwichtenberg et al. (in 2018) [5,6] shows that NIR video alone is enough for effective screening of OSA. Manual analysis from NIR videos can result in high correlation to PSG based diagnosis. Automatic video analysis is then proposed for sleep-wake detection [7–10] and sleep behavior analysis [11–16]. The NIR video is analyzed to extract subject's motion information by the methods such as background subtraction, optical flow, image difference and edge filter. Classification methods are then employed to inference sleep states and body parts. However, robust methods for stable analysis remains a necessary concern.

Challenges of robust sleep video analysis come from the characteristics of NIR videos and sleep pose. Capturing sleep behavior using NIR camera in dark environment has the problems of non-uniform illuminance and bad image quality. NIR camera needs to actively project a near-infrared light source on objects. An unevenly illuminated image is usually obtained because the projected area is over-exposure but the other area is under-exposure. Moreover, NIR images have poor imaging quality because they has low resolution, low signal-to-noise ratio (SNR) and low contrast. In addition, noise is inevitably introduced to NIR images because of the low-light situation for sleep. Low contrast, high noise and uneven illumination degrade the distinctiveness of motion and edge features that are usually applied in existing studies. Therefore, extracting body movement from IR video suffers from the image degradation problem.

Sleep pose recognition from videos is highly challenging for the nonrigid characteristics of the human body. Deformable and partially occluded postures plus with irregular movements induce high variation and inconsistency of appearance and shape features of human body, and make it difficult to classify postures.

This paper proposes a nonintrusive method to recognize sleep body positions. The joint-based approach is adopted for our sleep pose recognition, including joint detection and pose recognition. The joint detection step finds body joints using keypoints extraction and matching, and builds human models from these joints. The tracking step updates the human model by an online learning approach to consider the constraint of sequential change of viewpoint of joints. The recognition step includes a Bayesian network and statistical inference algorithm to deal with the problems of self-occlusion and pose variations. A special scheme is developed for the detection of joints to conquer poor image quality and self-occlusion problems. A special design, called IR-sensitive pajamas, which attaches visual markers on human joints is proposed. Joint markers contain visual patterns distinguished with each other and each marker corresponds only to one specific joint. A human joint model is constructed from the detected joint markers within a sleep image and is recognized to the sleep pose being supine or lateral. An earlier version of this paper appeared in [11]. Compared to the prior paper, this study contains (1) a substantial number of additional survey, explanations and analysis, and (2) various additional experiments to investigate the impact an accuracy of infrared image enhancement for sleep analysis.

The rest of this paper is organized as follows. Section 2 reviews state-of-the-art sleep behavior analysis with contact- and noncontact-based approaches. Section 3 describes our method that includes three components: NIR image enhancement, joint detection and tracking, and sleep pose recognition. Section 4 presents the experimental evaluation compared with different methods. Finally, Section 5 concludes the characteristics and advantages of the proposed method.

2. Related Works

The medical foundation of sleep analysis from videos is the physiological interpretation of body movement during sleep, that is first reviewed and explained. Existing contact and noncontact methods for sleep pose recognition are also discussed. The final subsection introduces general posture and action recognition methods been developed in computer vision, and identify the importance of feature representation for detection and recognition problems.

2.1. The Relation between Sleep Behavior and Sleep Disorder

Several studies of sleep medicine [5,17] show that body movements are an important behavioral aspect during sleep. They can be associated to sleep states and connected to the sleep state transitions. In particular, major body movements have been described in non-rapid eye movement (NREM) sleep, whereas small movements predominantly occur during REM phases. Therefore, the frequency and duration of body movements are important characteristics for sleep analysis. Moreover, some study [18] has found correlations between sleep body positions and sleep apnea. There is also some clinical evidence that the analysis of body pose is relevant to the diagnosis of OSA. A sleep monitoring system that detects body positions during sleep would help the automatic diagnosis of OSA.

Body positions in sleep posture can be classified into supine, lateral and prone positions. Supine and lateral positions are dominant postures in adults, but children and infants may have prone positions [19]. Many patients with OSA exhibit worsening event indices while supine. Since supine OSA has been recognized to be the dominant phenotype of the OSA syndrome [20], objective and automatic position monitoring becomes very important because of the unreliability of patient's self-report of positions [21,22].

2.2. Contact Sensors for Sleep Analysis

The screening of sleep is typically obtrusive using contact sensors, like biosensors, accelerometers, wrist watches, and headbands [5]. Contact sensors have to be worn on user's body, have possible skin irritations and may disturb sleep. Saturation signal of oxygen in the arteries obtained through oximetry measurement or pulse oximetry is very effective for OSA diagnosis. Another attempt has been carried out by considering thoracic and abdominal signals, e.g., the respiration waveform. The use of EEG and ECG signals for the detection of sleep-wake and breathing apnea is a well-known standard. Actigraphy is a commonly used technique for sleep monitoring that uses a watch-like accelerometer based device attached typically to the wrist. The device monitors activities and later labels periods of low activity as sleep. It is a headband that users need to wear each night so that it can detect sleep patterns through the electrical signals naturally produced by the brain. The pressure sensitive mattress is an interestingly alternative of contact-based approach to identify occurrence of sleep movements [23]. It can monitor change in body pressure on the pad to detect movements. The main advantage of the pressure sensitive mattress is that users do not need to wear any device. But, it is a high-cost device and in some cases it may be uncomfortable to sleep on the pad and thus, they can affect sleep quality.

Sleep pose can be recognized by a contact-based approach [24]. Accelerometer [25], RFID [26], and pressure sensors [27] are used to acquire raw motion data of human, and inference sleep state from the motion data. While these methods are appropriate for sleep healthcare, their raw motion data is insufficient for accurate classification of sleep pose. More abundant data of human motions acquired by imaging sensors with both spatial and temporal information should greatly benefit sleep pose recognition.

2.3. Noncontact Sensors for Sleep Behavior Analysis

Noncontact approach usually employs imaging sensors to noninvasively detect sleep behaviors. The methods with microwave [28] and thermal imaging system [29] are advantageous to see through the bed covering to detect body movement. However, these imaging modalities are expensive, not portable, and is unable to perform long-time nocturnal video recording. More works adopted NIR camera [30,31] and computer vision techniques to extract body movement and chest respiration. The use of a NIR video camera to analyze movement patterns of a sleeping subject promises an attractive alternative.

Sleep posture has been analyzed in some studies. The system [12] detects posture change of the subject in bed by observing chest or blanket movement, and uses optical flow to evaluate the frequency of posture change. Wang and Hunter [14,15] addressed the problem of detecting and segmenting the covered human body using infrared vision. Their aim was to specifically tailor their algorithms for sleep monitoring scenarios where head, torso and upper legs may be occluded. No high-level posture is automatically classified. Yang et al. [13] proposed a neural network method to recognize the sleep postures. However, only edges detected by linear filters are applied as movement features of human body for the neural classifier, and recognition results were not satisfied. Liao and Kuo [16] proposed a video-based sleep monitoring system with background modeling approaches for extracting movement data. Since a NIR camera is often employed to monitor night-time activities in low illumination environment without disturbing the sleeper, the image noise can be quite prominent especially in regions containing smooth textures. They investigated and modeled the lighting changes by proposing a local ternary pattern based background subtraction method. However, none of these methods recognize positions of sleep body, especially supine and lateral positions that are strongly related to OSA. High-level postures can be robustly recognized by the modeling of articulated human joints.

Motion and texture features used for sleep pose recognition are sensitive to image degradation. Enhancing images before feature extraction [32] by recovering illumination, reducing noise and increasing contrast, can greatly improve the distinctness of features and increase detection and recognition accuracy [33]. Nonlinear filters, for example Retinex, have been successfully applied on many computer vision tasks [34] instead of vision based sleep analysis.

2.4. Pose Recognition by Computer Vision

Computer vision-based methods have been proposed for human pose recognition as a non-intrusive approach to capture human behavior with broad applications ranging from human computer interfaces, video data mining, automated surveillance, and sport training to fall detection. Appearance-based approach that directly adopts color, edge and silhouettes features for the classification of human poses has been widely applied [35]. However, nonrigid variations produced by limbs movement and body deformation make it difficult to the classification by appearance features. Joint-based approach [36] on the other way builds a structured human model by detected joints and/or body parts from low-level features, and then recognize poses by the structured human model. This approach tolerates not only high deformation but also self-occlusion issues in human poses.

Sleep poses are also highly deformable and partial occlusion often occurs. They should be tackled by joint-based approach [14]. Apart from partial occlusion, it is likely that limited motion information is available from partial and irregular movements, which seriously affects the usability of traditional feature extraction methods.

Local features such as scale invariant feature transform (SIFT) [37] and Speeded Up Robust Features (SURF) [38] are a new design scheme for salient feature representation of human postures. Its success on numerous computer vision problems has been well demonstrated [39]. Here we give only some examples of applying SIFT on action recognition. Scovanner et al. [40] proposed a 3D SIFT feature to better represent human actions. Wang et al. and Zhang et al. [41,42] applied SIFT flow to extract keypoint-based movement features between image frames and obtain better classification results than the features such as histogram of oriented gradients and histogram of optical flows. Local features have superior representability not only for visible-band images but also for NIR images. The paper [43] gave a comprehensive study of the robustness of four keypoint detectors for the three spectra: near infrared, far infrared and visible spectra. Robustness are demonstrated that performance of the four detectors is remaining for all the three spectra, although these interest point detectors were originally proposed for visual-band images. While these papers show the advantages of local features, it is still not easy to get articulated structure of human joints by local features.

In summary, sleep behavior is important and can be analyzed by non-contact approaches to achieve unobtrusive methods. NIR video analysis for sleep posture is challenging but innovative. A summary table of the reviews from related works is given in Table 1.

Table 1. Summary of reviews from related works.

Critical Points	Arguments
Sleep behavior is important to OSA diagnosis	• Body movements are an important behavior for sleep diagnosis • Body position is correlated to sleep apnea • Sleep behavior including body movements and body positions are relevant to OSA • Supine position is a critical posture
Non-contact and unobtrusive analysis are advantageous but have challenges	• Contact sensros have been well developed for sleep diagnosis • Non-contact imaging sensors are unobtrusive and better than contact sensors • NIR is a good non-contact sensor with many advantages • Challenges of NIR video analysis for sleep analysis are nonuniform illumination processing and nonrigid body deformation
Motivation of this paper	• Retinex is a nonlinear filter that could be applied to improve the NIR videos with nonuniform illumination • Joint-based methods are an important approach to traditional posture recognition in computer vision • Keypoints methods such as SIFT could be applied to joint-based posture recogntion

3. Sleep Pose Recognition

The proposed method analyzes near-infrared videos to recognize sleep poses by body joint model. The near-infrared images are first enhanced by an illumination compensation algorithm to improve the quality of feature extraction. SIFT-based local features are employed to perform joint detection of human body. Poses are recognized with a Bayesian inference algorithm to solve the occlusion issue.

A novel idea is developed for the joint detection and modeling in our method. One basic idea is that it becomes usual to delicately customize some bedding materials to facilitate more accurate monitoring, such as the mattress pad sensor. Therefore, we propose an unobtrusive passive way by revamping pajamas with NIR sensitive fabrics around the joint positions of human body. The fabrics that is sensitive to NIR light source can reflect more lights and show high intensity values in NIR images. With the NIR-sensitive fabrics we get more visual information of body joints and are able to detect and recognize sleep poses. Figure 1 gives an illustration of our design. There are ten joints that are common for posture and action recognition. We make ten NIR-sensitive patches with special fabrics sewing on pajamas.

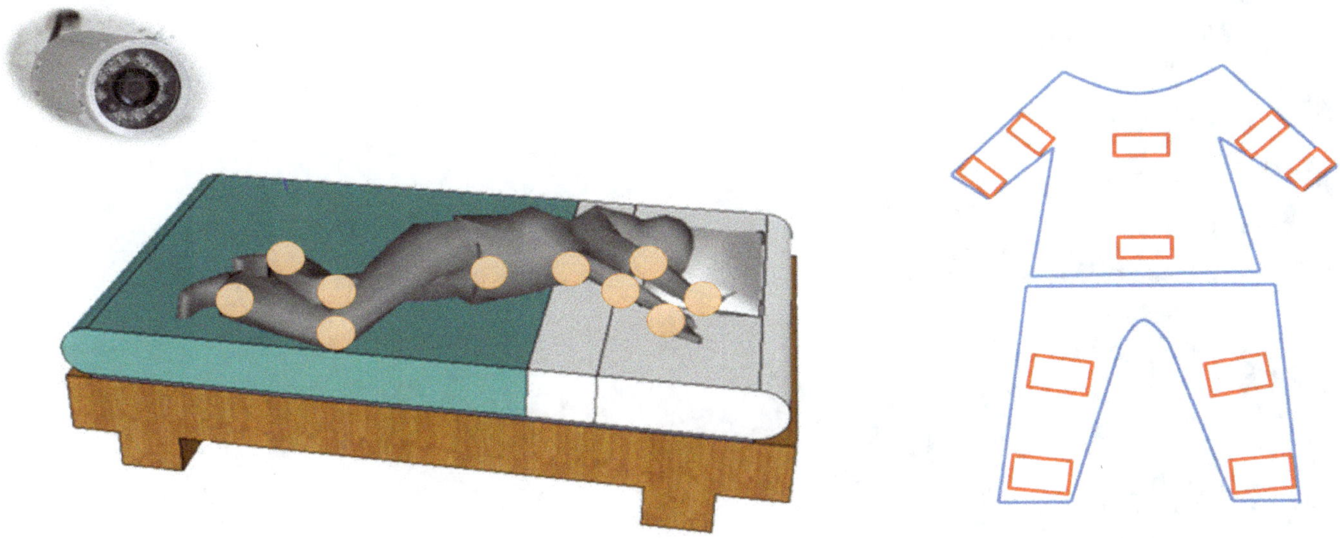

Figure 1. The proposed scheme for sleep pose recognition. (**a**) An infrared camera is used to acquire the sleep videos and analyze body joint positions. (**b**) Pajamas with ten near infrared (NIR)-sensitive patches are designed to facilitate the detection of body joints.

Another issue of the proposed method is to distinguish different joints. We apply the concept in augmented reality to design fiducial markers in order to not only reliably detect each joint, but also easily distinguish all joints. A fiducial marker supplements with image features originating in salient points of the image. However, we need to design a fiducial marker system that consists of a set of distinguishable markers to encode different joints. Desirable properties of the marker system are low false positive and false negative rates, as well as low inter-marker confusion rates. We adopt the markers designed in the paper [44] that derives the optimal design of fiducial markers specially for SIFT and SURF. Its markers are highly detectable even under dramatically varying imaging conditions.

3.1. *Near-Infrared Image Enhancement*

An illumination compensation algorithm [45] that includes single-scale Retinex and alpha-trimming histogram stretching is applied to enhance the NIR video. SSR is a nonlinear filter to improve lightness rendition of the images without uniform illumination. However, SSR does not improve contrast. The histogram stretching with alpha-trimming is then followed to improve contrast. Let I_t be an NIR image at time t and I'_t is the enhanced result, our image enhancement algorithm is a composition function of three successive steps as follows:

$$I' = m(f(R(I))), \text{ where } R(I) = \log(I) - \log(G(c) \otimes I). \tag{1}$$

$R(\cdot)$ is the SSR, $f(\cdot)$ is the alpha-trimming histogram stretching, and $m(\cdot)$ is a median filter for denoising. The SSR function $R(\cdot)$ uses a Gaussian convolution kernel $G(c)$ with size c to compute the scale of illuminant, and enhance the image by log-domain processing. The alpha-trimming histogram stretching applies a gray-level mapping that extends the range of gray levels into the whole dynamic range. Median filter is applied to eliminate the shot noise in the NIR images. The effect of the enhancement is majorly influenced by the size of Gaussian kernel size c. Figure 2 illustrates the influence with different kernel sizes. The original image has uneven illumination. The image in Figure 2b is still dark and the contrast of human body is low. It also has white artifact around image boundary. Figure 2f has better illumination compensation effect, better contrast on human body, and less artifact.

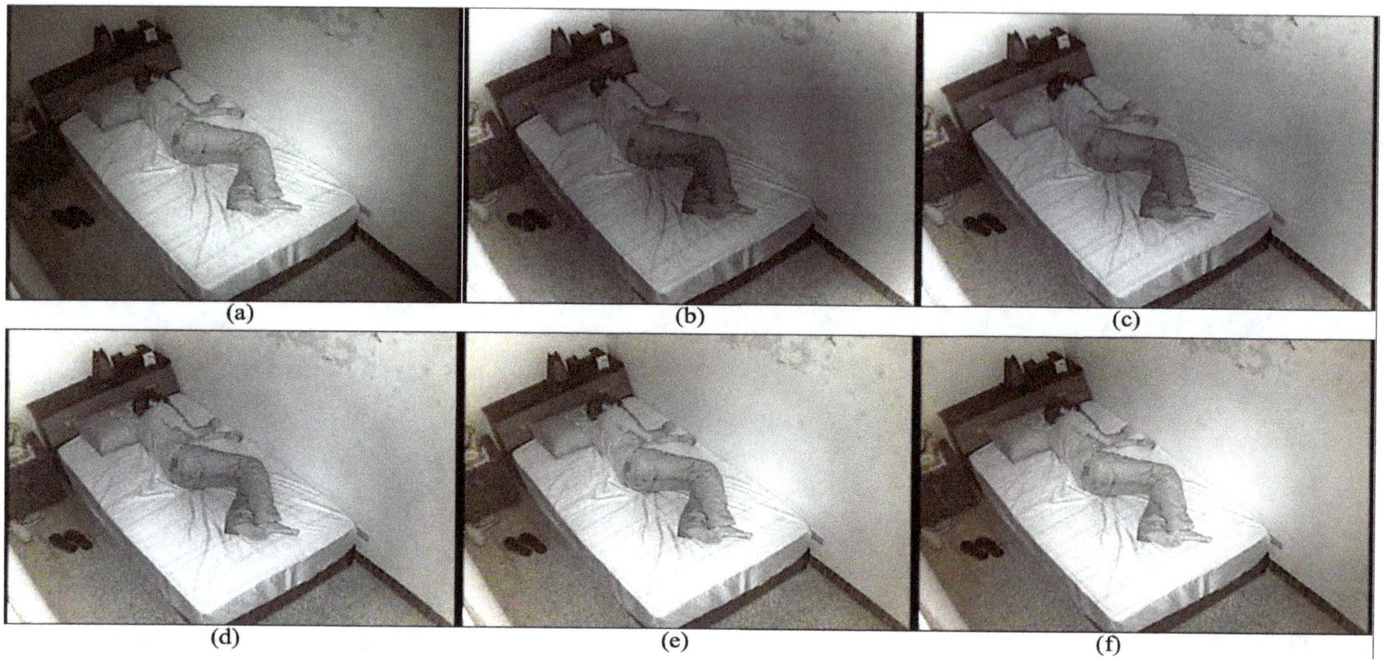

Figure 2. Enhanced NIR images with different Gaussian kernel sizes from 50 to 250. (**a**) Original image. (**b**) $c = 50$. (**c**) $c = 100$. (**d**) $c = 150$. (**e**) $c = 200$. (**f**) $c = 250$.

3.2. Detection and Tracking of Human Joints by Distinctive Invariant Feature

We propose a SIFT-based joint detection algorithm to detect joints in the first image, and a structured online learning to track those detected joints in the video. The SIFT analyzes an input image at multiple scales in order to repeatedly find characteristic blob-like structures independently of their actual size in an image. It first applies multiscale detection operators to analyze the so called scale space representation of an image. In a second step, detected features are assigned a rotation-invariant descriptor computed from the surrounding pixel neighborhood. The detail of applying SIFT to detect human joints is described in the following.

Given an enhanced image I'_t at time t and a set of joint markers M_i, i = 1~10, we apply SIFT to extract keypoint features of I'_t and M_i, and compute the correspondence set C_i to find all joints. The keypoints of I'_t is represented as a sparse set $X_t = \{x_t^j\}$ that is called image descriptor. The keypoints of M_i is a set $Y_i = \{y_i^k\}$ that is called a joint model descriptor. A correspondence set $C_i = \{(x_t^j, y_i^k) | s(x_t^j, y_i^k) > \tau\}$ is obtained for each joint marker M_i, where $s(\cdot,\cdot)$ is the matching score and τ is a matching threshold. The matching between X_t and Y_i is done by a best-bin-first search that returns the closest neighbor with the highest probability with pairwise geometric constraints. The set of matched joints $\widehat{J}$ is a set of joint coordinates J_i defined as follows:

$$\widehat{J} = \{J_i \mid J_i = median(C_i) \ and \ |C_i| > \alpha\} \tag{2}$$

where σ is a threshold of minimum number of matched keypoints. A matched joint requires enough matched keypoints, i.e., $|C_i| > \sigma$. The coordinates of the ith are calculated as the median coordinates from $x_t^j \in C_i$ to screen outlier of keypoint-based joint detection, which can reduce the distance error of joint. While the keypoint-based matching is robust to illumination, rotation and scale variance, some joints may not be detected because of occlusion. That is, some joints are not detected if $|\widehat{J}| < 10$.

An example of keypoint detection is shown in Figure 3a. Most detected keypoints are clustered together around joint markers, that demonstrates the image descriptor X_t is a salient representation of the set of joint markers. Figure 3b shows an example of joint detection. The joint marker is shown at the left top of the image. These lines represent matched keypoints between the joint marker and the visual marker in the pajamas.

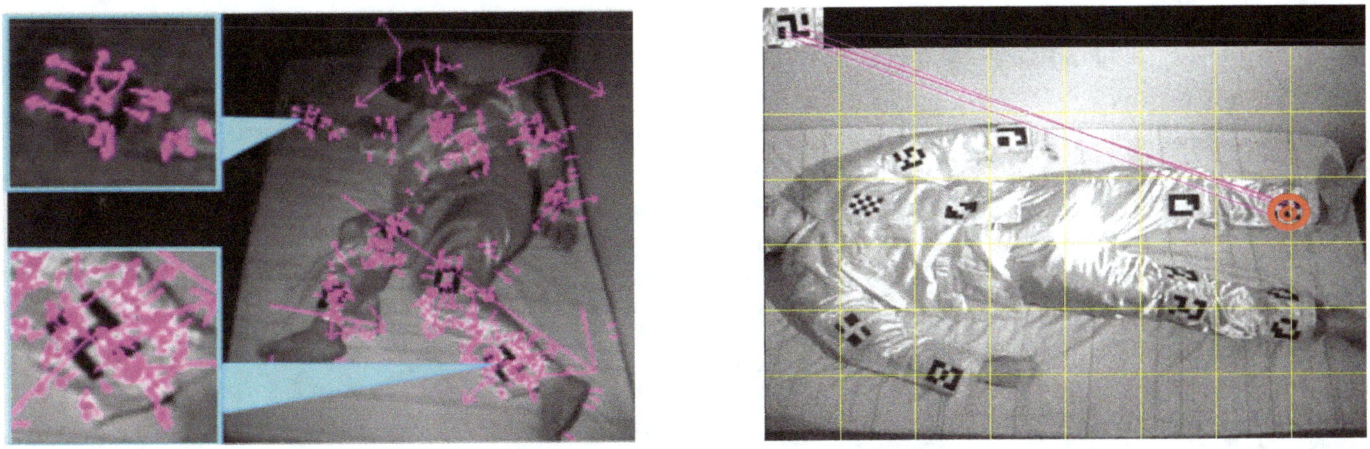

(a) (b)

Figure 3. Keypoint detection and joint detection. (**a**) Image descriptor of an original lateral-pose image overlaid with keypoints of length and orientation information. Each arrow represents one detected keypoint. (**b**) A joint detection example for left ankle. It is detected by matching a specific joint marker representing the left ankle with a visual marker in the sleep image.

A structured output prediction with online learning method [46] is applied to perform adaptive keypoint tracking of the human joints. It is used for homography estimation of correspondence between frames and binary approximation of model. Structured output prediction is handled by applying RANSAC to find the transformation of the correspondence. To speed up the detection and description process, we adopt SURF instead of SIFT. This is achieved by not only relying on integral images for image convolutions but applying a Hessian matrix-based measurement for the detector and a distribution-based descriptor.

3.3. Sleep Pose Estimation by Bayesian Inference

The sleep pose model is mathematically formulated as a Bayesian network, and the estimation of pose class is achieved by probabilistically inferencing the posterior distribution of the network.

Bayesian network combining probability theory and graphical model for statistical inference is employed in this paper because of its great robustness capability with missing information. That is, pose class can be inferred even when there are undetected joints.

Our sleep pose model is a Bayesian network G with one root node representing the state of pose and ten child nodes J_i, $1 \leq i \leq 10$, corresponding to the states of joints. This network gives a probabilistic model to represent the causal relationship between sleep pose and joint positions: a given pose affects the positions of joints, and thus the pose can be inferred by Bayesian theory from a given set of joint positions. The property of conditional independence exists in this naïve model and is helpful for the inference of poses.

Let the undetected and detected joint sets be individually represented by U and $\widehat{J}$. The conditional posterior distribution of p given $\widehat{J}$ can be derived as follows:

$$P(p|J_1, \cdots, J_{10}) = \pi \textstyle\sum_{J_i \in U} \prod_{J_i \in \widehat{J}} P(p|J_i), \tag{3}$$

where π is the prior probability $P(p, J_1, ..., J_{10})$ that is in the form of full joint probability. The estimated sleep pose $\widehat{p}$ is the maximum a posterior (MAP) estimate given by the following:

$$\widehat{p} = arg\ max\ P(p|J_1, \cdots, J_{10}), \tag{4}$$

Both approximate and exact inference algorithms can be applied for the MAP calculation of our sleep pose model. While approximate inference algorithms are usually more efficient than exact inference algorithms, our sleep pose model could be solved more efficiently with exact inference approach. We employ clique-tree propagation algorithm [47] that first transforms the Bayesian model into undirected graph, then use query-driven message passing to update the statistical distribution of each node.

An example of sleep pose estimation is shown in Figure 4, which is a lateral pose with fully detected joints. The reconstructed human model is depicted with a cardboard representation.

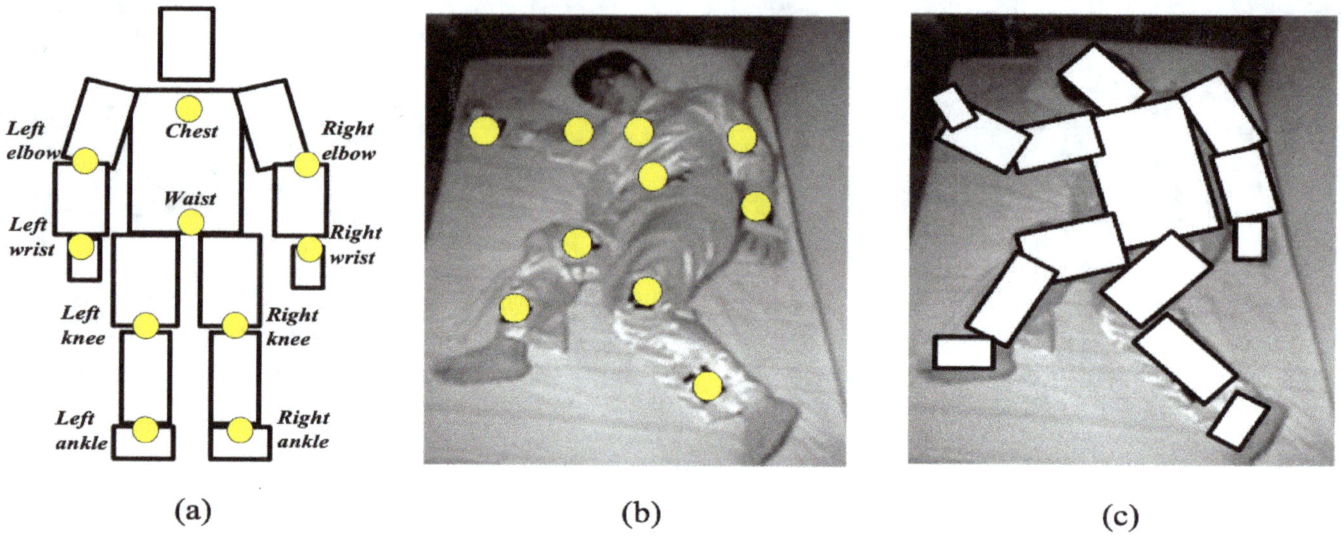

Figure 4. An example of reconstructed human model by fully detected joints. (**a**) A standard model with a standing pose. (**b**) A sleep image overlaid with the detected/tracked joints found by keypoint match and structured learning. (**c**) Reconstructed model of the lateral pose.

4. Experimental Results

We evaluated these components in our method: near-infrared image enhancement, joint detection and pose recognition. Accuracy and performance compared with existing methods are conducted and discussed. Two individual setups of experiments were established. The first setup was established to evaluate the efficacy of near-infrared image enhancement, whose accuracy was assessed by total sleep time (TST) measured from the sleep–wake detection results obtained after the enhancing of images. The second setup is built for joint detection and pose recognition. The detection of ten joints is assessed by pixel difference of joint positions, and the recognition of supine/lateral poses are assessed by classification precision.

The experimental setups were conducted in a sleep laboratory equipped with a PSG, near-infrared cameras and related instruments. The PSG was adopted to obtain ground truth. A full-channel PSG (E-Series, Compumedics Ltd., Melbourne, Australia) was employed to record overnight brain wave activity (electroencephalography from C3-M2, C4-M1), eye movements (left and right electrooculogram), electrocardiography, leg movements (left and right piezoelectric leg paddles), and airflow (oral/nasal thermister). The near-infrared video has the resolution of 640 * 480 pixels with the frame rate of 20 fps.

4.1. *Effectiveness of Near-Infrared Image Enhancement*

In this subsection, the assessment of image enhancement is carefully created from sleep experiments, because there is still no objective criteria to evaluate the quality of near-infrared images. Since our goal is to build a computer-vision based sleep evaluation system, it is reasonable to adopt a sleep quality criteria, TST, obtained in a sleep experiment to evaluate our image enhancement component. TST is the amount of actual sleep time including REM and NREM phases in a sleep episode; this time is equal to the total sleep episode less the awake time.

In this first sleep setup, eighteen subjects involved in the experiments are divided into two groups, including a normal group without a sleep disorder and an OSA group with sleep disorder. Table 2 gives statistics of the subjects in the two groups. From the data we confirmed that these subjects have only OSA symptom and have no PLM problems, because the means of body mass index and PLM are statistically identical, and the OSA group has higher RDI and lower sleep efficiency.

Table 2. Statistics of the two groups in the sleep-wake detection experiment. SD means standard deviation. RDI (respiratory disturbance index) is the number of abnormal breathing events per hour of sleep. PLM (periodic leg movements) is the number during nocturnal sleep and wakefulness. Sleep efficiency is the proportion of sleep in the episode, i.e., the ratio of total sleep time (TST) to the time in bed.

		Age	Body Mass Index	RDI	PLM	Sleep Efficiency
Normal group	Mean	42.63	24.39	4.23	1.28	91.44
	SD	14.37	4.18	2.44	1.61	4.7
OSA group	Mean	51.1	24.99	35.85	1.43	84.22
	SD	15.25	2.69	21.68	3.03	12.3

Both PSG data and IR videos were recorded overnight for each subject. Sleep stages were scored using the standard AASM criteria with thirty-second epochs. Obstructive apneas were identified if the airflow amplitude was absent or nearly absent for the duration at least eight seconds and two breaths cycles. A well-trained sleep technician was responsible for configuring the PSG for each subject. The ground truth of sleep state is manually labeled by the sleep experts working in hospital. The ground truth of the TST is obtained by the total sleep time calculated from the manual annotation.

Estimated TST is obtained from near-infrared videos by a process including the proposed image enhancement, followed by background subtraction and sleep-wake detection. We extract body movement information from the motion feature obtained from background subtraction. A statistical differencing operator is applied to measure the distance d_t between the enhanced infrared image I'_t and the previous background model B_{t-1} as follows:

$$d_t = |I'_t - B_{t-1}| \tag{5}$$

The background model B_{t-1} was recursively updated by the Gaussian mixture background subtraction method [48], and can successfully approximate the background of a given image which has a time-evolving model. The body movement BM_t at time t is obtained by accumulating the total motion pixels in d_t:

$$\begin{aligned} &BM_t = \textstyle\sum_x \sum_y M_t \\ &where\ M_t(x,y) = \begin{cases} 1, & if\ d_t(x,y) > threshold \\ 0, & otherwise \end{cases} \end{aligned} \tag{6}$$

Sleep activity feature was then calculated from BM_t by descriptive statistics such as mean, standard deviation and maximum, defined over an epoch of 30 s. Sleep activity is obtained by the sleep-wake detection algorithm that is modeled by the linear regression [49] of the sleep activity feature.

The proposed image enhancement algorithm is first qualitatively compared with four classical methods: histogram stretching, histogram equlization, gamma correction and single-scale Retinex, with regard to illumination uniformity and contrast. Figure 5b–d show the results of three global enhancement methods with raised image contrast, but the middle of these images is over-exposed. Figure 5e is the result of SSR filtering with uniform illumination but low image contrast. Figure 5f show the result of the proposed method that can solve both non-uniform illumination and low contrast issues.

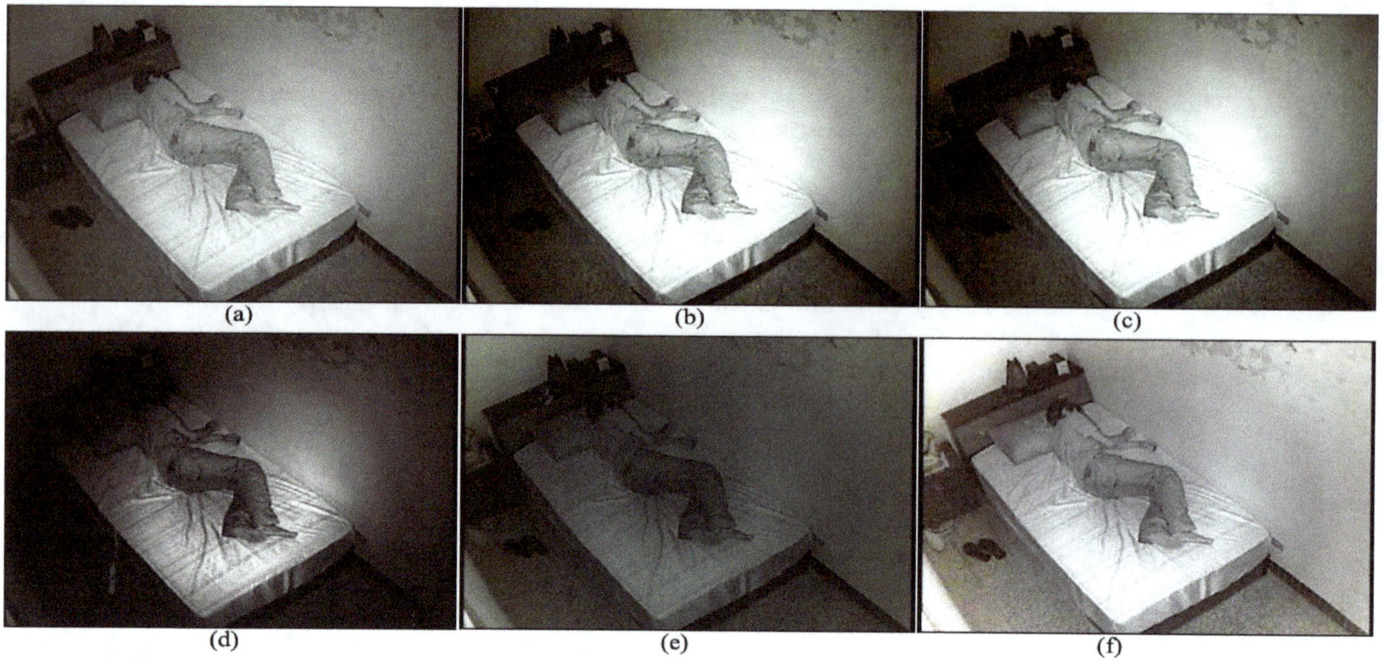

Figure 5. Enhancement of NIR images. (**a**) Original image. (**b**) Histogram stretching. (**c**) Histogram equalization. (**d**) Gamma correction. (**e**) Single-scale Retinex. (**f**) The proposed illumination compensation method.

Quantitative assessment of the proposed method was achieved by an index called TST error E_{TST}, that is defined as the normalized difference between estimated TST and ground truth of TST.

$$E_{TST} = \frac{|Estimated\ TST - Ground\ truth\ TST|}{Ground\ truth\ TST} \quad (7)$$

Its value is between [0,1]. Lower E_{TST} means better performance of our method.

The performance for a normal group with respect to three different sleep activity features, MA (moving average), MS (moving standard deviation), and MM (moving maximum), is shown in Figure 6. The three performances without image enhancement are not statistically differential. However, the performances with image enhancement are consistently lower than those without enhancement, and MA with image enhancement has the best performance.

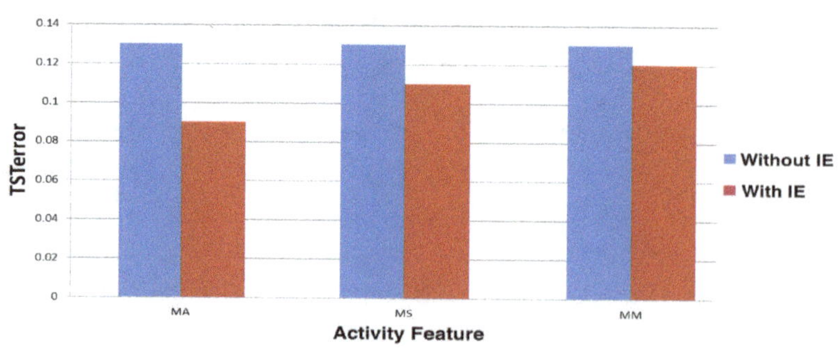

Figure 6. Effect of image enhancement (IE) for the performance improvement of the error of total sleep time.

The performance comparison of using image enhancement with respect to normal and OSA groups is shown in Table 3. MA is adopted as the only sleep activity feature in this comparison. Specificity (SPC) and negative predictive value (NPC) are also calculated for performance comparison. We can observe that while normal group has better performances with less standard deviation, OSA group still has good performances.

Table 3. Effect of image enhancement (IE) for the performance improvement of the error of total sleep time.

		E_{TST}	SPC	NPV
Normal group	Mean	0.09	0.95	0.91
	STD	0.16	0.04	0.10
OSA group	Mean	0.15	0.93	0.84
	STD	0.18	0.19	0.21

4.2. Evaluation of Pose Recognition

The second experiment has five subjects of various gender, height and weight wearing the custom pajamas and sleeping with free postures. Ten video clips were recorded with respect to the episodes of supine and lateral poses of various limb angles and occlusion. Half clips are randomly chosen for training of the classifier, and the remaining half for test. Ground truth of body positions and joint positions are manually labeled. The pose recognition in this experiment will not detect sleep and wake states. Therefore, background subtraction and sleep-wake detection algorithms are excluded, and the method in this experiment will include the three components in Section 3: image enhancement, joint detection and pose recognition. However, only the effectiveness of joint detection and pose recognition is validated here.

Figure 7 gives some example results of joint detection with respect to various poses. The positions of IR-markers are marked on the original image to evaluate the effectiveness of the proposed method. Some quantitative experiments are conducted to evaluate the localization accuracy of the proposed method. Figure 8a shows the effect of the threshold of matched keypoint numbers (σ) on detected joint numbers. High precision can be obtained with $\sigma = 1$. This result indicates that the design of joint markers is distinctive and so the joint localization does not need to match more numbers of keypoints. Figure 8b shows average detection rate of each joint position with mostly achieving high accuracy. The detection of right knee joint is a little not satisfactory because of perspective variations. Euclidean distance errors of each joint position is shown in Figure 8c. The average error of all joints is 6.57 pixels. The result indicates higher error in both ankle joints.

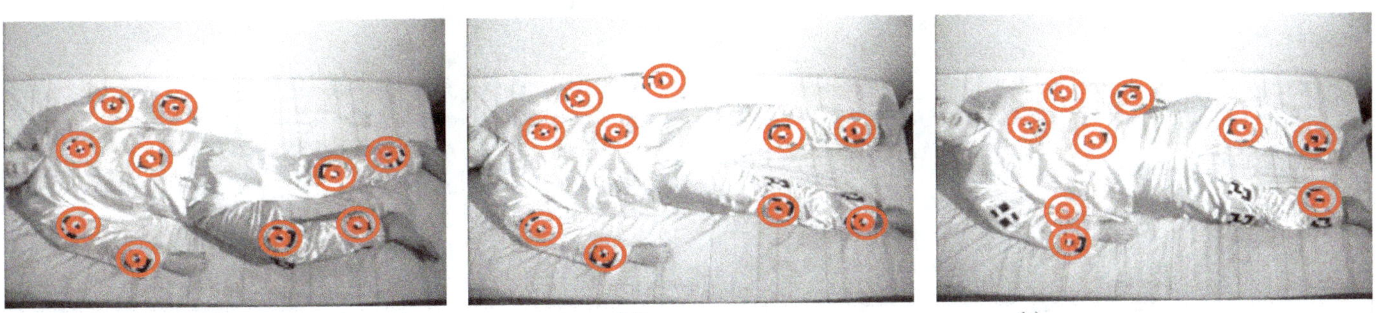

(a) (b) (c)

Figure 7. Examples of joint detection results. Each double-red circle represents a detected joint. (**a**) Lateral pose with ten successful detections. (**b**) Supine pose with ten successful detections. (**c**) Supine pose with eight successful detections. The right-knee and right-elbow joints are missed because of great distortion induced by perspective and cloth's wrinkles.

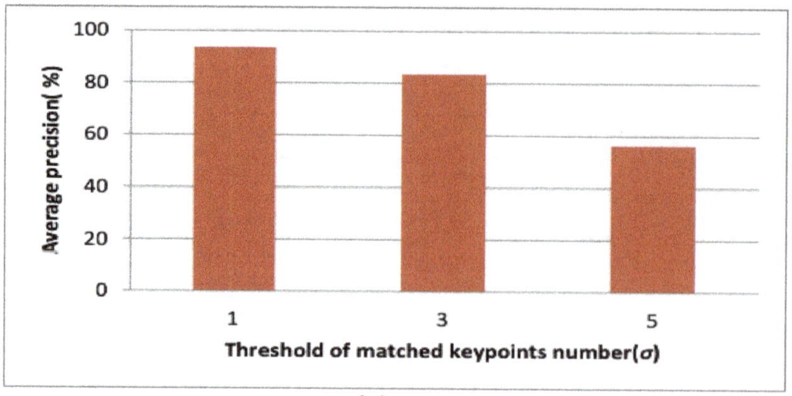

(a)

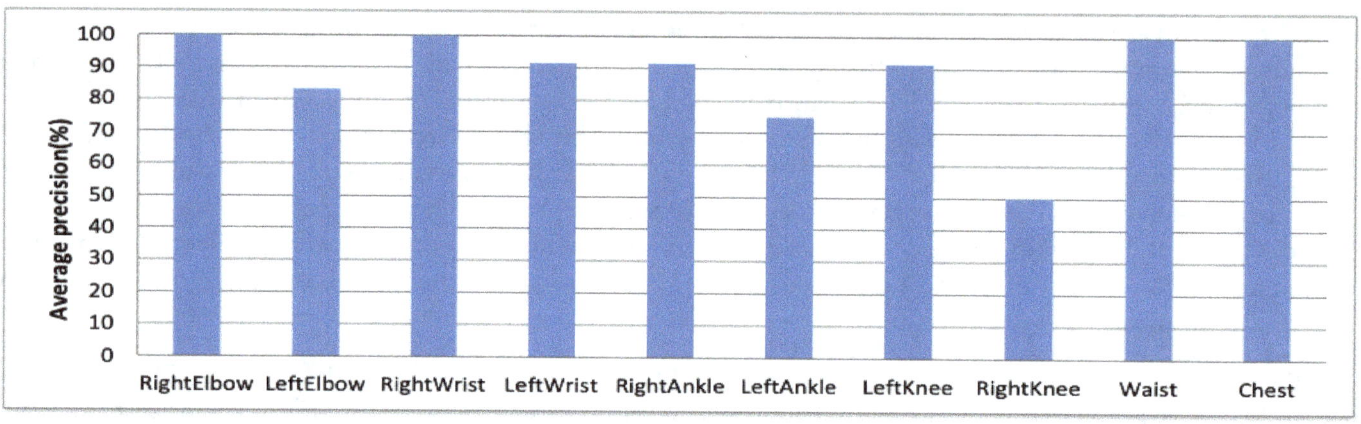

(b)

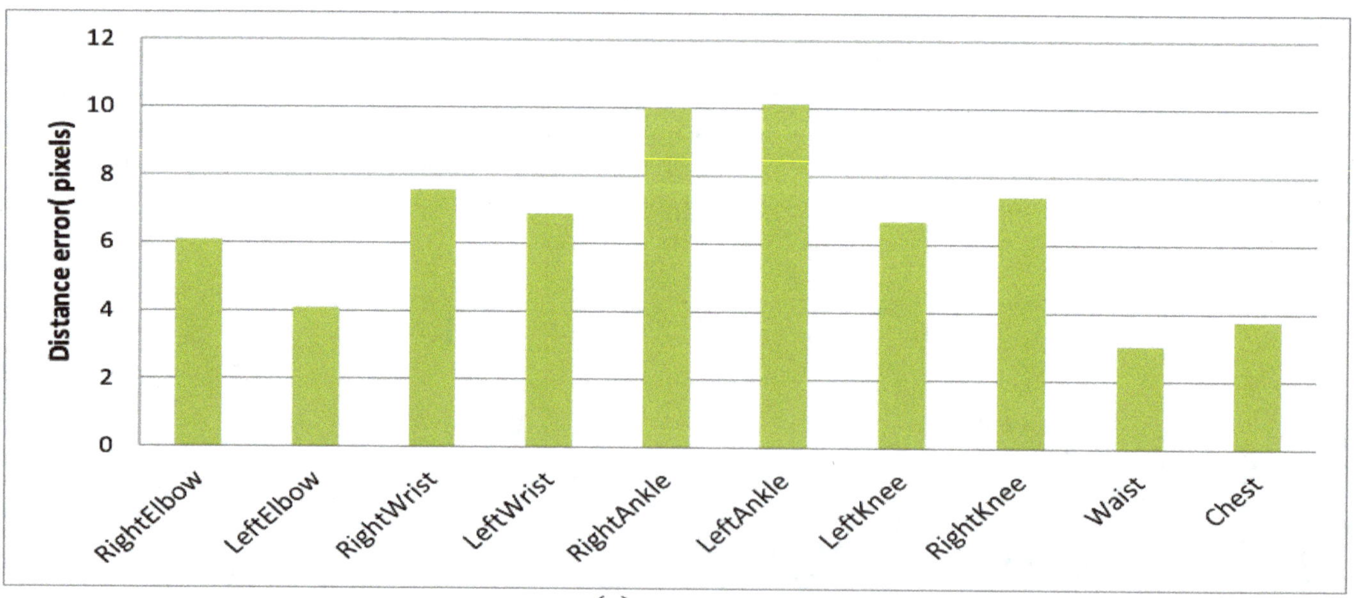

(c)

Figure 8. Accuracy evaluation. (**a**) The effect of the threshold of matched keypoint numbers. (**b**) Average precision of joint localization. (**c**) Average distance error of joint localization.

The performance of the proposed sleep pose model with clique-tree propagation inference was evaluated by comparing with five inference algorithms. Four are approximate algorithms: stochastic sampling, likelihood sampling, self-importance sampling, and backward sampling, and one exact algorithm: loop cutset conditioning. Figure 9 show execution and precision of the six algorithms. The result shows that clique-tree propagation algorithm takes the least time to achieve the best precision.

The positive predictive value, negative predictive value, specificity and sensitivity of the proposed method are 80%, 71%, 63% and 86%.

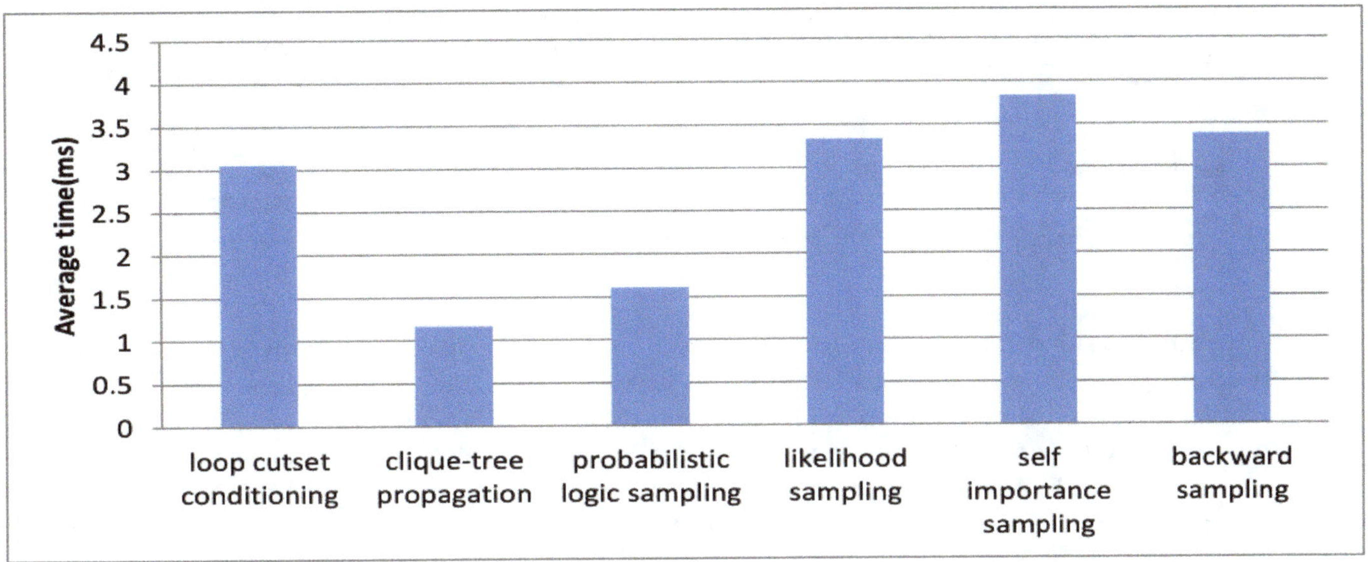

(a)

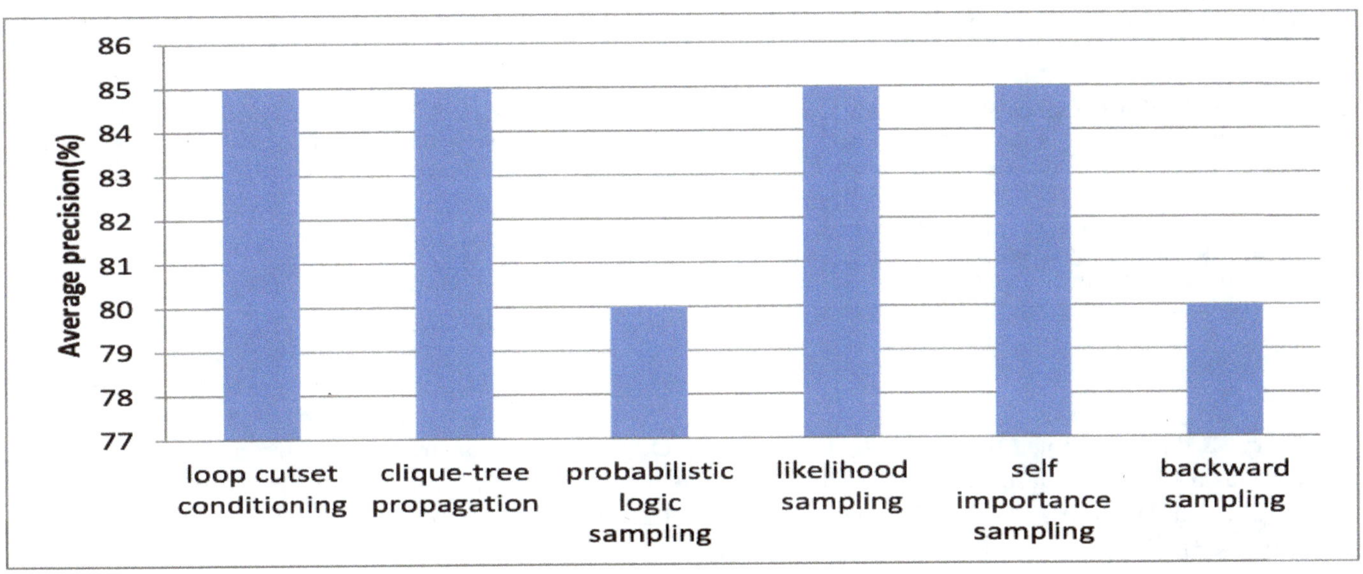

(b)

Figure 9. Comparison of six inference algorithms with respect to (**a**) execution time, and (**b**) accuracy.

The experimental results are compared with previous results: RTPose [14], MatchPose [15] and Ramanan [50]. The comparison is shown in Table 4. The previous results are obtained from their published publications. The results of our method were always superior than previous results except to right knee. Note that the accuracy of torso and head of our method are obtained from chest and waist, and the accuracy of ankles and knees in the table correspond to the lower legs and upper legs in previous publications.

Table 4. Comparisons with previous results. The numbers represent accuracy in percentage. N/A means the data are not available from their methods.

	Torso	Right Ankle	Left Ankle	Right Knee	Left Knee	Right Elbow	Left Elbow	Right Wrist	Left Wrist	Head
Ramanan	80	60	53	60	37	N/A	N/A	N/A	N/A	53
RTPose	93	N/A	N/A	70	80	N/A	N/A	N/A	N/A	80
MatchPose	97	45	69	75	80	N/A	N/A	N/A	N/A	94
Our	100	92	75	50	92	100	83	100	92	100

5. Conclusions

An automatic sleep pose recognition method from NIR videos is proposed in this paper. The method proposes keypoint-based joint detection and online tracking to persistently locate joint positions. Sleep poses are recognized from located joints by statistical inference with the proposed Bayesian network. Our method detects and tracks the human joints of great variations and occlusions with high precision. Experimental results validate the accuracy of the method for both supine and lateral poses. Further studies could incorporate more non-invasive sensors to develop a cheap and convenient sleep monitoring system for home care with long-term stability. With the reliable method proposed in this paper, an enhanced pajamas for home sleep monitoring can be further developed by costume designers.

Author Contributions: Conceptualization, Y.-K.W.; Funding acquisition, Y.-K.W.; Investigation, H.-Y.C.; Project administration, Y.-K.W.; Resources, Y.-K.W.; Software, J.-R.C.; Supervision, H.-Y.C.; Validation, H.-Y.C.; Visualization, H.-Y.C.; Writing—original draft, J.-R.C. and H.-Y.C.; Writing—review and editing, Y.-K.W.

Acknowledgments: This research is jointly supported by the Sleep Center at Shin Kong Wu Ho-Su Memorial Hospital, Taiwan. The authors gratefully acknowledge the support of Chia-Mo Lin and Hou-Chang Chiu for their valuable comments in obstructive sleep apnea.

References

1. Berry, R.B.; Budhiraja, R.; Gottlieb, D.J.; Gozal, D.; Iber, C.; Kapur, V.K.; Marcus, C.L.; Mehra, R.; Parthasarathy, S.; Quan, S.F.; et al. Rules for scoring respiratory events in sleep: Update of the 2007 AASM manual for the scoring of sleep and associated events. *J. Clin. Sleep Med.* **2012**, *8*, 597–619. [CrossRef] [PubMed]
2. Procházka, A. Sleep scoring using polysomnography data features. *Signal Image Video Process.* **2018**, *12*, 1043–1051.
3. Roebuck, A.; Monasterio, V.; Gederi, E.; Osipov, M.; Behar, J.; Malhotra, A.; Penzel, T.; Clifford, G.D. A review of signals used in sleep analysis. *Physiol. Meas.* **2014**, *35*, 1–57. [CrossRef] [PubMed]
4. Park, K.S.; Choi, S.H. Smart Technologies Toward Sleep Monitoring at Home. *Biomed. Eng. Lett.* **2019**, *9*, 73–85. [CrossRef] [PubMed]
5. Sivan, Y.; Kornecki, A.; Schonfeld, T. Screening obstructive sleep apnoea syndrome by home videotape recording in children. *Eur. Respir. J.* **1996**, *9*, 2127–2131. [CrossRef] [PubMed]
6. Schwichtenberg, A.J.; Choe, J.; Kellerman, A.; Abel, E.; Delp, E.J. Pediatric videosomnography: Can signal/video processing distinguish sleep and wake states? *Front. Pediatr.* **2018**, *6*, 158. [CrossRef] [PubMed]
7. Scatena, M. An integrated video-analysis software system de-signed for movement detection and sleep analysis. Validation of a tool for the behavioural study of sleep. *Clin. Neurophysiol.* **2012**, *123*, 318–323. [CrossRef] [PubMed]
8. Kuo, Y.M.; Lee, J.S.; Chung, P.C. A visual context-awareness-based sleeping-respiration measurement system. *IEEE Trans. Inf. Technol. Biomed.* **2010**, *14*, 255–265. [PubMed]

9. Cuppens, K.; Lagae, L.; Ceulemans, B.; Huffel, S.V.; Vanrumste, B. Automatic video detection of body movement during sleep based on optical flow in pediatric patients with epilepsy. *Med. Biol. Eng. Comput.* **2010**, *48*, 923–931. [CrossRef]
10. Choe, J.; Schwichtenberg, A.J.; Delp, E.J. Classification of sleep videos using deep learning. In Proceedings of the IEEE Conference on Multimedia Information Processing and Retrieval, San Jose, CA, USA, 28–30 March 2019; pp. 115–120.
11. Wang, Y.K.; Chen, J.R.; Chen, H.Y. Sleep pose recognition by feature matching and Bayesian inference. In Proceedings of the International Conference on Pattern Recognition, Stockholm, Sweden, 24–28 August 2014; pp. 24–28.
12. Nakajima, K.; Matsumoto, Y.; Tamura, T. Development of real-time image sequence analysis for evaluating posture change and respiratory rate of a subject in bed. *Physiol. Meas.* **2001**, *22*, 21–28. [CrossRef]
13. Yang, F.C.; Kuo, C.H.; Tsai, M.Y.; Huang, S.C. Image-based sleep motion recognition using artificial neural networks. In Proceedings of the International Conference on Machine Learning and Cybernetics, Xi'an, China, 5 November 2003; pp. 2775–2780.
14. Wang, C.W.; Hunter, A. Robust pose recognition of the obscured human body. *Int. J. Comput. Vis.* **2010**, *90*, 313–330. [CrossRef]
15. Wang, C.W.; Hunter, A.; Gravill, N.; Matusiewicz, S. Real time pose recognition of covered human for diagnosis of sleep apnoea. *Comput. Med. Imaging Graph.* **2010**, *34*, 523–533. [CrossRef] [PubMed]
16. Liao, W.H.; Kuo, J.H. Sleep monitoring system in real bedroom environment using texture-based background modeling approaches. *J. Ambient Intell. Humaniz. Comput.* **2013**, *4*, 57–66. [CrossRef]
17. Okada, S.; Ohno, Y.; Kenmizaki, K.; Tsutsui, A.; Wang, Y. Development of non-restrained sleep-monitoring method by using difference image processing. In Proceedings of the European Conference of the International Federation for Medical and Biological Engineering, Antwerp, Belgium, 23–27 November 2009; pp. 1765–1768.
18. Oksenberg, A.; Silverberg, D.S. The effect of body posture on sleep-related breathing disorders: Facts and therapeutic implications. *Sleep Med. Rev.* **1998**, *2*, 139–162. [CrossRef]
19. Isaiah, A.; Pereira, K.D. The effect of body position on sleep apnea in children. In *Positional Therapy in Obstructive Sleep Apnea*; Springer Nature Switzerland: Basel, Switzerland, 2014; Volume 14, pp. 151–161.
20. Joosten, S.A.; O'Driscoll, D.M.; Berger, P.J.; Hamilton, G.S. Supine position related obstructive sleep apnea in adults: Pathogenesis and treatment. *Sleep Med. Rev.* **2014**, *18*, 7–17. [CrossRef] [PubMed]
21. Russo, K.; Bianchi, M.T. How reliable is self-reported body position during sleep? *Sleep Med.* **2016**, *12*, 127–128. [CrossRef] [PubMed]
22. Ravesloot, M.J.L.; Maanen, J.P.V.; Dun, L.; de Vries, N. The undervalued potential of positional therapy in position-dependent snoring and obstructive sleep apnea—A review of the literature. *Sleep Breath.* **2013**, *17*, 39–49. [CrossRef] [PubMed]
23. Liu, J.J.; Xu, W.; Huang, M.C.; Alshurafa, N.; Sarrafzadeh, M.; Raut, N.; Yadegar, B. Sleep posture analysis using a dense pressure sensitive bedsheet. *Pervasive Mob. Comput.* **2014**, *10*, 34–50. [CrossRef]
24. Hossain, H.M.S.; Ramamurthy, S.R.; Khan, M.A.A.H.; Roy, N. An active sleep monitoring framework using wearables. *ACM Trans. Interact. Intell. Syst.* **2018**, *8*, 22. [CrossRef]
25. Foerster, F.; Smeja, M.; Fahrenberg, J. Detection of posture and motion by accelerometry: A validation study in ambulatory monitoring. *Comput. Hum. Behav.* **1999**, *15*, 571–583. [CrossRef]
26. Hoque, E.; Dickerson, R.F.; Stankovic, J.A. Monitoring body positions and movements during sleep using WISPs. In *Wireless Health*; ACM: New York, NY, USA, 2010; pp. 44–53.
27. van Der Loos, H.; Kobayashi, H.; Liu, G. Unobtrusive vital signs monitoring from a multisensor bed sheet. In Proceedings of the RESNA Conference, Reno, NV, USA, 22–26 June 2001.
28. Xiao, Y.; Lin, J.; Boric-Lubecke, O.; Lubecke, V.M. A Ka-band low power doppler radar system for remote de-tection of cardiopulmonary motion. In Proceedings of the 2005 IEEE Engineering in Medicine and Biology 27th Annual Conference, Shanghai, China, 17–18 January 2005; pp. 7151–7154.
29. Bak, J.U.; Giakoumidis, N.; Kim, G.; Dong, H.; Mavridis, N. An intelligent sensing system for sleep motion and stage analysis. *Procedia Eng.* **2012**, *41*, 1128–1134. [CrossRef]
30. Sadeh, A. Sleep assessment methods. *Monogr. Soc. Res. Child Dev.* **2015**, *80*, 33–48. [CrossRef] [PubMed]
31. Deng, F.; Dong, J.; Wang, X.; Fang, Y.; Liu, Y.; Yu, Z.; Liu, J.; Chen, F. Design and implementation of a noncontact sleep monitoring system using infrared cameras and motion sensor. *IEEE Trans. Instrum. Meas.* **2018**, *67*, 1555–1563. [CrossRef]

32. Gao, Z.; Ma, Z.; Chen, X.; Liu, H. Enhancement and de-noising of near-infrared Image with multiscale Morphology. In Proceedings of the 2011 5th International Conference on Bioinformatics and Biomedical Engineering, Wuhan, China, 10–12 May 2011; pp. 1–4.
33. Holtzhausen, P.J.; Crnojevic, V.; Herbst, B.M. An illumina-tion invariant framework for real-time foreground detection. *J. Real-Time Image Process.* **2015**, *10*, 423–433. [CrossRef]
34. Park, Y.K.; Park, S.L.; Kim, J.K. Retinex method based on adaptive smoothing for illumination invariant face recognition. *Signal Process.* **2008**, *88*, 1929–1945. [CrossRef]
35. Maik, V.; Paik, D.T.; Lim, J.; Park, K.; Paik, J. Hierarchical pose classification based on human physiology for behaviour analysis. *IET Comput. Vis.* **2010**, *4*, 12–24. [CrossRef]
36. Wang, Y.K.; Cheng, K.Y. A two-stage Bayesian network method for 3D human pose sstimation from monocular image sequences. *EURASIP J. Adv. Signal Process.* **2010**, *2010*, 761460. [CrossRef]
37. Lowe, D.G. Distinctive image features from scale-invariant keypoints. *Int. J. Comput. Vis.* **2004**, *60*, 91–110. [CrossRef]
38. Bay, H.; Ess, A.; Tuytelaars, T.; Gool, L.V. Speeded-up robust features (SURF). *Comput. Vis. Image Underst.* **2008**, *110*, 346–359. [CrossRef]
39. Ouyang, W.; Tombari, F.; Mattoccia, S.; Stefano, L.D.; Cham, W.K. Performance evaluation of full search equivalent pattern matching algorithms. *IEEE Trans. Circuits Syst. II Analog Digit. Signal Process.* **2012**, *34*, 127–143.
40. Scovanner, P.; Ali, S.; Shah, M. A 3-dimensional SIFT descriptor and its application to action recognition. In Proceedings of the 15th ACM international conference on Multimedia, Augsburg, Germany, 25–29 September 2007; pp. 357–360.
41. Wang, H.; Yi, Y. Tracking salient keypoints for human action recognition. In Proceedings of the IEEE International Conference on Systems, Man, and Cybernetics, Kowloon, China, 9–12 October 2015; pp. 3048–3053.
42. Zhang, J.T.; Tsoi, A.C.; Lo, S.L. Scale Invariant feature transform flow trajectory approach with applications to human action recognition. In Proceedings of the International Joint Conference on Neural Networks, Beijing, China, 6–11 July 2014; pp. 1197–1204.
43. Molina, A.; Ramirez, T.; Diaz, G.M. Robustness of interest point detectors in near infrared, far infrared and visible spectral images. In Proceedings of the 2016 XXI Symposium on Signal Processing, Images and Artificial Vision (STSIVA), Bucaramanga, Colombia, 31 August–2 September 2016; pp. 1–6.
44. Schweiger, F.; Zeisl, B.; Georgel, P.F.; Schroth, G. Maximum detector response markers for SIFT and SURF. In Proceedings of the Workshop on Vision, Modeling and Visualization, Braunschweig, Germany, 16 November 2009; pp. 145–154.
45. Wang, Y.K.; Huang, W.B. A CUDA-enabled parallel algorithm for accelerating retinex. *J. Real-Time Image Process.* **2012**, *9*, 407–425. [CrossRef]
46. Hare, S.; Saffari, A.; Torr, P.H.S. Efficient online structured output learning for keypoint-based object tracking. In Proceedings of the IEEE Conference on Computer Vision and Pattern Recognition, Providence, RI, USA, 16–21 June 2012; pp. 1894–1901.
47. Huang, C.; Darwiche, A. Inference in belief networks: A procedural guide. *Int. J. Approx. Reason.* **1996**, *15*, 225–263. [CrossRef]
48. Wang, Y.K.; Su, C.H. Illuminant-invariant Bayesian detection of moving video objects. In Proceedings of the International Conference on Signal and Image Processing, Honolulu, HI, USA, 14–16 August 2006; pp. 57–62.
49. Cole, R.J.; Kripke, D.F.; Gruen, W.; Mullaney, D.J.; Gillin, J.C. Automatic sleep/wake identification from wrist activity. *Sleep* **1992**, *15*, 461–469. [CrossRef] [PubMed]
50. Ramanan, D.; Forsyth, D.A.; Zisserman, A. Tracking people by learning their appearance. *IEEE Trans. Pattern Anal. Mach. Intell.* **2007**, *29*, 65–81. [CrossRef] [PubMed]

13

Data-Adaptive Coherent Demodulator for High Dynamics Pulse-Wave Ultrasound Applications

Stefano Ricci * and Valentino Meacci

Information Engineering Department (DINFO), University of Florence, Florence 50139, Italy; valentino.meacci@unifi.it

* Correspondence: stefano.ricci@unifi.it

Abstract: Pulse-Wave Doppler (PWD) ultrasound has been applied to the detection of blood flow for a long time; recently the same method was also proven effective in the monitoring of industrial fluids and suspensions flowing in pipes. In a PWD investigation, bursts of ultrasounds at 0.5–10 MHz are periodically transmitted in the medium under test. The received signal is amplified, sampled at tens of MHz, and digitally processed in a Field Programmable Gate Array (FPGA). First processing step is a coherent demodulation. Unfortunately, the weak echoes reflected from the fluid particles are received together with the echoes from the high-reflective pipe walls, whose amplitude can be 30–40 dB higher. This represents a challenge for the input dynamics of the system and the demodulator, which should clearly detect the weak fluid signal while not saturating at the pipe wall components. In this paper, a numerical demodulator architecture is presented capable of auto-tuning its internal dynamics to adapt to the feature of the actual input signal. The proposed demodulator is integrated into a system for the detection of the velocity profile of fluids flowing in pipes. Simulations and experiments with the system connected to a flow-rig show that the data-adaptive demodulator produces a noise reduction of at least of 20 dB with respect to different approaches, and recovers a correct velocity profile even when the input data are sampled at 8 bits only instead of the typical 12–16 bits.

Keywords: Cascaded-Integrator-Comb (CIC) filter; FPGA; fixed point math; data adaptive demodulator

---

1. Introduction

The velocity of blood flowing in an artery can be investigated by detecting the Doppler frequency shift that the moving particles produce on the energy pulses of 0.5–10 MHz periodically transmitted in the medium. This is a technique normally exploited by biomedical echographs for echo-Doppler exams [1]. Modern Pulse-Wave Doppler (PWD) electronics systems (including most of the clinical echographs) are nowadays based on the numerical approach for data processing. In these systems, the signal is converted to the digital domain as near as possible to the signal source, i.e., directly at the receiver front-end [2–5], while the analog conditioning is maintained at a minimum. This trend is common to most modern electronics [6,7]. The availability of relatively economic high-speed Analog-to-Digital (AD) converters working at several hundreds of MHz, and digital devices like Field Programmable Gate Arrays (FPGAs) [8] capable of in-line processing the high amount of data produced by the AD converters, foster the full-digital approach. In a PWD system, after the AD conversion, the signal is processed through coherent demodulation [9]. In the digital approach, a perfect match of the in-phase (I) and quadrature (Q) channels is easily achieved, with no need for compensation [10]. After demodulation, the signal is further processed through spectral analysis to detect the Doppler shift and, finally, the fluid velocity [1].

Fostered by the successful application in clinical echographs, the Doppler velocimetry [11] has been applied in detecting the velocity profile of industrial fluids flowing in pipes. The final application ranges from the accurate volume flow monitoring to the in-line rheological characterization of the fluids [12,13]. In industrial applications, the weak echoes produced by the fluid are acquired together with the strong reflections generated by the interface between the pipe wall and the fluid. This problem is similar to that present in a biomedical application with respect to blood and the vessel wall [14]. The pipe echoes are typically 30–40 dB stronger than the fluids', and this ratio can be even higher for special ultrasound transducers that investigate the fluid through the steel pipe surface [15,16]. This technique, which avoids cutting the pipe steel for creating an access "window", is employed in the food or pharmaceutical industries [17] where windows are not usable due to hygienic constraints.

The simultaneous presence of the high echo from the wall and the weak signal from flow imposes severe constraints to the dynamics of the processing chain in the PWD system. Moreover, the correct detection of both signals is necessary for assessing the Wall Shear Rate. Wall Shear Rate represents the velocity gradient in the radial direction evaluated at the wall position. It is a parameter widely used in rheology and in biomedical application [18].

Further challenges are imposed by the industrial environment: The PWD system is supposed to operate autonomously or with minimum intervention of operators. The system should be as robust as possible at the different conditions that can arise, for example, from the use of fluids with different ultrasound attenuation. In summary, the demodulator should not saturate at the high amplitude signal from the pipe, it should feature high dynamics, and should work in different conditions. The architecture of the demodulator should be carefully designed to accommodate these constraints.

In this paper, we present a coherent demodulator designed for high dynamics and suitable to be efficiently integrated into FPGA [19]. It is based on a modified Cascaded-Integrator-Comb (CIC) filter architecture [20]. The CIC, employing no multipliers but adders only, is attractive for FPGA implementation [21]. The proposed architecture includes barrel-shifters in the strategic positions where the dynamics of data bus-widths must be reduced. The barrel-shifters scale-down the bus-width by translating the most suitable section of the original bus, so that the resulting signal is maintained below but near the saturation. The barrel-shifter settings are automatically selected by a simple and quick procedure that occurs immediately before the PWD measurement. This procedure is based on the analysis of the actual data stream, therefore the demodulator is "data-adaptive" since its internal dynamics settings depend on the data to be processed [22].

The proposed data-adaptive demodulator was implemented in a PWD ultrasound system designed for the detection of the velocity profile of fluids moving in industrial pipes [23], whose final aim is the rheological characterization of industrial fluids [24]. The performance of the proposed demodulator was compared to the performance attainable by non-data adaptive approaches in simulation and experiments on flow-rig. Results show that the data-adaptive approach outperforms the other methods in the presence of high pipe wall echoes and for signals with reduced input dynamics.

This paper is organized as follows: Section 2 clarifies the processing chain of the PWD Doppler signal and presents the basics of the CIC filter architecture; Section 3 describes the proposed method, details the filter architecture, reports the procedure for the management of the dynamics in the filter stages; in Section 4 the error produced by the fixed-point numerical representation is evaluated and it is shown how the error affects the detection of the velocity profiles in fluids; Section 5 discusses and concludes the work.

2. Background and Motivation

2.1. *Pulse Wave Signals in Industrial Echo-Doppler Applications and Their Processing*

In PWD measurements a burst of ultrasounds with a central frequency F_T is transmitted in the medium to be investigated every Pulse Repetition Interval (PRI) through a suitable transducer [1]. The ultrasonic burst travels in the medium at velocity c, and when it encounters a scatter, part of its energy is reflected towards the transducer. If the scatter moves at velocity v, the echoes from subsequent transmissions are returned from slightly different positions. Thus, they are affected by a phase-shift. The echo signal sampled at the same distance from the transducer and from subsequent pulses presents a phase variation that corresponds to the frequency f_d described by the Doppler equation [1]:

$$f_d = 2\frac{v}{c} \cdot F_T \cdot cos(\theta) \tag{1}$$

where θ is the angle between the directions of the ultrasound wave and the scatter velocity, and the factor 2 in front of the formula accounts for the forth-back path the sound travels between the transducer and the target. Figure 1a reports an example of the signal acquired at 100 Ms/s, 16 bits resolution, from a fluid moving in an 8 mm diameter pipe and investigated with 5-cycle, 6 MHz ultrasound bursts. The 2 strong echoes located at 5 µs and 16 µs are the reflections of the static pipe walls, while the weak signal in-between, barely discernible from noise, is the echo of the moving fluid. In this example, the fluid signal is 27 dB below the pipe echoes. As the pipe is relatively still with respect to the transducer, the pipe echoes are stationary or quasi-stationary in the PRI sequence, at least for a temporal interval of several minutes. This is an important feature that will be exploited later to optimize the data-adaptive strategy (See Section 3.2).

The received signal feeds a coherent demodulator that removes the carrier frequency F_T. For example, Figure 1b reports in blue and red the I/Q components produced after coherent demodulation of the signal shown in Figure 1a.

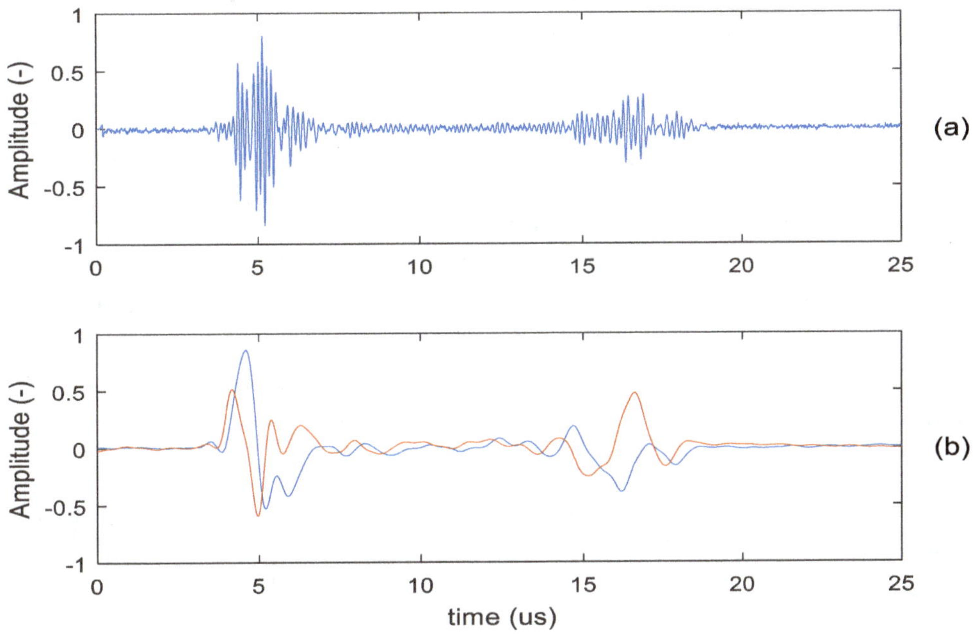

Figure 1. Raw signal (**a**) and I/Q demodulated signal (**b**) acquired from a fluid flowing in an 8 mm diameter pipe investigated with 6 MHz bursts. The strong echoes visible at 5 µs and 16 us are the reflections of the pipe walls; the useful signal of the moving fluid is barely visible in-between the pipe echoes.

As stated before, the acquisition system, and in particular the analog front-end, the AD converter, and the first step of the numerical data processing chain should accommodate the high signal from the wall and, simultaneously, the low echoes from the fluid. If the dynamics management of the demodulator is not appropriate, the low useful signal fades below the mathematical noise generated by the internal data truncations. This makes the demodulator a critical element in this application.

After demodulation, the I/Q components are processed through spectral estimation to detect f_d. The spectral analysis is performed through the efficient Fast Fourier Transform (FFT) [25–27] or more sophisticated adaptive estimators [28–30]. The demodulated ultrasound echoes are typically organized in the memory of the processing system along the columns of a matrix. The spectral analysis correlates the signal sampled at the same depth, i.e., proceeding along the rows of such a matrix and producing the power spectra matrix. The latter, color-coded, represents an intuitive picture of the flow profile in the pipe. Its rows report the Doppler shifts, which are proportional to the flow velocity through Equation (1); the columns report the depths inside the pipe. Some examples of spectral matrices are reported later in the experimental section of this paper.

2.2. Coherent Demodulator and CIC Filter Basics

The coherent demodulation [9] is typically obtained by multiplying the input signal $s_i(t)$ with two sinusoids of frequency F_T, affected by a 90° phase difference. In PWD applications the frequency F_T typically matches the transmission carrier. Each multiplier is followed by a low-pass filter that eliminates the spectral replica generated by the multiplication. The filtered signals, I(t) and Q(t), represent the phase and quadrature components of the complex output.

The two low-pass filters, implemented in FPGA, process the input signal at the AD converter rate, which can be up to 100 Ms/s. In this condition, the CIC architecture [20] has clear implementation advantages with respect to the standard Finite Impulse Response (FIR) filter [9]. With reference to the Z-domain [9], the basic CIC filter unit is a single integrator-comb (IC) cell, that can be realized as depicted in the graph reported in Figure 2a, where Z^{-i} represents an i-position delay. Basically, the integrator accumulates all of the input samples, while the comb removes from the accumulation the sample delayed of K-positions. The result is the summation of the latest K-samples. The IC cell is described with the following time-discrete equation, corresponding to the Z-domain transfer function $H(Z)$:

$$y(n) = y(n-1) + x(n) - x(n-K) \Leftrightarrow H(Z) = \frac{Y(Z)}{X(Z)} = \frac{1-Z^{-K}}{1-Z^{-1}} \quad (2)$$

From Equation (2) it is apparent that the filter cell features a low-pass behavior with transmission zeroes in $1 - Z^{-K} = 0$, i.e., where the normalized frequency f_N is i/K, with I = 1,2,3, etc. The side lobes have an amplitude of −13 dB. An example of the cell filter mask is reported in Figure 3b for a cut-off normalized frequency of F_L = 0.04, obtained with K = 15.

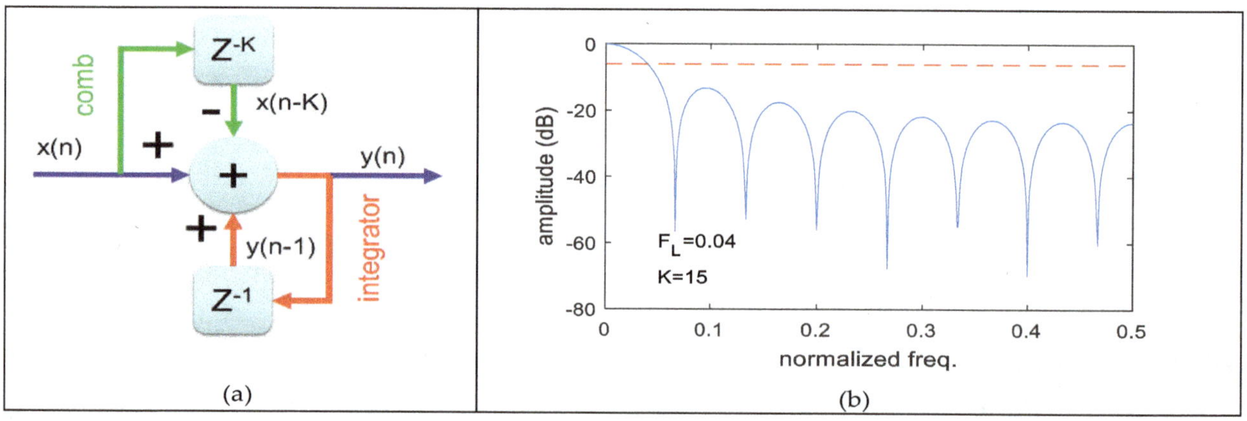

Figure 2. (**a**) Integrated-comb (IC) cell of cascaded-IC (CIC) filter and (**b**) an example of frequency mask obtained for K = 15, which corresponds to normalized cut-off frequency F_L = 0.04. Horizontal dashed line represents the −6 dB level.

In order to overcome the limited performance attainable by a single cell, the decimator CIC filter is normally based on several cells. It is typically realized by separating the integrator and the comb of the single IC cell and rearranging the sequence by cascading several integrators/combs separated by a decimator. The graph of the filter is reported in Figure 3a.

An example of the frequency mask referred to the normalized input frequency, i.e., before applying the spectrum folding due to the decimation, is shown in Figure 3b. For a better comparison, the cut-off frequency is the same as the previous example, i.e., $F_L = 0.04$, now obtained with D·K = 8. The transfer function is:

$$H(Z) = \frac{\left(1 - Z^{-DK}\right)^N}{\left(1 - Z^{-1}\right)^N} \tag{3}$$

As demonstrated in reference [20], the filter mathematics should allow a word-growth that corresponds to the gain of the filter, i.e., $(D \cdot K)^N$. In other words, if n is the number of bits used in input to the filter, all of the filter calculations and delay registers should work with a number of bits of:

$$m = n + \text{ceil}[N \cdot \log_2(D \cdot K)] \tag{4}$$

where ceil(x) is the nearest integer higher than x. For example, the resources for a 4-section complex CIC with K = 64, D = 16 and input data at $n = 28$ bits include 8 adders at 54 bits and 64·4·54 = 13824 bits of memory employed by the delay registers. Although this architecture can be realized in modern FPGA, it is onerous. In fact, the adders of the integrator sections work at the front-end clock frequency that can reach hundreds of MHz. Hogenauer in reference [20] describes how the number of bits can be safely reduced by truncating the least-significant part of the word. However, the method depends on the specific filter parameters (like K, D, F_L, etc.) and is not suitable for a programmable CIC whose FPGA architecture should work with different parameter sets.

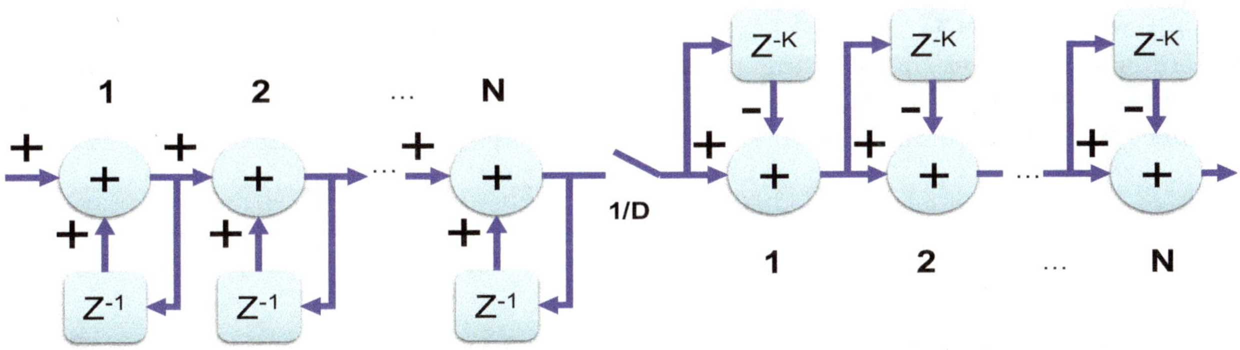

(a)

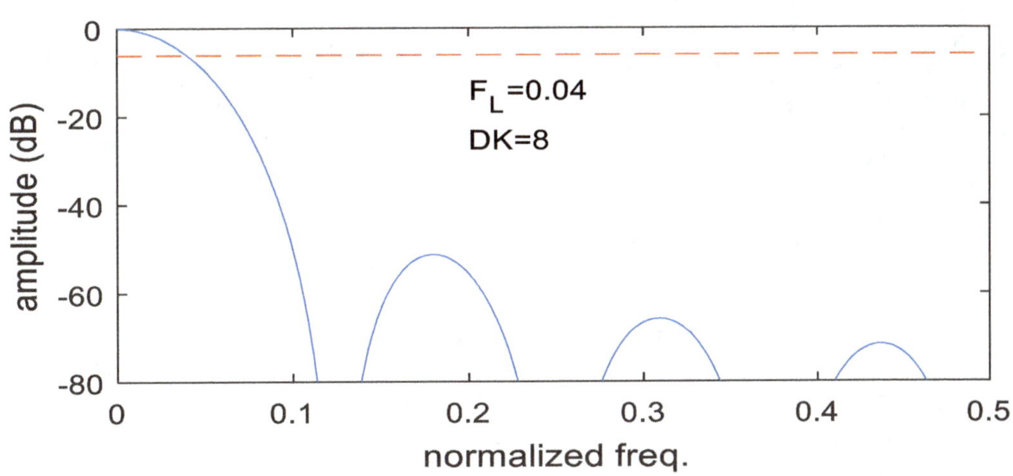

(b)

Figure 3. (**a**) 4-cell CIC filter and (**b**) an example of filter masks with DK = 8 for cut-off frequency $F_L = 0.04$. Horizontal dashed line represents the −6 dB level.

2.3. Demodulator Desired Features

The target for the numerical demodulator is the detection of the velocity profiles of fluids flowing in industrial pipes. In general, the demodulator includes the multiplication section and the following filter. However, in practice, the multiplication section is almost ideal and not critical, and all of the complexity resides in the filter. The filter should feature:

- Cut-off frequency programmable in a wide range of frequencies;
- Input dynamic range sufficient for accommodating both the strong pipe echoes and weak fluid signal;
- Low mathematical noise;
- Reasonable FPGA resource utilization;
- Up to 100 MHz working frequency.

3. Methods

3.1. Modified-CIC FilterAarchitecture

In order to face the aforementioned challenges, in this work, we implemented a slightly different CIC filter architecture, as reported in Figure 4. The filter employs 4 single IC cells numbered C_1–C_4, which include both the integrator and the comb, alternated to 4 decimators. At the output of each cell, a barrel shifter is added. The "Settings Manager" block sets the $K_{0\text{–}3}$ and $D_{1\text{–}4}$ values which establish the mask filter shape; while the "Dynamics Manager" block monitors the data amplitude at every cell output and sets the barrel-shifter according to a control strategy that is detailed in the next section. The transfer function of the modified filter, referred to the input frequency, is:

$$H(z) = \frac{1-z^{-K_0}}{1-z^{-1}} \cdot \frac{1-z^{-K_1 D_1}}{1-z^{-D_1}} \cdot \frac{1-z^{-K_2 D_1 D_2}}{1-z^{-D_1 D_2}} \cdot \frac{1-z^{-K_3 D_1 D_2 D_3}}{1-z^{-D_1 D_2 D_3}} \tag{5}$$

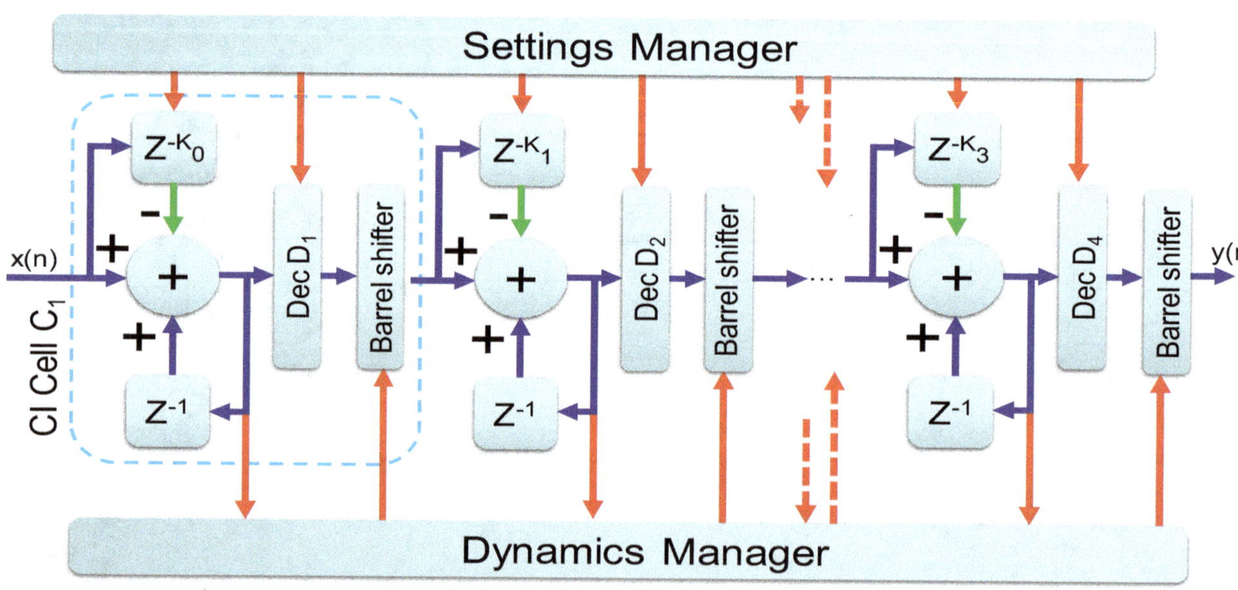

Figure 4. Modified CIC architecture based on Combo-Integrator sections interconnected by a barrel-shifter and a decimator. A dynamics manager monitors the dynamics in output of every section and operates the barrel-shifters.

An example of a filter mask is reported in Figure 5. It is obtained with $K_0 = 9$, $K_1 = 5$, $K_2 = 10$, $K_3 = 3$, $D_1 = 1$, $D_2 = 1$, $D_3 = 2$, $D_4 = 1$. The normalized cut-off frequency is $F_L = 0.04$ and it can be compared with the corresponding filter mask shown in Figure 3b produced by the standard CIC with 4 cells and $B{\cdot}K = 8$. Both filters achieve an attenuation higher than 50 dB outside the main lobes.

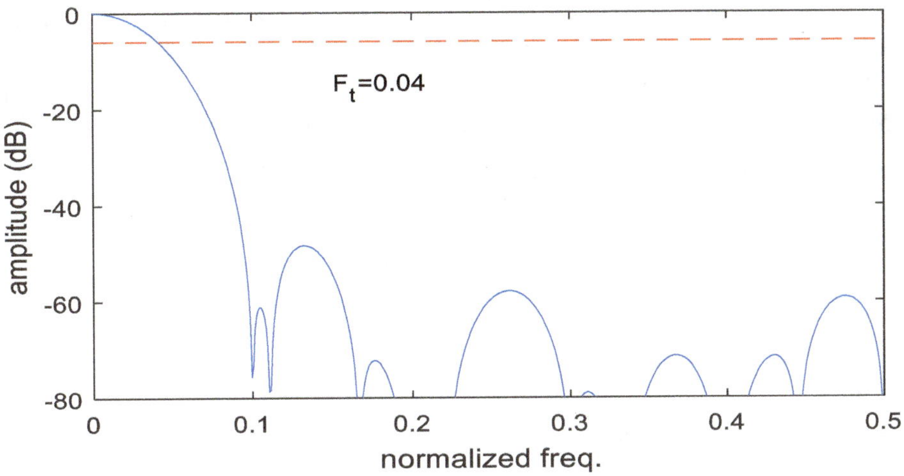

Figure 5. Filter mask obtained by the CIC architecture of Figure 6 with $K_0 = 9$, $K_1 = 5$, $K_2 = 10$, $K_3 = 3$, $D_1 = 1$, $D_2 = 1$, $D_3 = 2$, $D_4 = 1$. The cut-off normalized frequency is $F_L = 0.04$. Horizontal dashed line represents the –6 dB level.

3.2. Dynamics Management

The dynamics of the filter is one of the key-points for this application. The dynamics management is performed by setting the positions of the barrel-shifters inserted after each IC cell. The goal is to optimize the signal dynamics before the reduction of the bus-width operated on the output of each IC cell. This optimization is in charge of the "Dynamics Manager" block, which can operate according to the 3 different strategies described below. Although the data-adaptive is clearly the approach that grants the best result, coefficient-adaptive and non-adaptive approaches are described as well because they are typically employed in standard CIC and are used in this work for comparison. The strategies are:

(a) Non-adaptive

The most significant bits of the accumulator are selected in output. This is the simplest strategy, and the barrel shifters can be totally removed to save resources in the FPGA. However, bad performance is expected.

(b) Coefficient-adaptive

The barrel shifter position is selected according to the number of accumulations K programmed in the IC cell, i.e., the DC gain of the cell. The maximum word-growth for each cell in bit is ceil(log2(K)). The barrel-shifter is set to accommodate this growth regardless of the dynamics of the actual input data.

(c) Data-adaptive

The barrel-shifters are positioned to accommodate the effective dynamics of the data that are processed. However, the barrel-shifter positions must not change during the PWD measurement session in order to avoid gain steps. Fortunately, the dynamics of the input signal can be considered constant (see Section 2.1) during the duration of a measurement session (typically up to a few minutes). A quick training session was added before the measurement session. First of all the "Settings Manager" block sets the filter parameters (K_i and D_i) to establish the filter mask, gain, etc. Then the training session starts. During the first 10 PRIs, the "Dynamics manager" block monitors the data amplitude at the output of the first IC cell, i.e., C_1, and saves the maximum value. The "Dynamics manager" block uses the read value to tune the first barrel-shifter at the output of C_1. Then, the next 10 PRIs are acquired, and now the "Dynamics manager" block observes the data out of C_2, saves the maximum amplitude, and sets the second barrel-shifter. The procedure is repeated in sequence for C_3 and C_4 and, after 40 PRIs all the barrel-shifters are set for optimal performance. These first PRIs, corrupted by gain steps, are not suitable for Doppler analysis and thus are discarded, but the following are acquired and processed without even stopping the PRIs sequence between the training and acquisition sessions. In a typical set-up, a single PRI lasts about 100–1000 μs, while a complete Doppler measurement involves the acquisition and processing of several thousands of PRIs. Thus, the training session takes no more than 0.1 s of the several hundreds of second that take the whole measurement. The delay due to the filter training is negligible and not perceivable by the final user.

For reader convenience the training procedure is summarized below:

1) "Setting Manager" block program K_0, K_1, K_2, K_3, and D_1, D_2, D_3, D_4
2) Repeat for IC_i cells I = 1 to 4:
   a. Detect the maximum data amplitude on 10 PRIs, M=max(abs(Data))
   b. Calculate the bits necessary to represent data: J=ceil(log2(M))+1
   c. Set the shifter so that J is the most significant bit
   d. Discard the PRIs used for training
3) Start normal data acquisition and processing

3.3. FPGA Implementation

The demodulator with the modified-CIC architecture was implemented in an FPGA of the Cyclone V family (Intel/Altera, San Jose, CA). The architecture of the single IC cell is detailed in Figure 6. The IC cell is designed to accommodate the worst case of K_i = 64, although the cell can be set for a lower K_i value. The input data bus of width BI_i bits feeds a First Input First Output (FIFO) memory and an adder that constitutes the accumulator together with the following register. The delay of K-sample is obtained by generating with the suitable clock-delay the "write" and "read" commands of the FIFO memory that holds the data stream. The adder sums up the input data to the accumulator register value and subtracts the delayed samples coming from the FIFO.

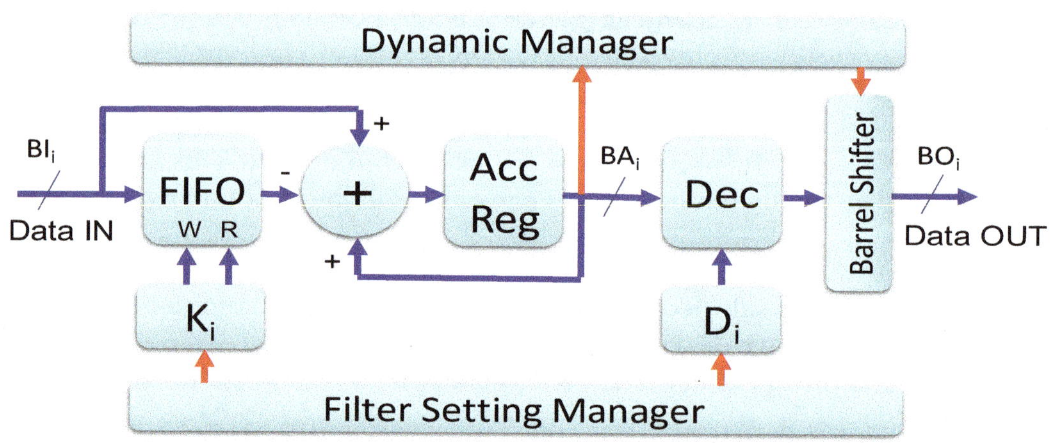

Figure 6. Details of the IC cell as implemented in the field programmable gate array (FPGA).

The FIFO is sized for holding, in the worst case, 64·BI_i bits of input data. An integration factor of K corresponds to a maximum gain of the same value K. The maximum data word-growth is 6 bits. Thus, the adder and the accumulation register work with a bit-width of:

$$BA_i = BI_i + 6 \tag{6}$$

The output of the accumulator is decimated by a programmable factor D_i.

In each stage of the filter the IC_i cell is designed to reduce the input-to-output bus width of 3 bits, i.e.,:

$$BO_i = BI_i - 3 \tag{7}$$

where BO_i is the bus-width in output. The combination of Equations (6) and (7) produces:

$$BO_i = BA_i - 9 \tag{8}$$

Thus, a barrel-shifter with 10 positions covers all of the possible shifts between the accumulator and the output bus. For reader convenience, Figure 7 summarizes the relation among the accumulator, the output bus, and the possible barrel-shifter positions for the three dynamics management strategies reported in Section 3.2.

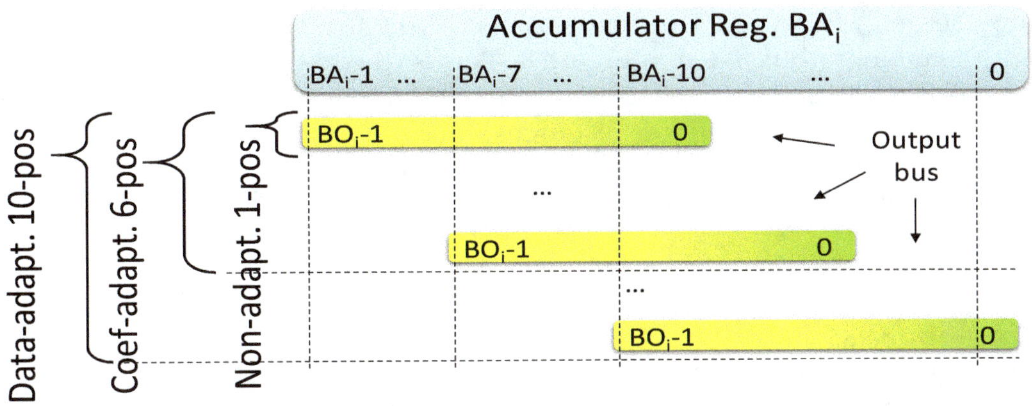

Figure 7. Barrel-shifter positions for the three different dynamics management strategies. The accumulator of the cell C_i features BA_i bits numbered from $BA_i - 1$ to 0. The output bus features BO_i bits numbered from $BO_i - 1$ to 0. The shifter has 1, 6, 10 positions for non-, coeff-, data- adaptive strategies, respectively.

The IC cell is integrated into the demodulator with the bus-widths reported in Figure 8. The data stream $s_i(t)$ sampled up to 100 Ms/s at 16-bit enters the demodulator. The coherent sin/cos sources are represented at 13-bit. The 2 multipliers produce an output at $16 + 13 - 1 = 28$ bits that feed the 2 identical filters composed by 4 sections for the phase and quadrature channels. The filters take in input the 2 buses at 28 bits, and, since each IC stage decreases the bus width of 3 bits, the I/Q signals are outputted at 16 bits. The number of words in FIFO (Mw), the total memory bits in FIFO (Mb), the adder, and accumulator width (BA), and the barrel-shifter positions for data-adaptive strategy (BS) are reported in Figure 8 inside the graphical blocks of each specific IC cell in the filter chain.

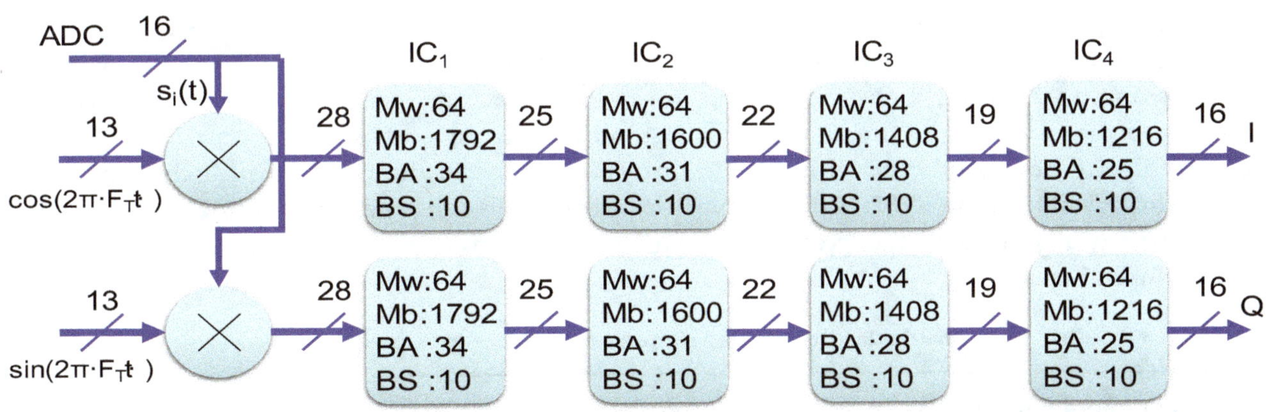

Figure 8. Architecture of the data-adaptive demodulator. IC cells report the memory words (Mw), the memory bits (Mb), the accumulator width (BA), and the barrel-shifter (BS) positions. The bus-widths in input and output of each IC cell are reported as well.

4. Experiments and Results

4.1. Resources Utilization

The first experiment aimed at evaluating the resource utilization of the proposed solutions. The demodulator of Figure 8 was implemented in an FPGA of the Cyclone V family (Altera/Intel,

San Jose, CA, USA) in all of the three configurations for dynamics management described in Section 3.2. The design was targeted for a clock up to 100 MHz, a goal easily reached for all of the implementations. The results are listed in Table 1, distinguished for Adaptive Logic Modules (ALM), Adaptive Look-up-Tables (ALUT), Registers (REG), Memory bits, and Digital Signal Processors (DSP) blocks. In all of the implementations two DSP blocks are employed for the two multipliers of the demodulator (see, e.g., Figure 8). The memory bits (17,700 for the proposed architecture) are more than the sum of the memory bits listed in Figure 8. This is due to the internal organization of FPGA memory. The data-adaptive and coeff-adaptive approaches have a similar resource utilization, while the non-adaptive approach employs fewer resources since the barrel-shifters are removed.

Table 1. Demodulator resources utilization in FPGA implementation.

Device	Cyclone V				
	ALM	ALUT	Reg	Memory Bits	DSP
data-adaptive demodulator	831	1271	871	17700	2
coeff-adaptive demodulator	818	1056	869	17700	2
non-adaptive demodulator	523	758	803	17700	2

4.2. Demodulator Noise Performance

This experiment aimed to evaluate the noise produced by the finite number representation in the mathematical calculations of the filter. The system for rheological fluid characterization described in reference [23] was connected to a flow-rig. A fluid composed by demineralized water with added specific ultrasonic scatters flowed in an 8 mm diameter pipe moved by a gear pump. The pipe was immersed in a water tank where a cylindrical ultrasound transducer was directed towards the pipe at an angle of 60° with respect to the pipe axis. The transducer was excited by the system with bursts composed by 5 cycles at 6 MHz, repeated with a PRIs of 200 μs. The received echoes were sampled at 16 bits 100 Ms/s. The analog gain of the front-end of the system was accurately tuned with a manual try-and-check procedure to exploit the full 16 bits dynamic range of the AD converter. An example of the signal acquired in a PRI is shown in Figure 1a.

The acquired signal was used to generate three different test signals. The first, hereafter named 'S_{16}' was the original signal itself, the second and the third signals, named 'S_{12}' and 'S_{08}' were obtained by reducing the dynamics of the original signal to 12 and 8 bits, respectively. This was obtained by dividing the data to 2^4 and 2^8 but maintaining the 16 bits word representation. These last two signals mimic a non-optimal tuning of the analog input gain of the front-end of the system.

The demodulators were coded in VHDL language and implemented in Modelsim® (Mentor Graphics Corp. Wilsonville 97070 OR). The filter parameters were set to obtain $F_L = 0.01$, that, for a 100 MHz sampling frequency, corresponds to a 1 MHz bandwidth. The employed parameters are detailed in Table 2.

Table 2. Filter parameter employed in experiments.

Parameters K_i	Parameters D_i	Cut-off Frequency (Normalized)	Cut-off Frequency
$K_0 = 32, K_1 = 17, K_2 = 9, K_3 = 14$	$D_1 = 1, D_2 = 3, D_3 = 1, D_4 = 1$	$F_L = 0.01$	1 MHz

The 3 test signals were processed according to all of the 3 strategies for dynamics management. The corresponding demodulated outputs were named SDxx, where xx is 16, 12, and 08 and indicate the corresponding input signal. The demodulator was implemented in Matlab® (The Mathworks, Natick, MA, USA) as well, and used to process the test signals in double precision. These results were considered as reference and named SDRxx. The signals were compared in Matlab® by computing the Signal-to-Noise ratio with the following metric:

$$\text{SNR} = 10 \cdot \log_{10}\left[\frac{\sum_i SDxx^2(i)}{\sum_i (SDxx(i) - SDRxx(i))^2}\right] \tag{9}$$

Please note that the reference output signals SDRxx were generated by the ideal Matlab® demodulator with the Sxx signals quantized at 16, 12, 08 bits. Thus, the quantization input noise is not included in the SNR evaluated by (9). SNR calculated by Equation (9) accounts for the mathematical noise of the demodulator and the final 16-bit quantization noise. The results, expressed in dB, are listed in Table 3. In addition, the maximum SNR achievable for the signals present in this application was further calculated in Matlab®. The output of the ideal demodulator SDRxx with in input the S_{16} signal was normalized at full dynamics and quantized at 16 bits. The SNR due to this quantization was calculated and reported in the last column of Table 3 (Reference). Note that the typical formula 6.02·N + 1.76 (where N is the number of bits) [9] results in SNR = 98.1 dB instead of 85.0 dB for N = 16 bits. In fact, the aforementioned formula is valid for a full-dynamics sinusoidal signal, while the actual signal used here exploits the full dynamics only for a small part of the acquired period (see Figure 1a).

Table 3. Signal-to-noise ratio (SNR) Performance of the demodulator–input quantization excluded.

SNR (dB)	Non-Adaptive	Coeff-Adaptive	Data-Adaptive	Reference
S_{16}	24.7	60.2	83.4	85.0
S_{12}	5.7	36.3	83.4	85.0
S_{08}	0.0	14.2	83.4	85.0

The performance in non-adaptive approach (see Table 3) is particularly bad, being the maximum SNR = 25 dB only. Since that the ratio between pipe and fluid echoes is up to 30–40 dB, the non-adaptive approach is not suitable for the application. The coef-adaptive strategy grants much better performance and reaches SNR = 60 dB in the best condition. However, the SNR degrades quickly when the input data scales-down. The coef-adaptive strategy is sensitive to input data dynamics and thus it is not so robust for industrial applications. The data-adaptive approach produces the best performance achieving an SNR = 84 dB. Most importantly, the performance does not depend on the input dynamics even at 8 bits of input data. Moreover, the predominant noise is generated by the 16 bits quantization in output, and not from the finite numerical representation of the filter mathematics. This confirms that data-adaptive performance is quite close to the reference (see Table 3).

The noise performance of the demodulators is further confirmed by positions of the barrel shifter present during the experiment and listed in Table 4. Each BS_i column reports the position of the barrel-shifter at the end of the cell IC_i. A value of m in the table means that the shifter scales the signal by 2^{-m}.

Table 4. Scaling positions of the barrel shifters.

	Non-Adaptive				Coeff-Adaptive				Data-Adaptive			
	BS_1	BS_2	BS_3	BS_4	BS_1	BS_2	BS_3	BS_4	BS_1	BS_2	BS_3	BS_4
S_{16}	9	9	9	9	8	8	7	7	7	7	6	6
S_{12}	9	9	9	9	8	8	7	7	3	7	6	6
S_{08}	9	9	9	9	8	8	7	7	0	6	6	6

In non-adaptive strategy, the scaling is fixed to 2^{-9}, i.e., the 6 positions related to the maximum filter gain (K_i up to 64) plus 3 for the bus-width reduction (7). In the coeff-adaptive approach, the positions correspond to the actual filter settings, plus the 3 positions for bus-width reduction. For example, since K_0 = 32 (see Table 2), BS_1 = ceil (log2(32)) + 3 = 8. However, the settings are the same regardless of the input signal Sxx. In a data-adaptive approach the filter positions change for different rows of Table 4, i.e., they depend on the signal dynamics. BS_1 scales 7 positions for the strong signal S_{16}, but 0 positions for S_{08}, thus recovering 7 bits of dynamics. BS_2 scales 6 positions for S_{08} and 7 for the other signals. BS_3 and BS_4 have the same behavior for all the signals. This means that the dynamics of S_{08} is recovered mostly by BS_1 and BS_2. Then BS_3 and BS_4 scale 6 positions like for the other signals. This explains how the demodulator achieves the best performance of 83.4 dB when processing S_{08} (see Table 3).

4.3. Flow Simulation

The performance of the demodulator was tested in a flow simulation. The simulation was carried out in Matlab® through the Field II ultrasound simulator [31,32], freely available at https://field-ii.dk. Field II, given the position of a set of scattering particles, the transducer characteristics, and the TX pulse, simulates the echo data acquired in each PRI. In this test, a piston transducer transmitted bursts of 5 cycles at 6 MHz in a 45 mm diameter pipe. The positions of the scattering particles were updated every PRI to mimic the typical parabolic profile of a Newtonian fluid flowing in a straight pipe [33]. The peak velocity was set to 1 m/s. A 16-bit AD converter was simulated by scaling the amplitude of the data generated by Field II and by applying the 16 bits fixed point representation. Two data sets were generated: The first was composed by the echoes from the particles in the flow only, while the other included the echoes from the static pipe wall as well. The power ratio between echoes from pipe wall and from flow particles was 35 dB.

The two data sets were processed by both the non-adaptive and by the data-adaptive demodulators. The demodulators were programmed with the same integration and decimation parameters used in the previous experiment. Four power spectral matrices were obtained and reported in Figure 9 in color code. The vertical axes show the depth along the pipe diameter, while the horizontal axes report the velocity obtained by converting the Doppler shift through (1).

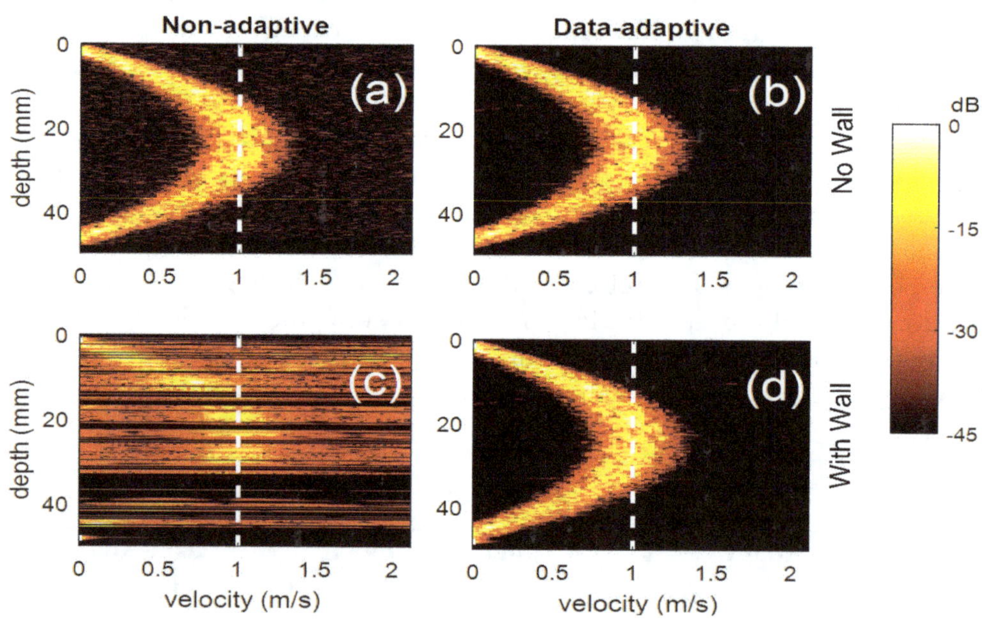

Figure 9. Power spectral matrices obtained for a simulated parabolic flow with 1 m/s peak velocity in a 45 mm diameter pipe. In (**c**,**d**) the signal from a static pipe-wall is added with a power 35 dB higher than the flow signal; in (**a**,**b**) the only flow signal is present. (**a**,**c**) are obtained with non-adaptive demodulator; (**b**,**d**) with data-adaptive demodulator. Horizontal axes report the Doppler shift converted to velocity. Vertical dashed lines correspond to the simulated peak velocity.

The simulated signal without the pipe wall echoes produces spectral matrices where the parabolic profile can be clearly detected (Figure 9a,b). When the pipe wall signal is added, the data-adaptive demodulator produces a spectral matrix (Figure 9d) that is identical to the case without the wall signal (Figure 9b). On the other hand, the non-adaptive demodulator does not produce a detectable profile when the pipe wall is added (Figure 9c). Background noise is quite high and several regions (black horizontal bands) are below the filter sensitivity. Moreover, whenever the velocity profile is detected (Figure 9a,b,d) the velocity that corresponds to the parabola peak is located with an accuracy of ±2.2%. For comparison, the reference velocity of 1 m/s is reported by the vertical dashed lines.

4.4. Example of Application

The proposed demodulator was included in the processing chain of the system for the detection of the velocity profile of fluids flowing in pipes described in reference [34]. The system was connected to the flow-rig as described in Section 4.2. The demodulator was programmed with the same integration and decimation parameters used in the previous experiment. The analog gain of the front-end was tuned to reproduce the 16, 12, 08 bits input signal dynamics, and the filter was set for non-, coeff-, data-adaptive approaches. Frames of power spectral matrices elaborated in real-time by the system were captured and reported in Figure 10.

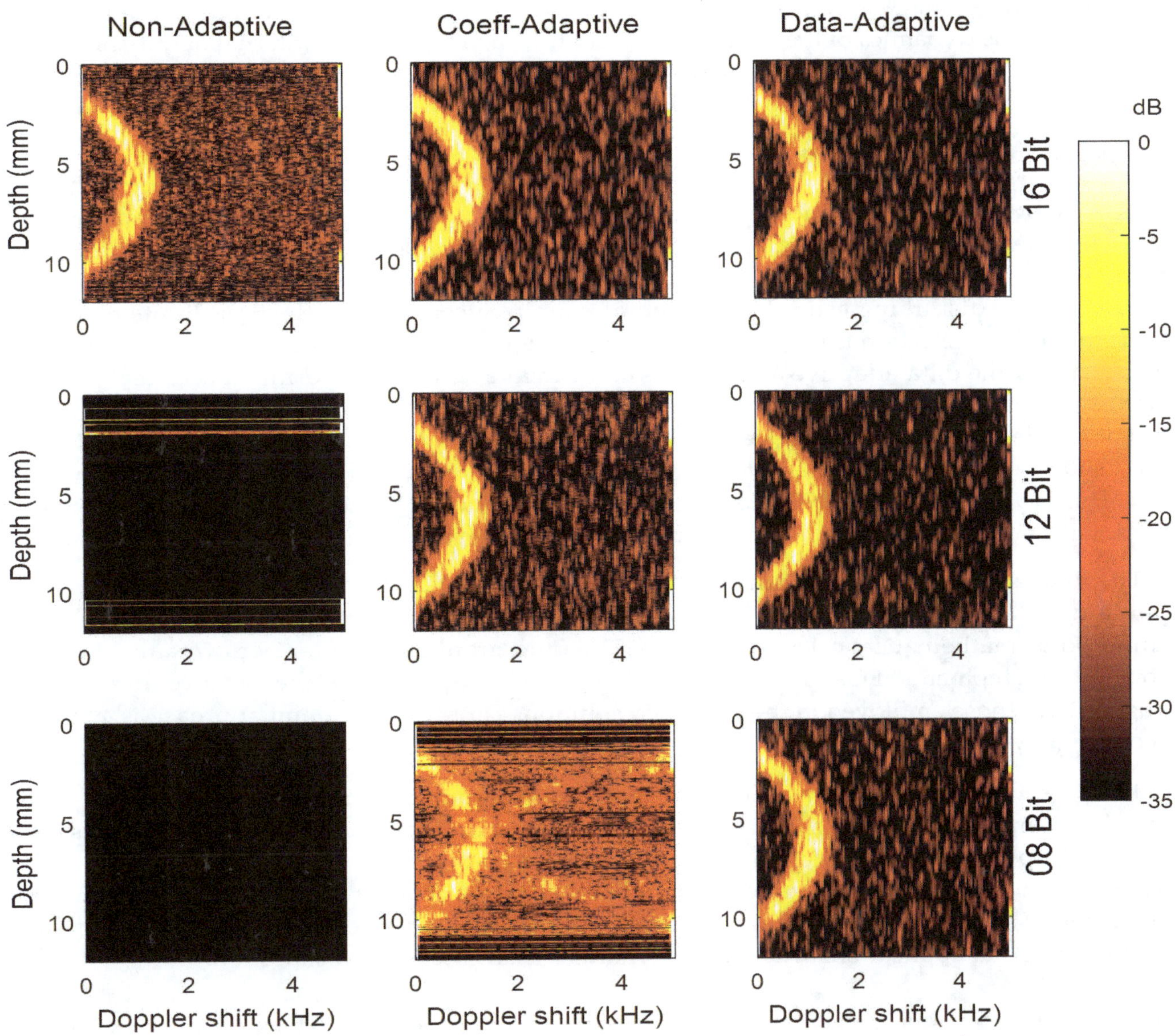

Figure 10. Power spectral matrices calculated by the system, including the proposed demodulator. Horizontal and vertical axes report Doppler shift and depth, respectively. Matrices processed with non-, coeff-, data- adaptive strategies are reported in columns; input signal equivalent to 16, 12, 08 bits are reported in rows.

The spectral matrices show the typical parabolic profile of a Newtonian fluid. When the input gain is tuned for exploiting the full dynamics of the AD converter (16 bits, first row in Figure 10), the parabolic profile is clearly detected regardless of the dynamic's management employed in the filter. The non-adaptive configuration features a higher noise level, the other two cases are similar. When the input signal covers 12 bits of the AD dynamics, coef- and data- adaptive approaches do not show appreciable deterioration, while a non-adaptive approach shows no usable signal. With input dynamics at 8 bits, coeff-adaptive approach features a very high noise level, while data-adaptive showed no visible difference with respect to previous analysis. In other words, non-adaptive demodulator produces a good signal only when the full input dynamics is exploited; data-adaptive demodulators produce the same high-quality signal even if the input dynamics is reduced to only 8 bits. The coeff-adaptive approach produces intermediate results.

5. Discussion and Conclusion

In this work, a data-adaptive demodulator for PWD applications is presented. A "training phase" is used to read the dynamics of the actual signal and tune accordingly the internal barrel-shifters. It is followed by the "running phase" where the signal is effectively processed with the gain parameters set in the training phase. The training phase is very quick and precedes the normal acquisition phase without impact to the final application.

The superior performance of the proposed method is evident in presence of strong pipe-wall echoes, as shown in the simulation of Section 4.3. The simulation highlights that the non-adaptive demodulator fails while the data-adaptive detects the correct velocity profile. In fact, in the presence of a strong pipe wall echo, the dynamics of the useful flow signal is reduced proportionally to the amplitude of the disturbing echo. If the dynamics are reduced beyond the SNR limits reported in Table 3, the profile detection is prevented because the signal is concealed in the noise. The high SNR performance of the data-adaptive approach is confirmed also in the experiment on a real pipe flow, whose results are shown in Figure 10. The data-adaptive approach allows us to recover the optimal signal at the demodulator output even when the signal at the AD converter input uses only 8 bits. In this condition, nor the coeff-adaptive, neither the non-adaptive approaches, can produce any usable signal. This is a very important feature in industrial applications, where the PWD system is expected to work with minimal tuning and to be robust to a wide range of conditions.

The data-adaptive approach can also be implemented with a single barrel-shifter at the end of a standard 4-stage CIC architecture, however, this approach would require more FPGA resources. Floating point mathematical calculations [35–37] would grant even better performance. However, although recent high-end FPGAs integrates floating-point hard-processors, the resources needed are by far higher than those employed in the proposed solution. Thus, floating point approach is, at present, not cost-effective.

The presented demodulator fulfils the requirements reported in Section 2.3. It includes a filter with a programmable mask, it can be easily implemented in low-cost FPGA, and it features a data throughput up to 100 Ms/s. Most importantly, the data-adaptive approach is not affected by the strong pipe echoes and is capable of auto-tuning for the widest range of input conditions, reducing the intervention of specialized workers. The proposed demodulator can represent a valuable processing block for industrial applications where high dynamics is an essential precondition.

Author Contributions: Conceptualization, methodology, writing paper, funding acquisition: S.R.; software, investigation, data curation: V.M.

Acknowledgments: Authors thank Johan Wiklund for his advice about fluid rheology.

References

1. Evans, D.H.; McDicken, W.N. *Doppler Ultrasound Physics, Instrumentation and Signal Processing*; Wiley: Chichester, UK, 2000; ISBN 978-0471970019.
2. Vogt, M. Direct sampling and baseband conversion in Doppler systems for high-frequency ultrasound blood flow measurements. *Electron. Lett.* **2005**, *41*, 189–790. [CrossRef]
3. Weibao, Q.; Zongying, Y.; Yanyan, Y.; Yan, C.; Liyang, C.; Peitian, M.; Guofeng, L.; Congzhi, W.; Yang, X.; Jiyan, D.; et al. A Digital Multigate Doppler Method for High Frequency Ultrasound. *Sensors* **2014**, *14*, 13348–13360. [CrossRef]
4. Boni, E.; Bassi, L.; Dallai, A.; Meacci, V.; Ramalli, A.; Scaringella, M.; Guidi, F.; Ricci, S.; Tortoli, P. Architecture of an Ultrasound System for Continuous Real-Time High Frame Rate Imaging. *IEEE Trans. Ultrason. Ferroelectr. Freq. Control* **2017**, *64*, 1276–1284. [CrossRef] [PubMed]
5. Jensen, J.A.; Nikolov, S.I.; Yu, A.C.H.; Garcia, D. Ultrasound Vector Flow Imaging-Part II: Parallel Systems. *IEEE Trans. Ultrason. Ferroelectr. Freq. Control* **2016**, *63*, 722–1732. [CrossRef] [PubMed]
6. Hervás, M.; Alsina-Pagès, R.M.; Salvador, M. An FPGA Scalable Software Defined Radio Platform Design for Educational and Research Purposes. *Electronics* **2016**, *5*, 27. [CrossRef]
7. Koulamas, C.; Lazarescu, M.T. Real-Time Embedded Systems: Present and Future. *Electronics* **2018**, *7*, 205. [CrossRef]
8. Rodriguez-Andina, J.J.; Moure, M.J.; Valdes, M.D. Features, design tools, and application domains of FPGAs. *IEEE Trans. Ind. Electron.* **2007**, *54*, 1810–1823. [CrossRef]
9. Richard, L. *Understanding Digital Signal Processing*, 2nd ed.; Prentice Hall: Upper Saddle River, NJ, USA, 2004; ISBN 978-0-13-702741-5.
10. Mohsin, A.; Fadhel, M.G.; Mohamed, H. Blind Compensation of I/Q Impairments in Wireless Transceivers. *Sensors* **2017**, *17*, 2948. [CrossRef]
11. Ricci, S.; Matera, R.; Tortoli, P. An improved Doppler model for obtaining accurate maximum blood velocities. *Ultrasonics* **2014**, *7*, 2006–2014. [CrossRef]
12. Wiklund, J.; Stading, M. Application of in-line ultrasound Doppler-based UVP–PD rheometry method to concentrated model and industrial suspensions. *Flow Meas. Instrum.* **2008**, *19*, 171–179. [CrossRef]
13. Birkhofer, B.; Debacker, A.; Russo, S.; Ricci, S.; Lootens, D. In-line rheometry based on ultrasonic velocity profiles: Comparison of data processing methods. *Appl. Rheol.* **2012**, *22*, 44701. [CrossRef]
14. Morganti, T.; Ricci, S.; Vittone, F.; Palombo, C.; Tortoli, P. Clinical validation of common carotid artery wall distension assessment based on multigate Doppler processing. *Ultras. Med. Biol.* **2005**, *31*, 937–945. [CrossRef] [PubMed]
15. Shamu, T.J.; Kotzé, R.; Wiklund, J. Characterization of acoustic beam propagation through high-grade stainless steel pipes for improved pulsed ultrasound velocimetry measurements in complex industrial fluids. *IEEE Sens. J.* **2016**, *16*, 5636–5647. [CrossRef]
16. Kotzé, R.; Ricci, S.; Birkhofer, B.; Wiklund, J. Performance tests of a new non-invasive sensor unit and ultrasound electronics. *Flow Meas. Instrum.* **2016**, *48*, 104–111. [CrossRef]
17. Qwist, P.K.; Sander, C.; Okkels, F.; Jessen, V.; Baldursdottir, S.; Rantanen, J. On-line rheological characterization of semi-solid formulations. *Eur. J. Pharm. Sci.* **2019**, *128*, 36–42. [CrossRef] [PubMed]
18. Ricci, S.; Swillens, A.; Ramalli, A.; Segers, P.; Tortoli, P. Wall Shear Rate Measurement: Validation of a new Method through Multi-physics Simulations. *IEEE Trans. Ultrason. Ferroelectr. Freq. Control* **2017**, *64*, 66–77. [CrossRef] [PubMed]
19. Meacci, V.; Matera, R.; Ricci, S. High dynamics adaptive demodulator for ultrasound applications: FPGA implementation. In Proceedings of the 1st New Generation of CAS, NGCAS, Genoa, Italy, 6–8 September 2017.
20. Hogenauer, E. An economical class of digital filters for decimation and interpolation. *IEEE Trans. Acoust. Speech Signal Process.* **1981**, *29*, 155–162. [CrossRef]
21. Peilu, L.; Xinghua, L.; Haopeng, L.; Zhikun, S.; Hongxu, Z. Implementation of High Time Delay Accuracy of Ultrasonic Phased Array Based on Interpolation CIC Filter. *Sensors* **2017**, *17*, 2322. [CrossRef]
22. Pilato, L.; Fanucci, L.; Saponara, S. Real-Time and High-Accuracy Arctangent Computation Using CORDIC and Fast Magnitude Estimation. *Electronics* **2017**, *6*, 22. [CrossRef]

23. Ricci, S.; Meacci, V.; Birkhofer, B.; Wiklund, J. FPGA-based System for In-Line Measurement of Velocity Profiles of Fluids in Industrial Pipe Flow. *IEEE Trans. Ind. Electron.* **2017**, *64*, 3997–4005. [CrossRef]
24. Ricci, S.; Liard, M.; Birkhofer, B.; Lootens, D.; Brühwiler, A.; Tortoli, P. Embedded Doppler System for Industrial in-Line Rheometry. *IEEE Trans. Ultrason. Ferroelectr. Freq. Control* **2012**, *59*, 1395–1401. [CrossRef]
25. Cooley, J.W.; Tukey, J.W. An algorithm for the machine calculation of complex Fourier series. *Math. Comput.* **1965**, *19*, 297–301. [CrossRef]
26. Minotta, F.; Jimenez, M.; Rodriguez, D. Automated Scalable Address Generation Patterns for 2-Dimensional Folding Schemes in Radix-2 FFT Implementations. *Electronics* **2018**, *7*, 33. [CrossRef]
27. Nguyen, H.N.; Khan, S.A.; Kim, C.H.; Kim, J.M. A Pipelined FFT Processor Using an Optimal Hybrid Rotation Scheme for Complex Multiplication: Design, FPGA Implementation and Analysis. *Electronics* **2018**, *7*, 137. [CrossRef]
28. Ricci, S. Adaptive Spectral Estimators for Fast Flow Profile Detection. *IEEE Trans. Ultrason. Ferroelectr. Freq. Control* **2013**, *60*, 421–427. [CrossRef] [PubMed]
29. Elif, D.Ü.; Hakan, I.; İnan, G. Application of FFT and Arma Spectral Analysis to Arterial Doppler Signals. *Math. Comput. Appl.* **2003**, *8*, 311–318. [CrossRef]
30. Larsson, E.; Stoica, P. Fast implementation of two-dimensional APES and Capon spectral estimators. *Multidimens. Syst. Signal Process.* **2002**, *13*, 35–54. [CrossRef]
31. Jensen, J.A.; Svendsen, N.B. Calculation of pressure fields from arbitrarily shaped, apodized, and excited ultrasound transducers. *IEEE Trans. Ultrason. Ferroelect. Freq. Control* **1992**, *39*, 262–267. [CrossRef] [PubMed]
32. Jensen, J.A. Field: A Program for Simulating Ultrasound Systems. *Med. Biol. Eng. Comp.* **1996**, *34*, 351–353.
33. Granger, R.A. *Fluid Mechanics*; Dover: Mineola, NY, USA, 1995; ISBN 978-0486683560.
34. Meacci, V.; Ricci, S.; Wiklund, J.; Birkhofer, B.; Kotze, R. Flow-Viz—An integrated digital in-line fluid characterization system for industrial applications. In Proceedings of the 11th IEEE Sensors Applications Symposium (SAS), Catania, Italy, 13–15 April 2016; pp. 128–133.
35. 754-2008—IEEE Standard for Floating-Point Arithmetic. 2008. Available online: https://doi.org/10.1109/IEEESTD.2008.4610935 (accessed on 12 December 2018).
36. Al Kadi, M.; Janssen, B.; Huebner, M. Floating-Point Arithmetic Using GPGPU on FPGAs. In Proceedings of the IEEE Computer Society Annual Symposium on VLSI, ISVLSI, Bochum, Germany, 3–5 July 2017; pp. 134–139.
37. Sanchez, A.; Todorovich, E.; De Castro, A. Exploring the Limits of Floating-Point Resolution for Hardware-In-the-Loop Implemented with FPGAs. *Electronics* **2018**, *7*, 219. [CrossRef]

14

Simplified Swarm Optimization-Based Function Module Detection in Protein–Protein Interaction Networks

Xianghan Zheng [1,2], Lingting Wu [1,2], Shaozhen Ye [1,*] and Riqing Chen [3]

1 College of Mathematics and Computer Science, Fuzhou University, Fuzhou 350116, China; xianghan.zheng@fzu.edu.cn (X.Z.); mjyw_wlt@163.com (L.W.)
2 Fujian Key Laboratory of Network Computing and Intelligent Information Processing, Fuzhou 350116, China
3 College of Computer and Information, Fujian Agriculture and Forestry University, Fuzhou 350002, China; riqing.chen@fafu.edu.cn
* Correspondence: yeshzh@fzu.edu.cn

Abstract: Proteomics research has become one of the most important topics in the field of life science and natural science. At present, research on protein–protein interaction networks (PPIN) mainly focuses on detecting protein complexes or function modules. However, existing approaches are either ineffective or incomplete. In this paper, we investigate detection mechanisms of functional modules in PPIN, including open database, existing detection algorithms, and recent solutions. After that, we describe the proposed approach based on the simplified swarm optimization (SSO) algorithm and the knowledge of Gene Ontology (GO). The proposed solution implements the SSO algorithm for clustering proteins with similar function, and imports biological gene ontology knowledge for further identifying function complexes and improving detection accuracy. Furthermore, we use four different categories of species datasets for experiment: fruitfly, mouse, scere, and human. The testing and analysis result show that the proposed solution is feasible, efficient, and could achieve a higher accuracy of prediction than existing approaches.

Keywords: protein–protein interaction networks; protein function module; simplified swarm optimization

---

1. Introduction

Proteomics is one of the most important topics in the fields of life science and natural science [1–5]. Considering that proteins alone rarely exhibit their biological functions in individuals, the understanding of protein–protein interactions (PPI) [6] is the basis of revealing the activity of protein and promotes the study of various diseases and development of new drugs.

In the past 10 years, substantial work was conducted to promote the research in the field of PPI, such as publications in Nature [2] and Science [3], proceedings of the National Academy of Sciences [3], and nucleic acid research [7]. Available data on PPI are greatly enriched because of the fast development of high-throughput screening [7] and data mining technologies [8]. Some widely used and most complete open datasets are also released, for instance, the Biomolecular Interaction Network Database (BIND) [9], Database of Interaction Proteins (DIP) [10], IntAct [11], Human Protein Reference Database (HPRD) [12], and Molecular Interaction Database (MINT) [13,14].

However, the existing solution is incomplete or inaccurate due to the following technical challenges. On one hand, high-throughput screening technology generates a huge amount of noisy data and higher false positive rates, while the experimental method loses lots of real interactions (false negatives) [15]. On the other hand, the existing computation approaches (described in Section 2) are inefficient, computationally complex, or lack of convincing results. In this paper, we investigate protein function module detection and propose a lightweight and efficient simplified swarm optimization-based protein function module detection with the following contributions:

1. We investigate PPI datasets and existing function module detection methods and select four typical species of protein-protein interaction data from the DIP database for the experiment. A specific data crawler is developed to extract data features from these datasets.
2. The proposed PPIN function module detection is described from a few aspects: system model, feature selection, mathematical description, model optimization, etc. The proposed solution implements an SSO algorithm for clustering proteins with similar function and imports biological gene ontology knowledge for further identification.
3. Experiments are conducted to validate feasibility and efficiency of the proposed approaches. The evaluation of "degree of polymerization" and "similarity between classes" further proves the precision improvement and correctness of our proposed solution.

The paper is organized as follows. Section 2 introduces the existing research, including the graph theory-, machine learning-, and intelligent algorithm-based approaches. Section 3 describes our solution, including the system model, feature extraction, and SSO-based approach. The dataset and result evaluation are explained in Section 4. Finally, experiment conclusions are presented in Section 5.

2. Related Works

2.1. Protein–Protein Interaction Datasets

There are a few protein–protein interaction datasets described in the following:

BIND (Biomolecular Interaction Network Database) contains the known interactions among biological molecules, not only among proteins but also between proteins and DNA, RNA, small molecules, lipids, and carbohydrate substances. BIND is updated daily and has extensive coverage, including human, fruit flies, yeast, nematodes, and other species. DIP was created to establish a simple, easy-to-use, and highly credible PPI public database. It specializes in storing binary PPIs from the literature conf irmed by experiments, as well as the protein complexes from Protein Data Bank (PDB).

IntAct (Molecular Interaction Database) mainly records binary interactions and their experiment methods, experimental conditions, and interaction domain structures in people, yeast, fruit flies, escherichia coli, and other species. IntAct query is divided into basic query and advanced query (more accurate).

HPRD (Human Protein Reference Database) contains protein annotations, PPIs, posttranslational modifications, subcellular localizations, and other comprehensive information.

MINT (Molecular Interaction Database) mainly stores physical interaction of proteins, particularly PPIs of mammals. Besides, it also contains the PPIs of yeast, fruit flies, and viruses. Considering the deviation of definition and the promiscuity in different databases, Gene Ontology (GO), which is developed and maintained by the GO Consortium, should be introduced for the sharing and interoperability among bioinformatics data. Therefore, the retrieval results among different databases could be unified.

2.2. Existing Works

Existing works in the detection of protein function modules could be divided into three categories:

Graph theory-based approach. Similar to a computer network, the graph theory is introduced to improve the detection of protein functional modules, mainly based on three approaches: hierarchical algorithm, partitioning algorithm, and density algorithm [16]. The hierarchical algorithm (such as, modularity division-based method [17], etc.) is based on similarity of the connections between each node. For the partitioning algorithm, the most representative method is based on restricted neighborhood search clustering (RNSC) [18]. Although both hierarchical and partitioning algorithms are easy to understand and implement, the clustering number should be determined beforehand and the function modules cannot be overlapped.

Machine learning-based approaches. Considering the disadvantages (poor scalability and low clustering) of original Markov Clustering (MCL) algorithm, Lei et al. (2015) proposed an improved MCL clustering algorithm for PPIN [19] via importing two parameters: punishment and mutation factors. This approach improves convergence speed but leads to substantial computation complexity. In literature [20], Deddy proposed a rapid and lightweight hidden layer neural network prediction algorithm based on the Extreme Learning Machine (ELM) algorithm. It uses the speed advantage of the ELM algorithm and achieves better protein function module prediction results.

Intelligence algorithm-based approaches. Swarm intelligence algorithms are also implemented for PPIN function module detection. Examples of these algorithms include Ant Colony Optimization (ACO) [21], Particle Swarm Optimization (PSO) [22], and Artificial Bee Colony (ABC) [23]. Sallim applied ACO algorithm to the PPIN complex clustering problem, and further proposed the optimization strategies in protein interaction networks [24]. In 2012, Ji introduced a novel ACO-based functional module detection (NACO–FDM) [25] algorithm to improve the efficiency in searching for an optimal path. However, this algorithm easily falls into the local optimum. In literature, another ACO-MAE mechanism that combines ACO with the idea of multi-agent evolution (MAE) was developed to achieve better prediction accuracy.

Besides, some other works have demonstrated higher performance with a mixture of graph-based approach and machine learning-based approaches [26,27]. The algorithm is based on prior calculation of parameters on the protein residue networks and later machine learning. However, this approach still needs a lot of noted samples for training.

2.3. Clustering Evaluation

In this paper, the clustering evaluation indices include the degree of polymerization (cohesion) inside protein function module, and the deviation degree between modules (separation). Cohesion refers to the similarity degree of each data object in the same category. The higher the degree of polymerization, the higher the similarity. Separation refers to the dissimilarity between two different protein function modules. The higher degree of separation between two categories, the higher the distance between two cluster centers. From mathematics, the cohesion and separation functions are described as follows:

$$Co = \begin{cases} S + \frac{1}{D}, & D \neq 0 \\ S, & D = 0 \end{cases} \tag{1}$$

$$Se = \begin{cases} D + \frac{1}{S}, & S \neq 0 \\ D, & S = 0 \end{cases} \tag{2}$$

where S and D represent the values of protein nodes in the functional similarity matrix and distance matrix, respectively.

2.4. Discussion

However, there are still a few disadvantages in existing research. Graph-based approaches are far from being precise (with a highest precision rate of 46% [16]) because some clusters may be too thin due to the considerable weights between loosely connected nodes. Existing machine/deep learning-based approaches need huge amount of denoted sample for training, and this is difficult to implement in PPIN field. On the contrary, although intelligence algorithms (mainly ACO-related approaches) implemented have shown better precision rates and efficiency than graph-based solutions, more intelligent algorithms should be considered and implemented.

The detection of protein function modules is an NP hard problem [28]. Since the PSO-related solution is efficient and has been implemented in different kinds of NP hard problems, we propose the enhancement of PSO, Simplified Swarm Optimization (SSO) algorithms, for implementation in the detection of protein function modules. Theoretically, an SSO-based solution is capable of achieving better precision than the PSO algorithm and reduces computing complexity.

3. Simplified Swarm Optimization-Based Detection

In this section, we describe the proposed SSO-based solution in four steps: system model, feature extraction, mathematical description, and model optimization.

3.1. Interaction Model

Figure 1a–e illustrates the evolution process of protein function module detection. First, the PPI network is abstracted into the format of a protein distance matrix. The structure model is built by the measure of distance between each protein. Afterwards, the SSO algorithm is imported to search the shortest path between each node. Finally, the cutting and filtering strategies are defined and implemented to generate a clustering result.

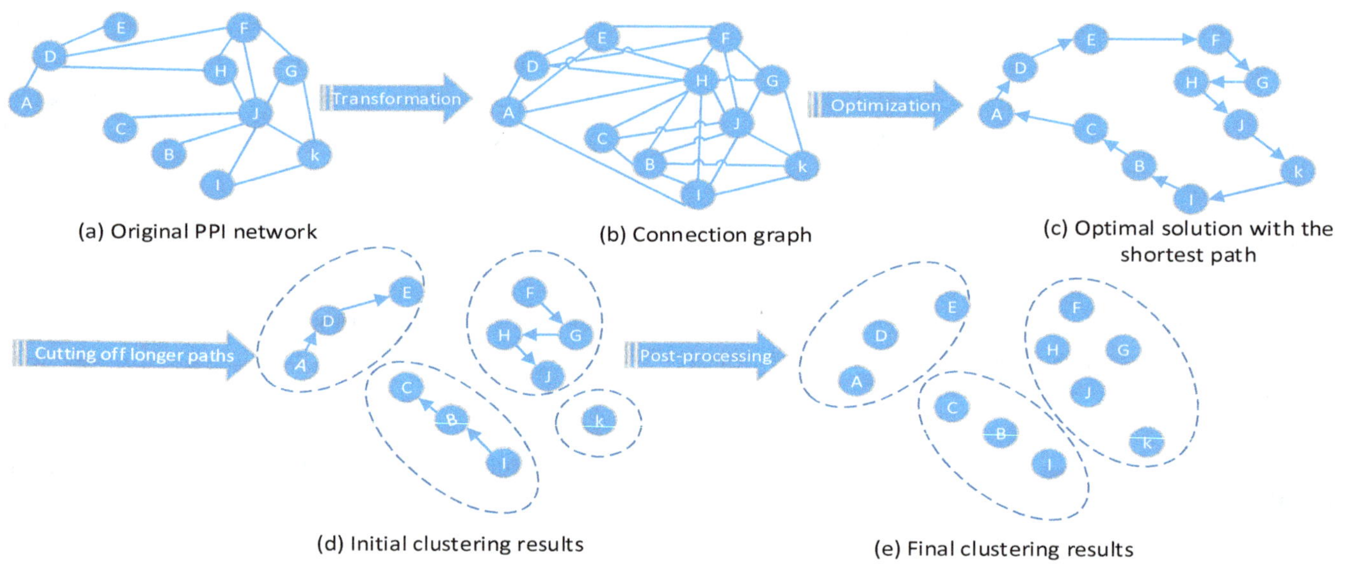

Figure 1. Interaction Model.

3.2. Feature Extraction

After acquiring a dataset from DIP and GO databases, features can be extracted in the following steps:

1. Noise Filter. Noise data refers to the existence of errors, redundant data, or abnormal data in crawled data. For example, in interaction.xml-based crawled data, the tag field "DIP-nnE" may be empty or not found. Therefore, eliminating noise and redundant data is the first step before the experiment.
2. Feature Selection. Feature selection is performed through the manual respection of protein xml data. For example, in the main part of the XML file, the tag names "interactorList" and "interactionList" indicate the interaction relationship among protein nodes. Therefore, feature data are selected through the manual inspection of protein data.
3. Feature Extraction and Reformat. After the feature selection, related data (e.g., protein id and interactor id) are extracted, reformatted, and stored in the structured database.

3.3. Mathematics Model

3.3.1. Model Establishment

Assume the initial particle swarm size n, the problem space dimensions m, the location $X_i^t = (x_{i1}^t, x_{i2}^t, \cdots, x_{im}^t)$, where $i = 1, 2, 3, \ldots n$, x_{im}^t is the value of i-th particle with respect to m-th dimension of feature space at time t; the particles in the search process reach the optimal location and are marked as $p^t{}_i$; the optimal location for the group is $g^t{}_i$. Therefore, the location of particle i in j dimension at time t is described in the following formulas:

$$x_{ij}^t = \begin{cases} X_{ij}^t, & if\ random \in [0, C_w); \\ p_{ij}^t, & if\ random \in [C_w, C_p); \\ g_{ij}^t, & if\ random \in [C_p, C_g); \\ X, & if\ random \in [C_g, 1). \end{cases} \tag{3}$$

In Equation (3), X represents the new value of the particle in every dimension randomly generated; the random number is between (0, 1); C_w, C_p, and C_g are the three predetermined positive constants with $C_w < C_p < C_g$.

In this study, we use the topological structure of a PPIN [29] as the basis, with the individual proteins as nodes and the interactions between proteins as lines, to construct a PPIN model (with interaction model shown in Figure 2, and adjacency matrix in Table 1). The interaction between the proteins is denoted as 1, whereas no relationship between proteins is denoted as 0.

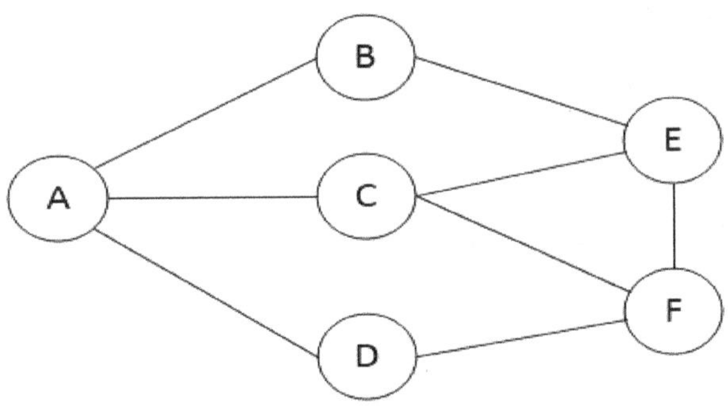

Figure 2. Protein interaction network.

Table 1. Adjacency matrix.

	A	B	C	D	E	F
A	0	1	1	1	0	0
B	1	0	0	0	1	0
C	1	0	0	0	1	1
D	1	0	0	0	0	1
E	0	1	1	0	0	1
F	0	0	1	1	1	0

Therefore, the distance between proteins d_{ij} (difference between two proteins), can be calculated according to Equation (4):

$$d_{ij} = \frac{|Int(i) \cup Int(j)| - |Int(i) \cap Int(j)|}{|Int(i) \cup Int(j)| + |Int(i) \cap Int(j)|} \tag{4}$$

where i and j express the two proteins. Normally, the value of d_{ij} is greater than 0; in some special cases, when proteins i and j are in completely different function modules, d_{ij} achieves the highest value 1.

3.3.2. Parameter Setting

Parameter setting plays a key important role in detecting function modules. In SSO algorithm, the initial location of a particle swarm set to be random. In addition, C_w, C_p, and C_g are set as 0.25, 0.5, and 0.75 respectively. The values of C_w, C_p, and C_g in this paper are set as 0.1, 0.55, and 0.8 to expand the search area to a global search at the beginning of the iteration. Table 2 shows the parameter setting of the SSO and PSO algorithms used in the experiments (t expresses t-th, Max_GEN expresses maximum number of iterations).

Table 2. Parameter setting for PSO and SSO algorithm [1].

Parameter Setting	PSO	SSO
MAX_GEN	500	500
Number of Particle	100	100
Maximum Fitness	1.0	1.0
C_w, C_p, C_g	-	0.1, 0.55, 0.8
Weight	0.9–0.4·t/MAX_GEN	-
c_1, c_2 [2]	2.0, t/MAX_GEN	-

[1] MAX_GEN: expresses maximum number of iterations; [2] c_1, c_2 expresses learning factor.

3.4. Model Optimization

Model optimization is divided into two main parts: module planning based on function information, module planning based on topology.

3.4.1. Module Planning Based on Function Information

The objective of this step is to merge the similar protein function modules (PFMs). The basic idea is to measure the similarity of two modules. When the similarity is greater than a certain threshold, two modules can be merged, based on Equation (5):

$$S(M_S, M_T) = \frac{\sum\limits_{i \in M_S, j \in M_T} s(i,j)}{\min(|M_S|, |M_T|)} \tag{5}$$

where M_S and M_T represent the size of the two protein function modules (including the number of proteins) respectively, and $s(i, j)$ is characterized by the following Equation (6):

$$s(i,j) = \begin{cases} 1, & if\ i = j; \\ f_{ij}, & if\ i \neq j. \end{cases} \tag{6}$$

Among these paramaters, f_{ij} is the similarity function based on gene topology and is characterized by the following Equation (7) [30]:

$$f_{ij} = \frac{|g^i \cap g^j|}{|g^i \cup g^j|} \tag{7}$$

In Equation (7), g^i and g^j represent the comment values of protein i and j in the Gene Ontology respectively [31]. The greater value of f_{ij} indicates higher similarity between two proteins.

3.4.2. Module Planning Based on Topology

This step measures the density of the initial protein function module and reduces the sparse protein module through filter setting. The density is calculated according to Equation (8):

$$D_s = \frac{e}{n \cdot (n-1)/2} \tag{8}$$

where n denotes the number of current protein function module and e represents the number of interactions in the module.

4. Experiments

4.1. Dataset Description

We select four different categories of species data sets for experiment: fruitfly, mouse, scere, and human. Additionally, we use the GO (Gene Ontology) for unifying the format of four species data. Via extracting and matching, the final data statistics are illustrated in Table 3.

Table 3. Matching statistics [1].

Species	Before Matching			After Matching
	Interaction	Interactor	GO Annotation	Interactor & GO Annotation
Human	8412	4823	20,201	3394
Scere	24,668	2340	4680	2325
Mouse	2498	2259	1480	1447
Fruitfly	680	607	3299	269

[1] GO: Gene Ontology.

4.2. Evaluations

4.2.1. Complexity and Running Times

First, we compare the complexity between SSO and PSO (a typical intelligent algorithm). Assuming that the iteration number of i particles was N_i, $i = 1, 2, ..., m$, m is the maximum number of iteration, $N_1 = N_2 = \cdots = N_m = N$. Assuming that each particle in each iteration requires the computational time T_t, the total execution time of PSO algorithm for optimal operation is $N \cdot m \cdot T_t$. As for SSO, assuming that each particle in each iteration requires the computational time D_t, the total execution time in optimal operation is $N \cdot m \cdot D_t$, where $D_t = \alpha \cdot D_1 + \beta \cdot D_2 + \gamma \cdot D_3 + \lambda \cdot D_4$, $\alpha = 0.1, \beta = 0.45, \gamma = 0.25, \lambda = 0.25$. Table 4 further illustrates the experimental comparison, and shows that the SSO algorithm is more efficient than the PSO algorithm.

Table 4. The average running time comparison.

Category	SSO				PSO			
Threshold	Fruitfly	Mouse	Scere	Human	Fruitfly	Mouse	Scere	Human
0.05	4.4	71.2	171.6	731.6	5.4	148.6	205.6	710.2
0.055	4	69.4	150.4	501.4	5	167.4	217.8	650
0.06	4	75.6	181.6	451.8	5	163.2	217.8	637.8
0.065	4	73.6	150.8	407.6	5	168	203.8	683.8
0.07	4	107.4	153	418.8	5	146	204.8	629.6
0.075	4	78	150.8	375.6	5	168	204.4	758.2
0.08	4	74.6	167.2	395.2	5	166.4	206	751.2
0.085	4	76.4	158.8	402	5	167.2	205	771.2

4.2.2. Results Analysis via Threshold Setting

Besides, for four species data, eight different threshold values were selected in the experiment: 0.05, 0.055, 0.06, 0.065, 0.07, 0.075, 0.08, and 0.085, with the result illustrated in Figures 3–5. Results show that when the threshold value increases to a certain extent, the unnecessary protein filtration is greatly reduced (illustrated in Figure 3b), and the size of the protein function module (PFM) increases (illustrated in Figure 3a). However, the other four aspects of the effect including degree of polymerization in the module, the deviation degree between modules, and so on (corresponding to Figures 4 and 5) remained nearly at the same level.

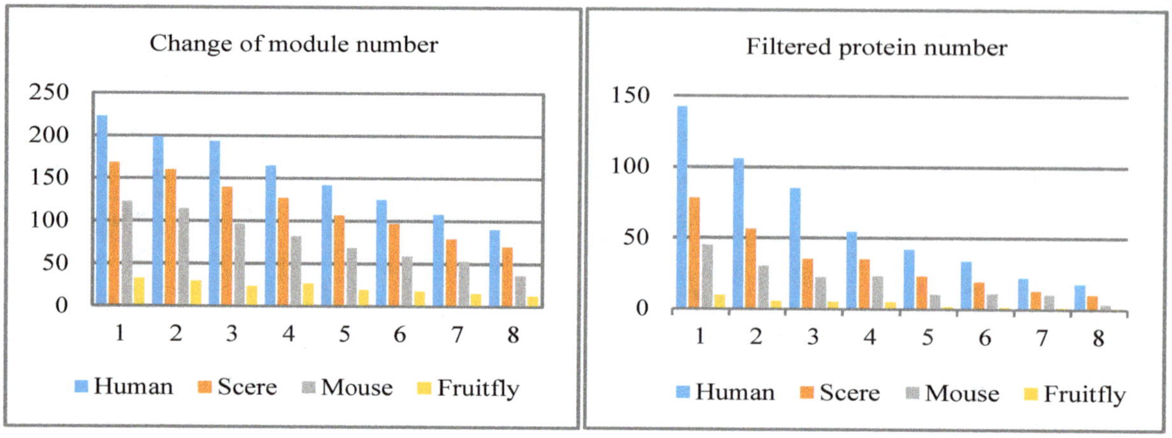

(a) (b)

Figure 3. Four species experimental results. Threshold value changes among 1 (0.05), 2 (0.055), 3 (0.06), 4 (0.065), 5 (0.07), 6 (0.075), 7 (0.08), 8 (0.085). (**a**) Change of module number; (**b**) filtered protein number.

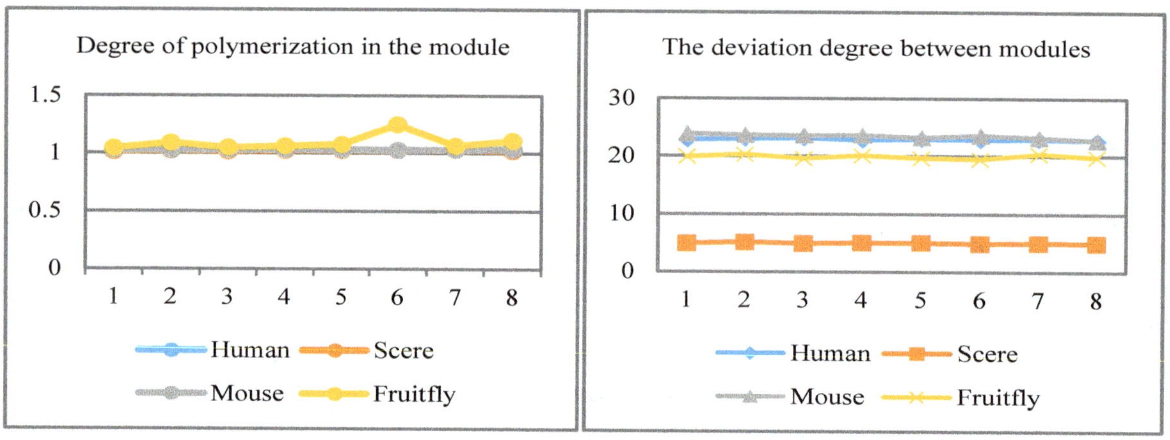

(a) (b)

Figure 4. (**a**) Degree of polymerization in the module; (**b**) deviation degree between modules.

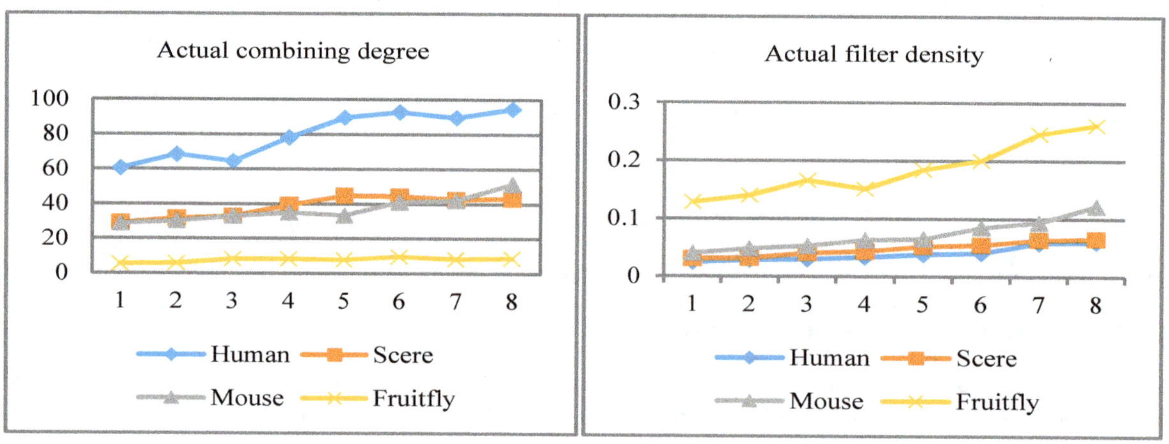

(a) (b)

Figure 5. (**a**) Actual combining degree in each threshold; (**b**) actual filter density during the experiment.

In order to evaluate the efficiency and feasibility of SSO algorithm for protein module detection, we take the human dataset and conduct experiments for evaluation (based on cluster indices described in Section 2.3). The reason for the selection of human species is that the number of nodes is more than other experimental data and the data integrity is better, which can better reflect the characteristics of the algorithm. Figure 6 shows the results under the detection strategy of PSO and SSO.

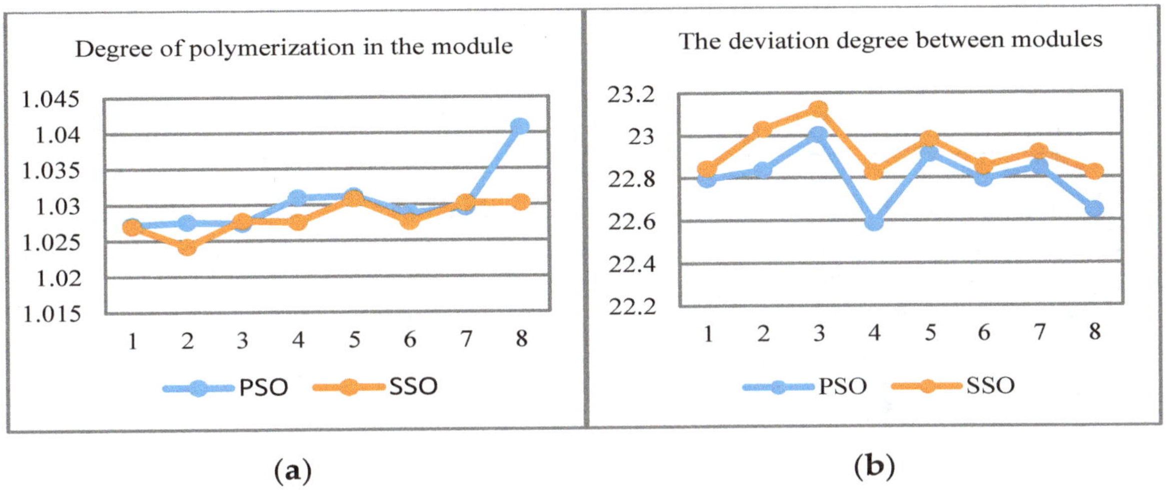

Figure 6. (**a**) Degree of polymerization in the module; (**b**) degree of deviation between modules.

In the Figure 6, we find that the curves of PSO and SSO strategies are more or less intertwined. The difference between PSO and SSO is not obvious in the index of "cohesion", however, the curve of SSO is more stable than PSO algorithm. This indicates that the SSO-based solution outperforms the PSO-based approach in "Separation".

Meanwhile, Table 5 indicates that the number of function module generated by SSO algorithm is a bit lower than PSO in fruitfly species. This may be because of the small number of protein nodes in fruitfly species. Table 6 shows the filtered protein number for PSO and SSO algorithms, which indicates that SSO is significantly better than those of PSO, especially when the number of protein increases. Table 7 shows the degree of polymerization in the module for both PSO and SSO algorithms. A higher value indicates higher similarity in the module. The result also reveals that the two algorithms are relatively close, however, the SSO algorithm has better stability.

Table 5. Change of module number for PSO and SSO algorithms.

Category	**SSO**				**PSO**			
Threshold	**Fruitfly**	**Mouse**	**Scere**	**Human**	**Fruitfly**	**Mouse**	**Scere**	**Human**
0.05	33	122.4	168.6	223	25.8	94.8	174.2	223.4
0.055	30	114	160	198.8	27	92.2	163.8	202.8
0.06	23.6	96.6	139.8	193.6	22.6	82.6	139.8	187.4
0.065	26.8	82.2	127	165.4	18	72.4	129.6	161.2
0.07	19.8	68.8	106.6	142	16.2	66	110.8	147
0.075	18.4	59	96.8	125	14.4	60.8	101.8	126
0.08	15.6	53.2	79.4	108	15.4	46.4	79.2	109
0.085	13.2	36.8	70.2	90.4	11.6	41.8	74.6	96.8

Table 6. Filtered protein number for PSO and SSO algorithm.

Category	SSO				PSO			
Threshold	Fruitfly	Mouse	Scere	Human	Fruitfly	Mouse	Scere	Human
0.05	9.8	45	77.8	142.4	10	280.2	342.4	706
0.055	5.6	30.4	56.2	106	9	172.6	205.2	432.8
0.06	5.2	22.4	35.4	84.8	6	95	102	270
0.065	5.2	23.2	35.4	54.6	4.4	56	64	234.4
0.07	2	10.4	23.2	42	3.4	45.6	35.8	157
0.075	1.6	11	19.4	33.8	4.4	17.8	33.8	100.8
0.08	1.4	10.4	13.2	22.2	1.4	12	18	70.2
0.085	0.8	3.6	10.4	17.8	1.4	6.4	13.8	48.2

Table 7. Degree of polymerization in the module for PSO and SSO algorithm.

Category	SSO				PSO			
Threshold	Fruitfly	Mouse	Scere	Human	Fruitfly	Mouse	Scere	Human
0.05	1.0448	1.028	1.016	1.027	1.0842	1.0288	1.0178	1.0272
0.055	1.0906	1.0298	1.0256	1.0242	1.0688	1.0278	1.0172	1.0276
0.06	1.0516	1.0296	1.0182	1.0278	1.0666	1.0334	1.0248	1.0274
0.065	1.0634	1.0326	1.0236	1.0276	1.071	1.031	1.025	1.031
0.07	1.0778	1.0306	1.0246	1.0308	1.0852	1.0356	1.0238	1.0312
0.075	1.2486	1.0274	1.025	1.0276	1.093	1.0296	1.0254	1.0288
0.08	1.0658	1.03	1.029	1.0302	1.098	1.0334	1.0244	1.0296
0.085	1.1094	1.0342	1.022	1.0302	1.105	1.0362	1.0282	1.0408

5. Conclusions

In this study, we introduce relevant research on protein interaction networks conducted in recent years, including the commonly used protein databases and existing detection methods. We then describe our proposed SSO algorithm for the detection problem of protein function module (PFM) in PPIN. Simultaneously, biological gene ontology knowledge is combined to improve the prediction accuracy. The performance of SSO is compared with existing work (typically PSO algorithm) through the analysis of the experimental results. Results show the feasibility and efficiency of our proposed SSO algorithm. All the datasets and code related with this paper are available from https://github.com/wulingting/PPIN-SSO-and-PSO-algorithms.

Acknowledgments: This work is supported by the National Natural Science Foundation of China under Grant No. 61502106; Fujian Major Project of Regional Industry 2014H4015.

Author Contributions: Xianghan Zheng and Lingting Wu conceived and designed the experiments; Lingting Wu performed the experiments; Xianghan Zheng and Shaozhen Ye analyzed the data; Riqing Chen contributed reagents, materials, and analysis tools; Lingting Wu wrote the paper; Xianghan Zheng participated in paper revision and made many suggestions. All authors read and approved the final manuscript.

References

1. Xu, B.; Guan, J. From function to interaction: A new paradigm for accurately predicting protein complexes based on protein-to-protein interaction networks. *IEEE/ACM Trans. Comput. Biol. Bioinform.* **2014**, *11*, 616–627. [PubMed]
2. Islam, M.F.; Hoque, M.M.; Banik, R.S.; Roy, S.; Sumi, S.S.; Hassan, F.M.N.; Tomal, M.T.S.; Ullah, A.; Rahman, K.M.T. Comparative analysis of differential network modularity in tissue specific normal and cancer protein interaction networks. *J. Clin. Bioinform.* **2013**, *3*, 19. [CrossRef] [PubMed]
3. Ahn, Y.Y.; Bagrow, J.P.; Lehmann, S. Link communities reveal multiscale complexity in networks. *Nature* **2010**, *435*, 761–764. [CrossRef] [PubMed]

4. Kachroo, A.H.; Laurent, J.M.; Yellman, C.M.; Meyer, A.G.; Wilke, C.O.; Marcotte, E.M. Systematic humanization of yeast genes reveals conserved functions and genetic modularity. *Science* **2015**, *348*, 921–925. [CrossRef] [PubMed]
5. Tanay, A.; Sharan, R.; Kupiec, M.; Shamir, R. Revealing modularity and organization in the yeast molecular network by integrated analysis of highly heterogeneous genomewide data. *Proc. Natl. Acad. Sci. USA* **2004**, *101*, 2981–2986. [CrossRef] [PubMed]
6. Szklarczyk, D.; Franceschini, A.; Wyder, S.; Forslund, K.; Heller, D.; Huerta-Cepas, J.; Simonovic, M.; Roth, A.; Santos, A.; Tsafou, K.P.; et al. Protein–protein interaction networks, integrated over the tree of life. *Nucleic Acids Res.* **2015**, *39*, D561–D568.
7. Ding, Y.; Tang, J.; Guo, F. Identification of Protein–Protein Interactions via a Novel Matrix-Based Sequence Representation Model with Amino Acid Contact Information. *Int. J. Mol. Sci.* **2016**, *17*, 1623. [CrossRef] [PubMed]
8. Szklarczyk, D.; Franceschini, A.; Kuhn, M.; Simonovic, M.; Roth, A.; Minguez, P.; Doerks, T.; Stark, M.; Muller, J.; Bork, P.; et al. The STRING database in 2011: Functional interaction networks of proteins, globally integrated and scored. *Nucleic Acids Res.* **2011**, *1093*, D561–D568. [CrossRef] [PubMed]
9. Xu, H.; Li, X.; Zhang, Z.; Song, J. Identifying Coevolution between Amino Acid Residues in Protein Families: Advances in the Improvement and Evaluation of Correlated Mutation Algorithms. *Curr. Bioinform.* **2013**, *8*, 148–160. [CrossRef]
10. Li, H.; Chang, Y.; Yang, L.; Bahar, I. The Gaussian network model database for biomolecular structural dynamics. *Nucleic Acids Res.* **2016**, *44*, D415–D422. [CrossRef] [PubMed]
11. Blohm, P.; Frishman, G.; Smialowski, P. A database of non-interacting proteins derived by literature mining, manual annotation and protein structure analysis. *Nucleic Acids Res.* **2014**, *42*, D396–D400. [CrossRef] [PubMed]
12. Orchard, S.; Ammari, M.; Aranda, B.; Breuza, L.; Briganti, L.; Broackes-Carter, F.; Nancy, H.; Campbell, G.C.; Chen, C.; del-Toro, N. The MIntAct project—IntAct as a common curation platform for 11 molecular interaction databases. *Nucleic Acids Res.* **2014**, *1093*, D358–D363. [CrossRef] [PubMed]
13. Motono, C.; Nakata, J.; Koike, R. A comprehensive database of predicted structures of all human proteins. *Nucleic Acids Res.* **2011**, *39*, D487–D493. [CrossRef] [PubMed]
14. Licata, L.; Briganti, L.; Peluso, D. MINT, the molecular interaction database: 2012 update. *Nucleic Acids Res.* **2012**, *40*, D857–D861. [CrossRef] [PubMed]
15. Ji, J.Z.; Jiao, L.; Yang, C.C.; Lv, J.W.; Zhang, A.D. MAE-FMD: Multi-agent evolutionary method for functional module detection in protein-protein interaction networks. *BMC Bioinform.* **2014**, *15*, 325. [CrossRef] [PubMed]
16. Ester, B.M.; Kriegel, H.P.; Sander, J.; Xu, X. A Density Based algorithm for discovering clusters in large spatial databases with Noise. In Proceedings of the International Conference on Knowledge Discovery and Data Mining, Chicago, IL, USA, 11–14 August 2013.
17. Newman, M.E. Fast algorithm for detecting community structure in networks. *Phys. Rev. E* **2004**, *69*, 066133. [CrossRef] [PubMed]
18. Hartuv, E.; Shamir, R. A clustering algorithm based on graph connectivity. *Inf. Proc. Lett.* **2000**, *76*, 175–181. [CrossRef]
19. Rujirapipat, S.; Mcgarry, K.; Nelson, D. Bioinformatic Analysis Using Complex Networks and Clustering Proteins Linked with Alzheimer's Disease. In *Advances in Computational Intelligence Systems*; Springer: Cham, Germany, 2017; pp. 219–230.
20. Ruan, P.; Hayashida, M.; Maruyama, O.; Akutsu, T. Prediction of heterotrimeric protein complexes by two-phase learning using neighboring kernels. *BMC Bioinform.* **2014**, *15*, S6. [CrossRef] [PubMed]
21. Lei, X.J. The Information Flow Clustering Model and Algorithm Based on the Artificial Bee Colony Mechanism of PPI Network. *Chin. J. Comput.* **2012**, *35*, 134–145. [CrossRef]
22. Dorigo, M. *Ant Colony Optimization*; MIT Press/Bradford Books: Cambridge, MA, USA, 2004.
23. Kennedy, J.; Eberhart, R. Particle swarm optimization. In Proceedings of the IEEE International Conference on Neural Networks, Perth, Australia, 27 November–1 December 1995; pp. 1942–1948.
24. Karaboga, D.; Basturk, B. On the performance of artificial bee colony (ABC) algorithm. *Appl. Soft Comput.* **2008**, *8*, 687–697. [CrossRef]

25. Ji, J.Z.; Liu, Z.J. Ant colony optimization with multi-agent evolution for detecting functional modules in protein-protein interaction networks. In Proceedings of the 3rd International Conference on Information Computing and Applications, Chengdu, China, 14–16 September 2012; pp. 445–453.
26. Rodriguez-Soca, Y.; Munteanu, C.R.; Dorado, J.; Pazos, A.; Prado-Prado, F.J.; González-Díaz, H. A web server for prediction of unique targets in trypanosome proteome by using electrostatic parameters of protein-protein interactions. *J. Proteome Res.* **2010**, *9*, 1182–1190. [CrossRef] [PubMed]
27. Rodriguez-Soca, Y.; Munteanu, C.R.; Dorado, J.; Rabuñal, J.; Pazos, A.; González-Díaz, H. A web-server predicting complex biopolymer targets in plasmodium with entropy measures of protein–protein interactions. *Polymer* **2010**, *51*, 264–273. [CrossRef]
28. Ji, J.; Liu, Z.; Zhang, A.; Jiao, L.; Liu, C. Improve ant colony optimization for detecting functional modules in protein-protein interaction networks. In Proceedings of the 3rd International Conference on Information Computing and Applications, Chengdu, China, 14–16 September 2012; pp. 404–413.
29. Debby, D.W.; Ran, W.; Hong, Y. Fast prediction of protein-protein interaction sites based on Extreme Learning Machines. *Neurocomputing* **2014**, *128*, 258–266.
30. Schlicker, A.; Albrecht, M. FunSimMat: A comprehensive functional similarity database. *Nucleic Acids Res.* **2008**, *36*, D434–D439. [CrossRef] [PubMed]
31. Ashburner, M.; Ball, C.A.; Blake, J.A.; Botstein, D.; Butler, H.; Cherry, J.M.; Davis, A.P.; Dolinski, K.; Dwight, S.S.; Eppig, J.T.; et al. Gene ontology: Tool for the unification of biology. The Gene Ontology Consortium. *Nat. Genet.* **2000**, *25*, 25–29. [CrossRef] [PubMed]

15

Electrochemical Nanobiosensors for Detection of Breast Cancer Biomarkers

Veronika Gajdosova [1], Lenka Lorencova [1], Peter Kasak [2,*] and Jan Tkac [1,*]

1 Institute of Chemistry, Slovak Academy of Sciences, Dubravska cesta 9, 845 38 Bratislava, Slovakia; Veronika.Gajdosova@savba.sk (V.G.); Lenka.Lorencova@savba.sk (L.L.)
2 Center for Advanced Materials, Qatar University, Doha 2713, Qatar
* Correspondence: peter.kasak@qu.edu.qa (P.K.); Jan.Tkac@savba.sk (J.T.)

Abstract: This comprehensive review paper describes recent advances made in the field of electrochemical nanobiosensors for the detection of breast cancer (BC) biomarkers such as specific genes, microRNA, proteins, circulating tumor cells, BC cell lines, and exosomes or exosome-derived biomarkers. Besides the description of key functional characteristics of electrochemical nanobiosensors, the reader can find basic statistic information about BC incidence and mortality, breast pathology, and current clinically used BC biomarkers. The final part of the review is focused on challenges that need to be addressed in order to apply electrochemical nanobiosensors in a clinical practice.

Keywords: breast cancer; nanobiosensors; biomarkers; electrochemistry; impedance; immobilization; nanomaterial; nanoparticles (NPs); magnetic NPs; self-assembled monolayers (SAMs); signal amplification

1. Introduction

According to the World Health Organization, the year of 2030 should witness roughly 12 million cancer-related deaths, making cancer one of the most prominent death-causing factors around the globe. In fact, the number of new cases of cancer (cancer incidence) is currently around 439 *per* 100,000 men and women *per* year [1]. Breast cancer (BC) has been considered the most frequent type of cancer disease worldwide among women, impacting 2.1 million women each year. In 2018, it was estimated that around 627,000 women died from BC; that is approximately 15% of all cancer deaths among women [2]. The highest incidence rates were observed in the United States and Western Europe. In the US, there were 101 new cases reported *per* 100,000 women, and in Europe, there were 85 [3]. East Asia has the lowest incidence with 21 cases *per* 100,000 women [3]. In Africa, the incidence is slightly higher with 23 cases *per* 100,000 women, but this amount can be undervalued due to a lack of accurate data [3].

BC is one of the leading causes of cancer-related mortality. The disease had always been common among women. That is supported by the fact that one of the first surgical treatments ever performed was BC treatment during the first surgical revolution at the end of the 19th century. BC rates are globally increasing and are higher among women in developed regions. The incidence and fatality increase with the increasing age of women as well. It was reported that statistically, women with an age 65 and above die with higher probability due to the disease [4–6]. The probability of the disease to develop within a woman's lifetime has grown over the past few decades from 1 in 11 in 1975 to 1 in 8 in 2016 [6]. There are several risk factors behind BC, including age, geographic location (country of origin), socioeconomic status, lifestyle risk factors (smoking, alcohol, diet, obesity, and physical activity), low rates of breastfeeding, family history of BC, mammographic density, ionizing radiation, etc. [5].

If the BC is diagnosed at an early stage, a 5-year survival rate can reach up to 90% in developed countries [7]. On the other hand, once a BC is metastatic, the patient's 5-year survival rate falls down to 27.4% [8]. Early diagnosis is needed for a successful treatment and high survival rate. T1 tumors with size less than 2 cm show a 10-year survival rate of approximately 85%, while T3 tumors show a 10-year survival of less than 60% mainly as the result of delayed accurate diagnosis [9]. Nowadays, mammography is used as a gold standard for early BC screening and detection, but it is less sensitive for young women (under 40 years old) with a sensitivity of 25–59%. A factor that is limiting the diagnosis of young women is a denser breast tissue compared to older women. Other limitations of mammography are high rates of false-positive and false-negative results which lead to biopsy, high cost of treatment, and procedural discomfort for the women [10].

To avoid development of the disease into advanced stages, there is clear need for early diagnostics, efficient treatment, and post-treatment monitoring. Therefore, there is an enormous demand for efficient less-invasive diagnosis i.e., analysis of cancer biomarkers in plasma/serum samples [11].

Although several review papers have been published recently describing the electrochemical biosensing of cancer biomarkers [12–16], such studies only partly covered the biosensing of BC biomarkers or the electrochemical biosensing of BC biomarkers. There are only two review papers specifically covering the electrochemical biosensing of BC biomarkers published in 2017 [17,18], but with only a minor coverage of beneficial properties of nanoparticles within electrochemical transducing schemes. To our best knowledge, this is the first review paper comprehensively covering the use of nanomaterials for enhanced electrochemical detection of breast cancer biomarkers.

2. Breast Pathology

In humans, the breast has a number of functions. The mammary gland is a distinguishing feature of mammals, and its primary role is to produce milk to nourish offspring. The breast develops in the superficial fascia. Until puberty, the breast includes only few ducts in both men and women. In females, true breast development begins at puberty due to the effect of estrogen and progesterone [19]. The breast consists of 12–15 major breast ducts, which lead to the formation of a nipple. These are connected to ducts ending in a duct lobular unit, which is the functional milk-producing unit of a breast [20]. Breast ducts are surrounded by myoepithelial cells supported by connective tissue stroma and a variable amount of fat [19]. The terminal duct lobular units spread during pregnancy. Milk is produced due to the secretion of prolactin and oxytocin. Imbalance in estrogen and progesterone concentrations *prior* to menopause results in atrophic changes of a breast tissue.

From a clinical point of view, the lymphatic drainage of a breast has a big importance. Approximately 5% of the lymph from the breast drains through the intercostal spaces to nodes along the internal mammary vessels. The remaining 95% of the lymph drains toward the axilla in one or two larger channels. As a result of this fact, all patients with invasive BC should go through some form of auxiliary surgery to find out whether there is lymph node involvement [21].

BC is a heterogeneous disease with various subtypes accompanied by a series of genetic changes. Breast tumors originate in the anatomical structures of the mammary gland that form the mammary gland, fibrous tissue, and adipose tissue. Mammary gland tumors can be benign such as papillomas and fibroadenomas. The most common malignant tumors are carcinomas. BC is most often caused by the terminal lobes (lobular) of the mammary gland and their ducts (ductal) (Figure 1). Globally, approximately 80% of all diagnosed BC cases are of the ductal subtype [22]. These two subtypes cover 40%–75% of all diagnosed cases [23]. Other types of cancer are present in 10% of cases where inflammatory BC, male BC, Paget's disease of breast, papillary carcinoma, and others are included [24]. BC can be classified by immunohistochemical examination into four subtypes: estrogen receptor (ER), progesterone receptor (PR), human receptor tyrosine-protein kinase erbB-2 (HER2), and antigen Ki-67 dependent [25].

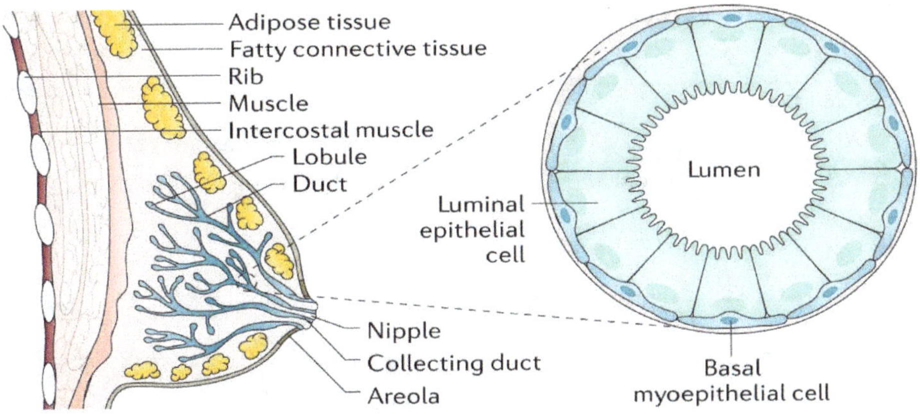

Figure 1. All breast cancers (BC) arise in the terminal duct lobular units (the functional unit of the breast) of the collecting duct. The histological and molecular characteristics have important implications for therapy. Several classifications based on molecular and histological characteristics have been developed.

3. BC Biomarkers

Due to progress in genomics, proteomics, and glycomics, various candidate biomarkers have been identified with a clinical potential for BC management [27]. A tumor marker was first discovered in 1847, and currently, there are more than 100 known different tumor markers [28]. Biomarkers have great potential for screening and diagnostics because they are present in blood and provide information about the health condition [7]. In healthy individuals, the tumor marker concentration is at a very low level or even in some cases absent, while increased values can reveal development and/or progression of a disease [29]. Serum biomarkers providing key information about the disease are important for the management of cancer patients, since blood aspiration is only a moderately invasive procedure.

The most relevant biomarkers that have occurred in BC include the presence of gene markers such as BReast CAncer Type (*BRCA1*, *BRCA2*), and protein-based biomarkers including cancer antigen CA 27.29, carcinoembryonic antigen (CEA), human epidermal growth factor receptor 2 (HER2), vascular endothelial growth factor (VEGF), polypeptide antigen (TPA), cytokeratin 19 fragment (CIFRA-21-1), platelet-derived growth factor (PDGF), and osteopontin (OPN). The basic characteristics of BC biomarkers are summarized in Table 1.

BC biomarkers (glycoproteins: mucin 1 (MUC1), HER2, carcinoembryonic antigen (CEA), epidermal growth factor receptor (EGFR), carbohydrate antigen 15-3 (CA15-3), CA 27-29, mammaglobin (MAM); DNA: *BRCA1*, *BRCA2*, proteins: Ki-67, OPN, microRNAs, and circulating tumor cells (CTC)) can be classified as diagnostic (healthy versus BC), prognostic (early BC versus advanced BC), predictive (provide information regarding whether a particular treatment will be beneficial for the BC patient) or therapeutic (a target biomolecule for therapeutics) based biomarkers [30,31].

Interestingly, although many studies have been published, only 9 biomarkers of cancer have been approved by the Food and Drug Administration (FDA) for clinical examinations so far. Since these biomarkers are all glycosylated proteins, changes in the glycan composition of these glycoproteins may serve as additional information for cancer diagnostics and/or prognosis. The following glycoprotein-based biomarkers have been published in the literature for BC management: HER2/NEU, CA15-3, CA27.29, MAM, galectin 3 binding protein, nectin 4, and fibronectin 1 with a typical concentration in human serum of 1–50 ng/mL [30]. The invasion, migration, and metastasis of cancer are caused by the deregulation of glycosylation related to an essential post-translational modification of proteins. In more than 90% of BC cases, there are observed changes in *O*-linked mucin-type glycosylation for example, expression of the Tn antigen, and the loss of core 2 *O*-glycans [32]. In BC, major glycan changes involve increased sialylation and fucosylation [33–36].

Table 1. Candidate breast cancer biomarkers (BRCA1, BRCA2, CA27.29, CA 15-3, CEA, HER-2, VEGF, tPA, CIFRA-21-1, PDGF, OPN).

Biomarker	Size/kDa	Incidence in Cancer	Level in Serum
BRCA1	207–220	breast, ovarian, prostate, pancreatic	ND
BRCA2	384	Fanconi anemia, breast, ovarian, lung, prostate, pancreatic	ND
CA27.29	250–1000	breast	≤37 U/mL
CA15-3	290–400	breast	3–30 U/mL
CEA	180–200	gastric, pancreatic, lung, breast, medullary thyroid	2–4 ng/mL
HER-2	185	breast, ovarian, gastric, prostate	15 ng/mL
VEGF	18–27	brain, lung, gastrointestinal, hepatobiliary, renal, breast, ovarian	~220 pg/mL
TPA	20–45	breast, lung, pancreatic	109 U/L
CIFRA-21-1	40	breast, lung, pancreatic	50 ng/mL
PDGF	35	glioblastoma, lung, colorectal, breast, liver and ovarian	(7.5 ± 3.1) ng/mL
OPN	41–75	breast, colon, liver, lung, ovarian, prostate	16 ng/mL

When new BC biomarkers are identified, it is of high importance to compare their clinical performance with already approved biomarkers in a form of AUC (area under curve) values in the receiver operating characteristic (ROC). The ROC curves calculated using the Youden index for the determination of CEA and CA15-3 showed AUC values of 0.616 or 0.678, respectively for CEA (cut-off value of 3.2 ng/mL) and CA15-3 (cut-off value of 13.3 ng/mL), when applied for disease-free survival examination [37]. We have found out clinical parameters for some of the novel BC biomarkers, showing significant advantage over already approved biomarkers. For example, Park et al. found out that the level of the human cytosolic thioredoxin correlated very well with the progress of BC [38]. At the cut-off value of 33.2 ng/mL, a sensitivity of 89.8%, a specificity of 78.0%, and an AUC value of 0.901 ± 0.025 were obtained by applying the ELISA format for thioredoxin analysis [38]. The ELISA method developed by Bernstein et al. resulted in an estimated AUC value of 0.892 using mammaglobin detection [39]. Thus, their method was able to distinguish healthy women from those having BC with high accuracy [39]. Yan et al. examined a clinical potential of the level of one type of fucosyltransferase (FUT4) determined in blood serum by ELISA for BC diagnostics [40]. AUC values of 0.784, 0.468, and 0.563 were determined for FUT4, CA15-3, and CEA, respectively. The results pointed out that FUT4 is in correlation with CA15-3 ($p < 0.05$). Moreover, FUT4 could be applied besides BC diagnostics also for BC prognosis [40].

4. Nanomaterials/Nanoparticles-Based Electrochemical Biosensors as Ultrasensitive Tools in Detection of BC Biomarkers

The speech of the physicist Richard Feynman entitled "There's plenty of room at the bottom", which took place at the Meeting of the American Physical Society in 1959 at CalTech, is considered to be the beginning of the nanotechnology era. Significant attention is currently being paid to nanomaterials. Nanomaterials are considered a pivotal tool for numerous applications in part due to their high surface area, compared to their respective bulk forms. Nanostructures with at least one dimension of size of 100 nm (1 nm = 1×10^{-9} m) or smaller are extremely useful in a number of areas, such as electronics, aerospace, military, pharmaceuticals, medicine, etc. Within last years, there has been an improvement in the synthesis and characterization of different nanomaterials, such as carbon-based nanomaterials, hydrogels, magnetic nanoparticles, metallic nanoparticles, polymer nanoparticles, and/or nanocomposites and two-dimensional nanomaterials [41,42].

One of the leading areas for practical application of the state-of-the-art nanoscience and nanotechnology is the development of various types of biosensors.

The application of nanomaterials to design biosensing platforms offers exceptional electronic, magnetic, mechanical, and optical properties for such devices. Nanomaterials can increase the surface of the transducing area of the sensors, which in turn provides enhanced catalytic activity. Electroactive properties of nanoparticles toward certain reactions have been widely exploited in biosensing applications. Nanometer-size structures have a large surface-to-volume ratio, controlled morphology, and structure that would scale down the characteristic size, which is a clear advantage when the sample volume is critical. The integration of advanced 2D nanomaterial MXene into biosensors architecture brings the advantage of hydrophilic character due to functional groups onto the nanoscale surface [43]. However, advances in nanomaterial biofunctionalization are crucial to achieve higher specificity in biosensing. To that end, nanomaterials can be "decorated" with different (bio)receptors offering specific recognition for biosensing [44–49]. There are basically two approaches applied to designing nanobiosensors: i.e., the application of nanoparticles for the modification of electrode surfaces (Approach 1, Figure 2), or the application of nanoparticles to make signal nanoprobes that enhance a generated signal (Approach 2, Figure 2). There are some nanobiosensors constructed using both amplification approaches (hybrid biosensing, i.e., Approach 3). In the forthcoming sections, when discussing particular nanobiosensors, amplification strategies are indicated as well.

Electrochemical biosensors (amperometric, potentiometric, conductometric, impedimetric, field-effect devices, etc.) are of particular interest for early-stage diagnostics of cancer diseases [15,50]. Electrochemical techniques such as cyclic voltammetry (CV), chronoamperometry (CA), differential pulse voltammetry (DPV), electrochemical impedance spectroscopy (EIS), and square wave voltammetry (SWV) offer an easy-to-use, affordable, highly sensitive, and reliable way for the ultrasensitive sensing of biomarkers related to such diseases [51,52]. Lab-on-chip biosensors presenting the compact and low-power portable miniaturized devices can be utilized in cancer biomarker discovery research, leading to potential clinical applications [53–57]. The surface architecture connecting the sensing element to the biological sample at the nanometer scale determines signal transduction and the general performance of electrochemical sensors. The eventual biosensor sensitivity is affected by the most common surface modification techniques with subsequent functionalization, various electrochemical transduction mechanisms, and by the choice of the recognition element (antibodies, nucleic acids, cells, micro-organisms, etc.). Electrochemical biosensors employing surface nanoarchitectures offer attractive features including robustness, easy miniaturization, excellent detection limits, as well as small analyte volumes and the ability to be used in turbid biofluids with optically absorbing and fluorescing compounds.

Nonetheless, there is still great room for improvement with regard to reproducibility, specificity, stability, and assay throughput of biosensing assay formats.

Regarding the sensitivity of detection by the biosensors, there is need to achieve a limit of detection (LOD) for the analytes that is at least comparable with ELISA assay format offering LODs of 0.75 ng/mL (HER2), 0.1 μg/L (kallikrein 5), and 0.17 ng/mL (thymidine kinase (TK1)). It is also important to outperform ELISA by the design of electrochemical biosensors offering to complete the whole assay procedure within 5 h and with a moderate throughput of analysis (up to 50 samples analyzed *per* run), which is typical for ELISA-based assay formats [58–60]. The novel generation of highly specific, sensitive, selective, and reliable micro (bio-)chemical sensors and sensor arrays can merge interdisciplinary knowledge in bio- and electrochemistry, solid-state chemistry, surface physics, bioengineering, integrated circuit silicon technology, and data processing. In the forthcoming sections, we discuss novel, nanoparticle-based approaches for the electrochemical detection of BC biomarkers.

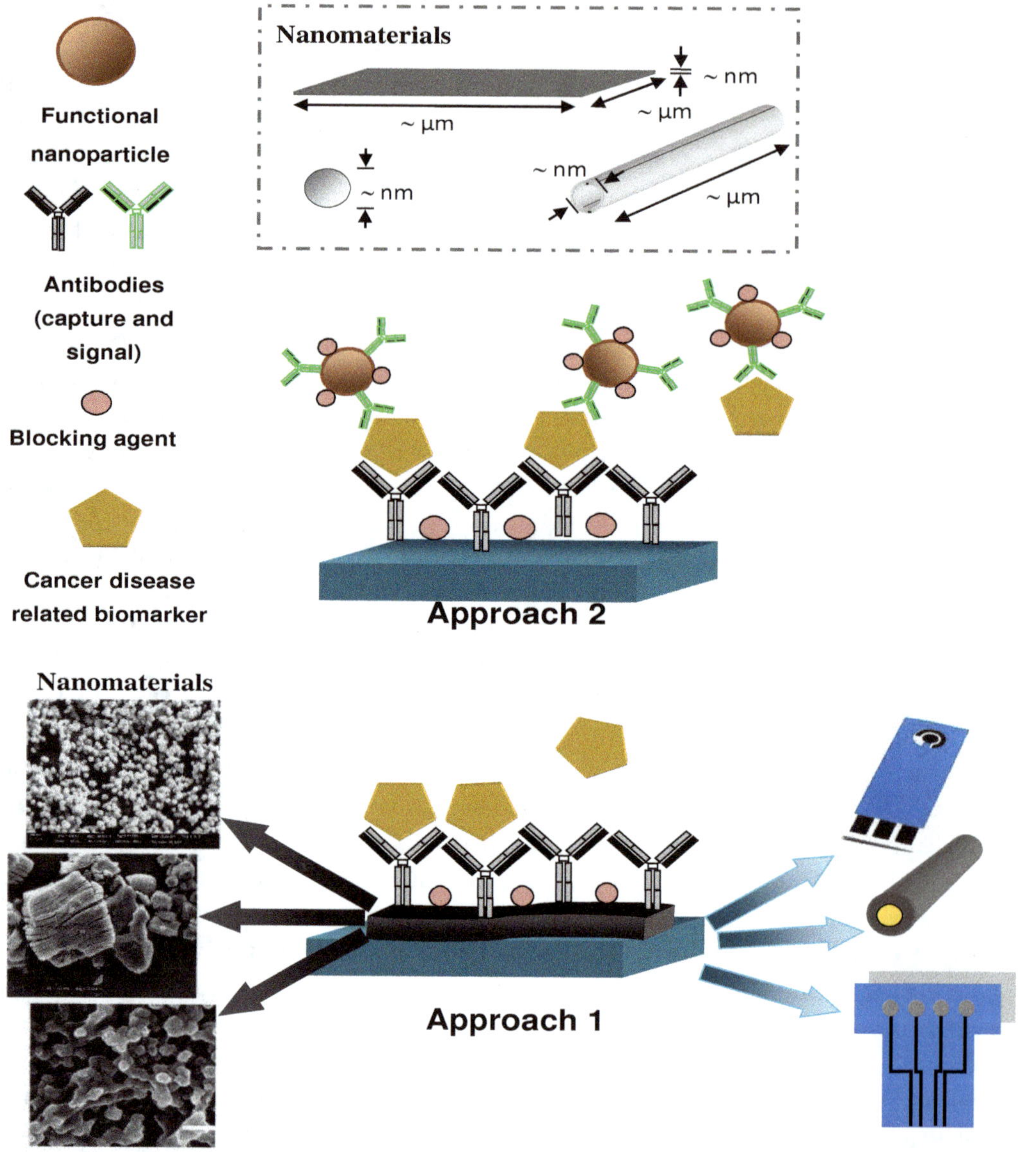

Figure 2. Schematic illustration of two different approaches applicable for the enhanced biosensing of cancer biomarkers using functional nanomaterials/nanoparticles either to enhance the electrode area, accessibility of analytes toward the interface, or interfacial properties with capture biorecognition elements (antibodies) immobilized (*Approach 1*) or for enhanced signal generation using a signal probe with biorecognition elements (antibodies) immobilized on the electrode (without being modified by nanoparticles) of a signal probe (*Approach 2*). Please note that we recognize *Approach 3* (not shown in the figure) applied to design biosensor devices by a combination of the nanomaterial/nanoparticle-modified electrode (*Approach 1*) with the use of a signal nanoprobe (*Approach 2*) within one biosensor device.

4.1. Detection of DNAs

The product of a BReast CAncer Type 1 (*BRCA1*) gene controls the cell cycle and ensures DNA repair. Mutation in the *BRCA1* gene leads to BC predisposition due to the loss of a gene function [61].

Benvidi and co-workers are topically focused on the development of DNA biosensors for the detection of *BRCA1* mutation at initial stages [62–65]. Benvidi and Jahanbani [63] applied a carbon paste electrode in combination with metallic nanocomposite, i.e., a magnetic bar carbon paste electrode decorated with magnetic iron oxide and silver nanoparticles by a physical method for label-free DNA detection. In the next step, the nanocomposite was modified with a self-assembled monolayer (SAM) of thiolated single-stranded DNA. The biosensor detected *BRCA1* 5382 mutation by the EIS method with an LOD of 3.0×10^{-17} M (a linear range from 1.0×10^{-16} M to 1.0×10^{-8} M) [63]

(Approach 1). Benvidi et al. [64] published results obtained with an improved strategy based on the application of glassy carbon electrode (GCE) modified by another type of carbon nanomaterial, e.g., reduced graphene oxide (RGO) or multi-walled carbon nanotubes (MWCNTs). 1-pyrenebutyric acid-*N*-hydroxysuccinimide ester was applied as a scaffold molecule for the immobilization of a *BRCA1* DNA probe for the detection of complementary DNA sequences. By applying this approach, the authors obtained a low LOD of 3.1×10^{-18} M and 3.5×10^{-19} M for a MWCNT-modified or RGO-modified device, respectively [64] (Approach 1). Other work from the same group of authors [65] was focused on an advanced coating of GCE with a dispersion of GO and a silk fibroin (SF) with subsequently electrochemically immobilized gold nanoparticles (AuNPs) for *BRCA1* 5382 mutation detection. In the next step, the analyte was incubated with the modified electrode and measured by CV and EIS techniques with complementary target DNA sequences. The impedimetric DNA sensor achieved an LOD of 3.3×10^{-17} M (a linear range from 1.0×10^{-16} M to 1.0×10^{-8} M) [65] (Approach 1).

A pre-treated GCE surface was coated with a hydrophilic material consisting of electrochemically deposited polydopamine, which was followed by the deposition of tannic acid assisted by Fe^{3+} ions [66]. In the next step, the branched structure of four-armed polyethyleneglycol was grafted onto a modified interface via a layer-by-layer technique. To enhance *BRCA1* gene detection, AuNPs with thiol-modified oligonucleotides were finally deposited onto the modified surface (Figure 3). An impedimetric biosensor detected *BRCA1* with an LOD of 0.05 fM in a linear range from 0.1 fM to 10 pM [66] (Approach 1). A carbon paste electrode (CPE) modified with electrospun ribbon conductive nanofibers of polyethersulfone and nanotubes were employed for *BRCA1* detection by Ehzari et al. [67]. DNA was detected with LOD of 2.4 pM with high selectivity, stability, reproducibility, and with a recovery index in the range from 101.5% to 105.2% [67] (Approach 1).

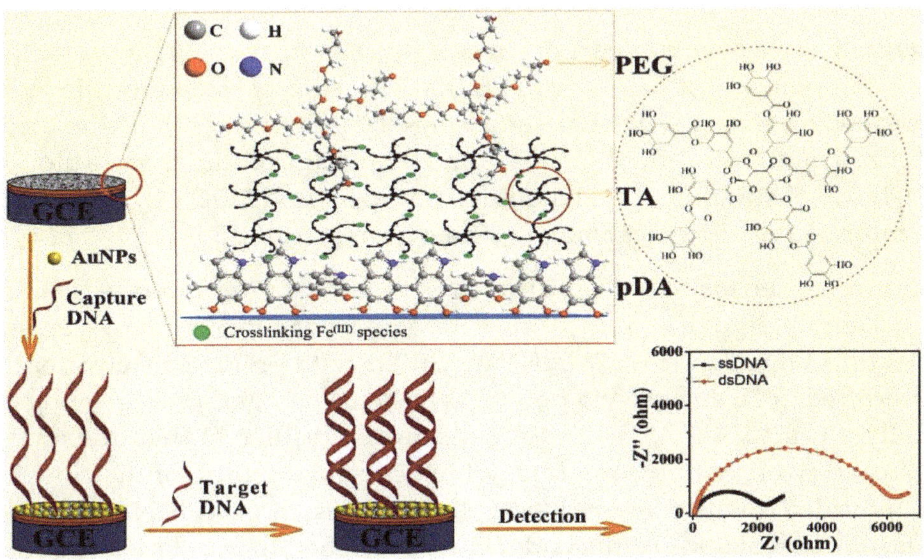

Figure 3. Fabrication process to design nanobiosensors for the detection of *BRCA1*.

Graphene oxide (GO) was successfully applied as a promising nanomaterial with high surface area for the detection of the *BRCA1* gene. Kazerooni and Nassernejad developed a biosensor for detection of *BRCA1* with LOD of 2 pM by applying supramolecular ionic liquids grafted on nitrogen-doped graphene aerogel-modified GCEs by electrochemical reading [68] (Approach 1). The single-stranded DNA probe for the detection of *BRCA1* 5382 insC mutation was immobilized onto GCE electrochemically patterned with RGO and gold nanoparticles (AuNPs) [69]. The impedimetric biosensor was able to specifically recognize targets with LOD of 1.0×10^{-20} M [69] (Approach 1). RGO was also applied in combination with polypyrrole polymer by Shahrokhiana et al. for *BRCA1* detection [70]. A pyrrole-3-carboxylic acid monomer was electrochemically polymerized and applied for probe immobilization. *BRCA1* was determined with LOD of 3 fM in a linear range of 10 fM–0.1 μM by DPV and EIS [70] (Approach 1).

In addition to the development of a biosensor for the detection of the *BRCA1* gene, a DNA biosensor for the detection of the ERBB2c gene (producing HER2 protein) and CD24c was also prepared [71]. GCE was modified by GO, to which 4-aminothiophenol as a linker was covalently attached via amine coupling. The linker was in the subsequent step applied for the attachment of AuNPs. Then, a DNA capture probe was deposited on AuNPs via SAM formation. Then, DNA for the ERBB2c target was hybridized with a surface-confined capture DNA probe. Finally, the electrochemical signal was generated by hybridization with a conjugation DNA probe linked to horseradish peroxidase (HRP). The biosensor detected the ERBB2c gene down to 0.16 nM and CD24 down to 0.23 nM [71] (Approach 1).

The phosphatidylinositol-4,5-bisphosphate 3-kinase catalytic subunit alpha gene (*PIK3CA* gene) as a circulating tumor DNA was detected by a biosensor employing a nanocomposite of MoS_2 and poly(indole-6-carboxylic acid) as a surface-confined mediator, which was also applied for the covalent immobilization of $-NH_2$-modified ssDNA [72]. First, the surface of CPE was modified with exfoliated MoS_2 nanosheets, and then, it was incubated with a mediator monomer via π–π stacking with a subsequent potentiostatic polymerization of the monomer. Afterwards, ssDNA probes were covalently immobilized to such a modified electrode. The DNA biosensor could detect analytes down to 15 aM [72] (Approach 1).

4.2. Detection of MicroRNAs (MiRNAs)

The miRNAs are biomolecules consisting of 18–24 nucleotides that have a key role in biological processes such as cell proliferation, apoptosis, and tumorigenesis [73–75]. Abnormal expression has been observed in BC as well as in other cancer types [74,76].

GO was exploited as an effective part of several biosensors for miRNA detection. For example, the electrochemical nanobiosensor based on GCE that was step-by-step modified with GO and gold nanorods was fabricated for the detection of a serum miR-199a-5p level [77]. A thiolated oligonucleotide probe was immobilized on the modified electrode, and unspecific bindings were blocked by incubation with 6-mercapto-1-hexanol solution. The nanobiosensor exhibited LOD of 4.5 fM, which is a standard deviation of 2.9% for miR-199a-5p detection and a linear range from 15 fM to 148 pM [77] (Approach 1).

An impedimetric biosensor based on ZrO_2–RGO nanohybrids-modified GCE coupled with a catalytic hairpin assembly signal amplification strategy determined miRNA-21 in the range from 10 fM to 100 pM with LOD of 4.3 fM [78]. H1 modified with $-NH_2$ was covalently attached onto the ZrO_2–RGO-modified GCE surface via poly(acrylic acid) using amine coupling chemistry. In the absence of the analyte (miRNA-21), H1 and H2 did not hybridize. When the analyte was present, the hairpin of H2 hybridized with the analyte, which caused opening of the closed structure of H2. Subsequently, H1 hybridized with the unfolded H2. After this, target miRNA was released due to the DNA strand displacement reaction. At the end, H2 was attached to the electrode surface, and targeted miRNA started another cycle. This caused the amplification of the detected signal, since several H2 molecules per one analyte molecule were attached to the electrode surface (Figure 4) [78] (Approach 1).

The miRNA sensor using methylene blue as a redox mediator was fabricated by Rafiee-Pour et al. with a linear range from 0.1 to 500 pM with LOD of 84.3 fM [79]. In the experiment, the GCE electrode was modified with the dispersion of oxidized MWCNTs. Afterwards, 1.0 μM ss-DNA was immobilized, and half of the modified electrodes were incubated with target miRNA. The second half of the electrodes was used as a control. Non-hybridized miRNA was removed from the surface with saline sodium citrate. Both types of electrodes were immersed into 4.0 μM methylene blue, which was intercalated into a double-stranded helix, and DPV was applied to evaluate the change of the electrochemical signal [79] (Approach 1).

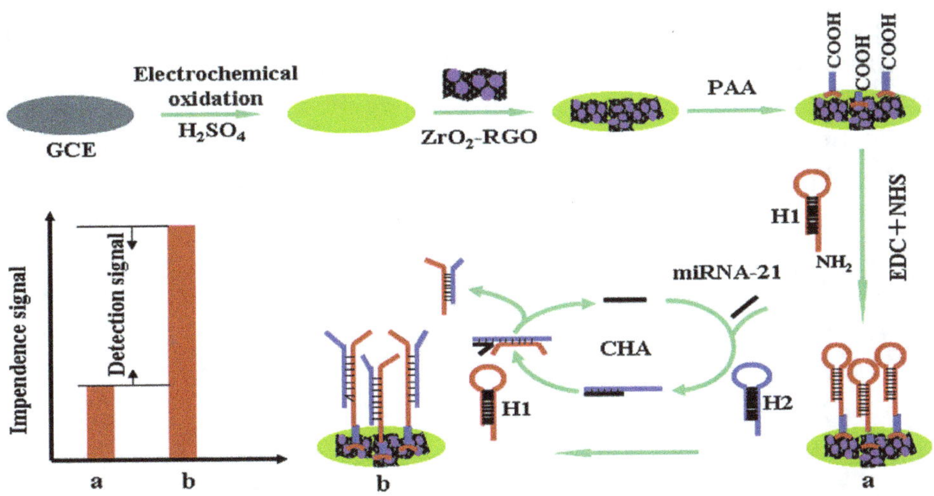

Figure 4. Immobilization of the capture probe H1 with subsequent miRNA-21 detection. For more information, please see the text. Published with permission by The Royal Society of Chemistry, Ref. [78].

Kilic et al. detected miRNA from cell lysates by using graphene-modified disposable pencil graphite electrodes [80]. The electrode was modified by an inosine substituted anti miRNA-2 probe. The analyte was detected with LOD of 2.1 μg/mL (EIS) or 5.8 μg/mL (DPV) [80] (Approach 1).

An enzyme-free biosensor based on a sandwich-type hybridization of two DNA probes with target miRNA was developed by Zouari et al. [81]. Thiol chemistry ensured the immobilization of a thiolated capture DNA onto the electrodes modified by a hybrid nanomaterial of RGO and AuNPs. Ferrocene-capped AuNPs were modified with streptavidin and conjugated with a biotinylated signal probe containing signal DNA. An enzymeless biosensor was able to determine the synthetic target miRNA with LOD of 5 fM (a linear range between 10 fM and 2 pM). Moreover, the biosensor was able to determine the target miRNA directly in diluted serum from BC patients. A 3-fold higher level of miRNA-21 was detected in serum samples of BC patients compared to a control [81] (Approach 3).

4.3. Detection of Mucins

Nowadays, there are more than 20 known types of mucins. They are encoded by MUC genes and represent high molecular weight glycoproteins expressed on epithelial cells. Aberrantly glycosylated mucins are expressed in cancer cells and serve as oncogenic molecules [82].

Nawaz et al. applied diazonium salt chemistry to modify single-walled carbon nanotubes (SWCNTs) for a biosensor development [83]. The MUC1 aptamer was immobilized onto modified SPCE via amine coupling. A DNA aptamer-based biosensor detected MUC1 with LOD of 0.02 U/mL with a linear range up to 2 U/mL [83] (Approach 1).

The MUC1 biosensor was also developed using GCE modified with core–shell nanofibers, MWCNTs, and AuNPs that were covalently modified with the anti MUC1-binding aptamer for the detection of MUC1 [84]. The impedimetric device using a soluble redox probe was able to detect MUC1 with LOD of 2.7 nM with a linear range up to 115 nM [84] (Approach 1).

Mouffouk together with colleagues applied bioconjugated self-assembled pH-responsive polymeric micelles loaded with ferrocene (Fc) and antiMUC1 antibodies as a signal probe [85]. The biosensor was able to detect MUC1 in a sample containing about 10 cells/mL [85] (Approach 2).

Nowadays, a novel 2D nanomaterial MXene (Ti_3C_2) due to its excellent electrical conductivity and large specific surface area with a large number of potential attachment binding sites is used as a conductive support for the immobilization of aptamer probes [53]. Wang et al. modified an electrode surface with MXene for the development of a MUC1 biosensor [86]. The Fc-labeled complementary DNA was bound onto MXene nanosheets to form a signal probe to amplify an electrochemical signal. GCE was modified by the electrodeposition of AuNPs with the MUC1 aptamer attached to the modified electrode via Au–S bonds. The modified electrode was blocked using bovine serum albumin (BSA) in order to resist non-specific interactions (Figure 5). Then, a signal probe was attached to the modified electrode via hybridization between complementary DNA and a MUC1 aptamer. Upon the interaction of MUC1 with such an electrode, the signal probe was detached from the working electrode, resulting in a decrease of an electrochemical signal (a signal-off response). This competitive aptasensor detected MUC1 with LOD of 0.33 pM with a linear range up to 10 mM [86] (Approach 3).

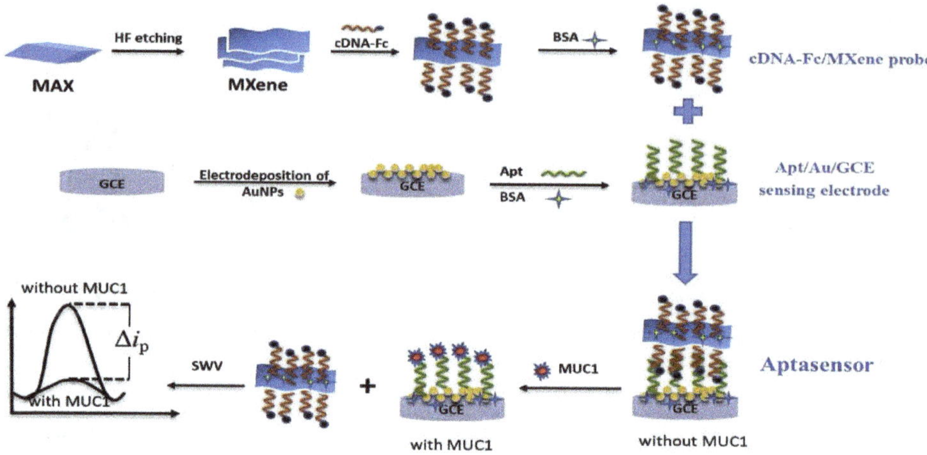

Figure 5. Procedure for fabrication of the competitive electrochemical aptasensor.

CA15-3 (290–400 kDa) represents a soluble form of mucin 1 (MUC1): a transmembrane protein on the apical cellular surface. MUC-1 is a glycoprotein with three domains. The association between BC and elevated expression of CA15-3 has been experimentally confirmed [87].

Santos et al. used imprinting technology with a CA15-3 imprint within an electropolymerized layer of polypyrrole for CA15-3 detection [88]. Polypyrrole was deposited on a fluorine-doped tin oxide conductive glass support in the presence of the analyte. Then, the analyte was removed from the imprinted layer with ethanol, and the biomimetic material was then incorporated in a polyvinylchloride plasticized membrane acting as a potentiometric ionophore. The best results were obtained with electrodes covered by the imprinted polymer without any lipophilic additive with LOD of 1.07 U/mL and a linear response from 1.44 to 13.2 U/mL for CA15-3 [88] (Approach 1).

A CA15-3 immunosensor based on RGO and CuS NPs was fabricated using gold screen-printed electrode [89]. Firstly, anti CA15-3 antibodies were immobilized on the electrode. Once the analyte CA15-3 was bound to the surface of the electrode, the electrochemical response toward catechol was decreased. The sensor reached LOD of 0.3 U/mL, a sensitivity of 1.88 $\mu A/(\mu M\ cm^2)$, and a linear response from 1.0 to 150 U/mL [89] (Approach 1).

Nakhjavani et al. prepared a sandwich-type of electrochemical immunosensor for the detection of CA15-3 [87]. Bare GE was incubated with streptavidin for 12 h with the subsequent immobilization of biotinylated anti-CA15-3 monoclonal antibodies. A considerable signal enhancement was reached due to the enhanced density of HRP delivered via streptavidin-coated magnetic beads (MBs) conjugated with biotinylated HRP and anti-CA15-3 antibodies. CA15-3 was detected employing the immunosensor in an electrolyte containing 0.1 M PBS pH 7.0 with a hydroquinone (HQ) as a redox mediator in the presence of H_2O_2 by CV and EIS techniques with LOD of 15×10^{-6} U/mL (a linear range from 50 to 15×10^{-6} U/mL). The lowest value of an electron-transfer resistance (R_{et}) at a bare electrode increased after the addition of streptavidin onto the surface, as well as after adding monoclonal antibodies and finally after CA15-3 addition. The R_{et} values decreased after the addition of a detection label, confirming attachment onto the electrode surface [87] (Approach 2).

The nanostructure-based immunosensor was developed by applying the non-covalent functionalization of GO with 1-pyrenecarboxylic acid as a modified electrode interface for the immobilization of a primary antibody (Ab_1) against the analyte [90]. Pre-treated GE were modified with a SAM of cysteamine, and the remaining empty places on the electrode were blocked with 2-mercaptoethanol. These electrodes were covalently patterned by GO already functionalized with 1-pyrenecarboxylic acid via amine coupling. Then, such modified electrodes were immobilized with monoclonal anti-CA15-3 Ab_1, blocked with BSA, incubated with CA15-3, and after immunoreaction took place, they were incubated with a signal probe (Figure 6). MWCNTs supporting a high density of ferritin molecules together with secondary antibody (Ab_2) against the analyte applied as a signal probe for the determination of CA15-3. MWCNTs were treated by a mixture of strong inorganic acids for the formation of carboxylic groups, for nanotube shortening, and for removing metallic and carbonaceous impurities. After the activation of MWCNTs, nanotubes were covalently modified by polyclonal anti-CA15-3 Ab_2 and ferritin. CA15-3 was detected through an enhanced bioelectrocatalytic reduction of H_2O_2 mediated by HQ at the immunosensor-offered LOD of 0.01 U/mL in human serum samples using DPV [90] (Approach 3).

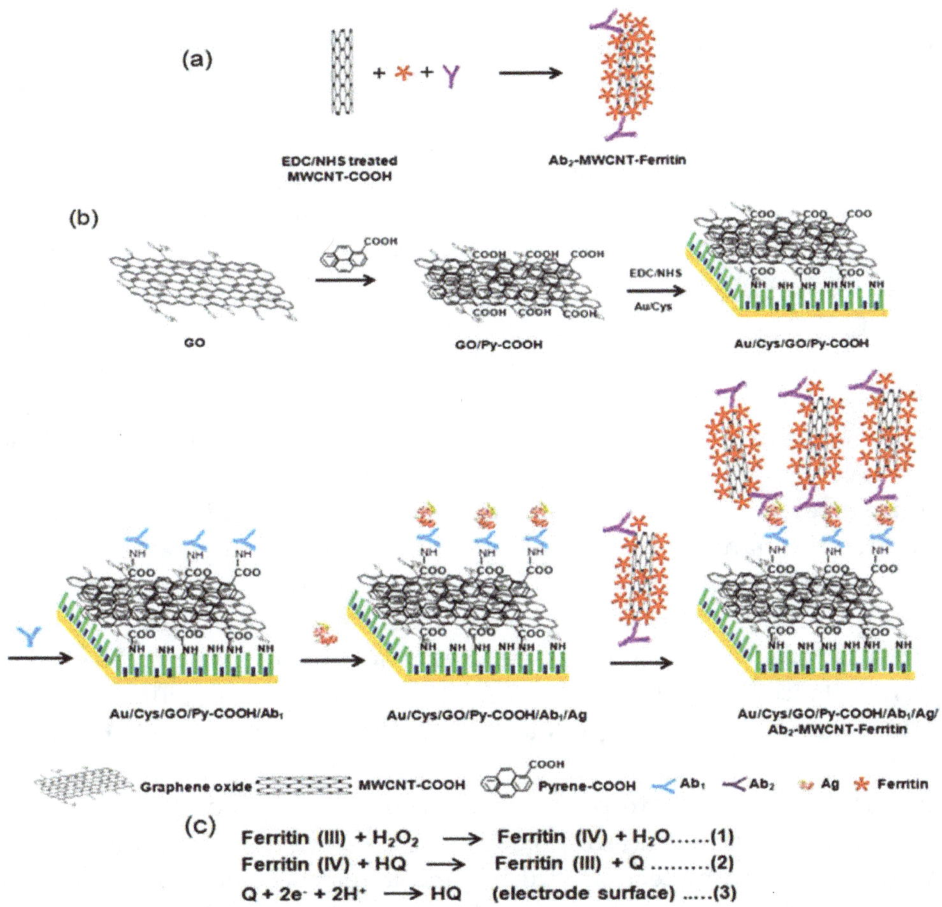

Figure 6. (**a**) Preparation of the Ab_2 conjugate applied as a signal probe, (**b**) fabrication of the interfacial layer of the immunosensor device, and (**c**) mechanism behind the generation of an electrochemical signal.

4.4. *Detection of Human Epidermal Growth Factor Receptor-2 (HER2)*

HER2 (185 kDa) i.e., human epidermal growth factor receptor-2, belongs to a family of receptor tyrosine kinases [91]. HER2 in BC is characterized by its high expression of growth factor receptor-related genes (*ERBB2*, *EGFR*, and/or *FGFR4*) and cell cycle-related genes [85].

There are several publications describing the development of biosensor platforms using various forms of graphene to enhance the selectivity and specificity of such devices. The in situ growth of 1D molybdenum trioxide anchored onto the 2D RGO via one-pot low-temperature hydrothermal synthesis and further functionalized using 3-aminopropyltriethoxysilane was fabricated as a suitable nanohybrid platform for HER2 detection [92]. In the following step, the surface conjugation of the monoclonal anti-HER2 antibodies onto the modified electrode was performed via amine coupling chemistry (Figure 7). The LOD of this nanohybrid-based immunosensor was 0.001 ng/mL, with a linear response in a concentration range of 0.001–500 ng/mL [92] (Approach 1).

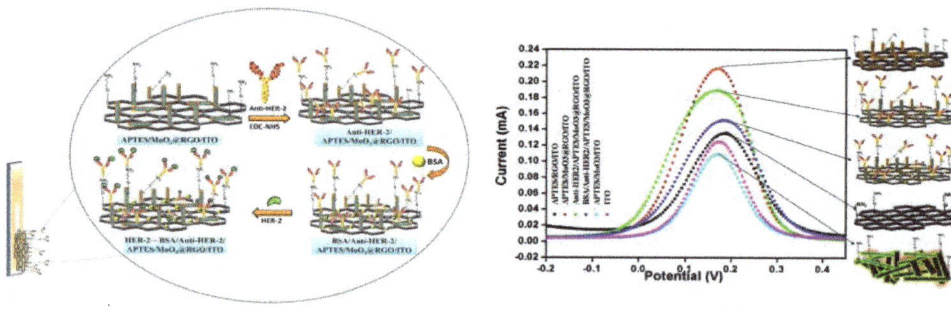

(a) (b)

Figure 7. Development of an immunoelectrode for BC biomarker detection (**a**). Electrochemical peak response obtained via differential pulse voltammetry (DPV) at each step of electrode modification (**b**).

An HER2 biosensor was prepared by the modification of GCE by a thin layer of RGO and SWCNTs to which a densely packed layer of AuNPs was deposited [93] (Approach 1). In the final step, the aptamer against HER2 was attached to the modified electrode and changes in the impedance were applied for the detection of HER2 with LOD of 50 fg/mL (a linear range from 0.1 pg/mL to 1 ng/mL). The recovery index of HER2 detection, when spiked into serum samples, was close to 100%, and the results of assaying HER2 levels in serum samples obtained by the biosensor device were in an excellent agreement with the ELISA method [93].

Arkan developed an impedimetric immunosensor using a hybrid nanomaterial modified electrode by the deposition of AuNPs and MWCNTs glued to the electrode by ionic liquid [94]. AuNPs were electrodeposited onto an electrode already patterned by MWCNTs and ionic liquid. Such an electrode was then immersed in an ethanol solution of 1,6-hexanedithiol. Then, another layer of AuNPs was deposited to which anti-HER2 antibodies were covalently grafted via amine coupling. It was found out that the charge transfer resistance increased linearly with increasing concentrations of HER2 antigen. The biosensor could detect HER2 in the linear range from 10 ng/mL to 110 ng/mL with LOD of 7.4 ng/mL. The results indicated the ability of HER2 detection in serum samples of BC patients, and such assays were in an excellent agreement with the results obtained by a commercial HER2 kit [94] (Approach 1).

An electrochemical molecularly imprinted polymer-based sensor (Figure 8) was developed for the detection of an extracellular domain of HER2 [95]. The sensor was prepared on a screen-printed gold electrode (AuSPE), where a molecularly imprinted layer was electropolymerized from a solution consisting of phenol and the analyte using the CV technique. The device exhibited a linear range for analyte detection from 10 to 70 ng/mL and LOD of 1.6 ng/mL, when DPV was applied as an electrochemical detection technique [95] (Approach 1).

Freitas et al. developed several biosensor devices for the detection of HER2 [96–99]. The first one was developed on SPCE modified either by AuNPs or combination of AuNPs with MWCNTs [96]. Such a modified electrode was then modified by primary anti-HER2 antibodies. Then, the biosensor was incubated with an analyte, and in the subsequent step, it was incubated with biotinylated secondary anti-HER2 antibodies. The electrochemical signal was generated by a final incubation of the biosensor by streptavidin-modified alkaline phosphatase, which catalytically reduced silver ions in the presence of 3-indoxyl phosphate. Under optimal conditions, the biosensors could detect HER2 in a concentration window of 7.5–50 ng/mL with LOD of 0.16 ng/mL (MWCNTs with AuNPs) or 8.5 ng/mL (AuNPs). The total assay time was 140 min, and the biosensor was applied for the analysis of HER2 spiked into serum samples [96] (Approach 1).

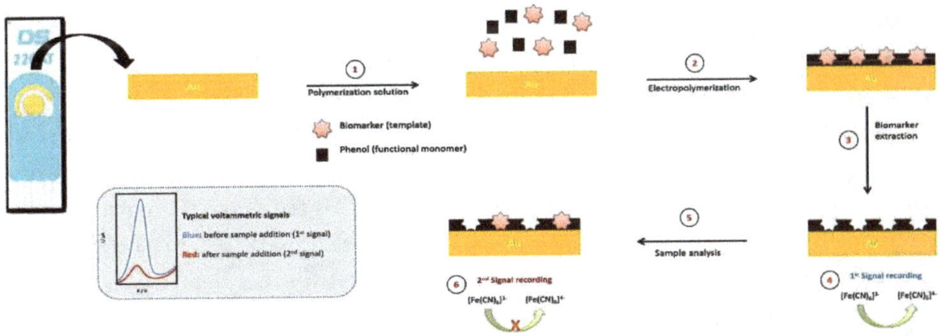

Figure 8. Fabrication and operation principles of the molecularly imprinted polymer-based sensor deposited on a gold screen-printed electrode (AuSPE).

Malecka with colleagues constructed a cellulase-linked sandwich assay based on magnetic beads for HER2 detection [100]. The principle behind detection is the formation of an insulating layer consisting of nitrocellulose film on spectroscopic graphite electrode. HER2 interacts with primary aptamer/antibody-modified magnetic beads with the subsequent formation of a sandwich configuration on MBs by secondary aptamers/antibodies conjugated to cellulose. Once MBs are incubated with the electrode surface, nitrocellulose film is digested with the formation of holes within the film, resulting in a decrease of electrode capacitance (Figure 9). The chronocoulometry was measured for the determination of an electric charge, which was proportional to HER2 in the concentration window of 10^{-15}–10^{-10} M HER2 with LOD of 1 fM and with an overall assay time within 3 h. HER2 spiked into serum samples was detected with a recovery index of (109 ± 3)% [100] (Approach 1).

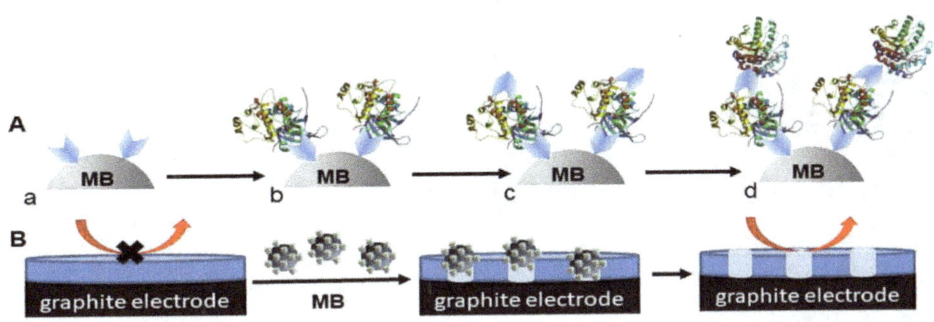

Figure 9. Schematic representation of (**A**) sandwich assembly on magnetic beads (MB) modified (**a**) with either an antibody or an aptamer, (**b**) binding of human epidermal growth factor receptor-2 (HER2)/neu via biorecognition to MB and the further reaction of MB (**c**) with a second antibody or an aptamer and (**d**) binding of the biotinylated cellulase label, through the biotin–streptavidin interaction. The protein structures' PDB (Protein Data Bank) IDs are: 3PP0 (HER-2/neu; DOI:10.2210/pdb3PP0/pdb) and 4IM4 (cellulase; DOI:10.2210/pdb4IM4/pdb). (**B**) Basic principle of the biosensor operation: electrochemically insulating nitrocellulose film on the surface of porous spectroscopic graphite is digested by MBs only when the analyte is present on the MB by cellulase, and that changes the electrochemical properties of the nitrocellulose-modified graphite surface.

A DNA-based biosensor for the detection of HER2 was designed by the modification of GE with a DNA tetrahedron containing an aptamer against HER2 [101]. An electrochemical signal was generated by a signal probe consisting of gold nanorods with deposited PdNPs (5 nm), anti-HER2 aptamer, and HRP. Upon interaction of the modified electrode with HER2, a sandwich configuration was completed by a final incubation of the electrode with the signal probe. The biosensor could detect the analyte with LOD of 0.15 ng/mL and within a linear range from 10 to 200 ng/mL. Finally, the biosensor was applied for the analysis of HER2 spiked into serum samples [101] (Approach 2).

Lah and co-workers constructed a sandwich immunosensor for HER2 detection based on PbS quantum dots (QDs)-conjugated secondary anti-HER2 antibody as a signal probe [102]. Firstly, PbS QDs were synthesized, and anti-HER2 antibodies were attached to them. The application of QDs provided advantageous features such as a straightforward synthesis and well-defined electrochemical stripping signal of Pb(II) through acid dissolution. Primary anti-HER2 antibodies were immobilized onto pre-treated activated SPCE to capture the analyte. In the final incubation step, the signal probe formed a sandwich configuration. The biosensor could detect analyte down to 0.28 ng/mL with a linear calibration range up to 100 ng/mL. The biosensor was tested for the analysis of HER2 spiked into serum samples with a recovery index in the range from 91% to 104% [102] (Approach 2).

In the next work of Freitas et al., primary anti-HER2 antibodies were immobilized on MBs (Figure 10) [97] (Approach 2). The whole immunocomplex sandwich was formed directly in the solution phase, and then it was magnetically transferred to the electrode surface. The total assay time was 205 min with LOD down to 2.8 ng/mL. The biosensor was applied for the analysis of HER2 spiked into serum samples with a recovery index of 95%–99% [97].

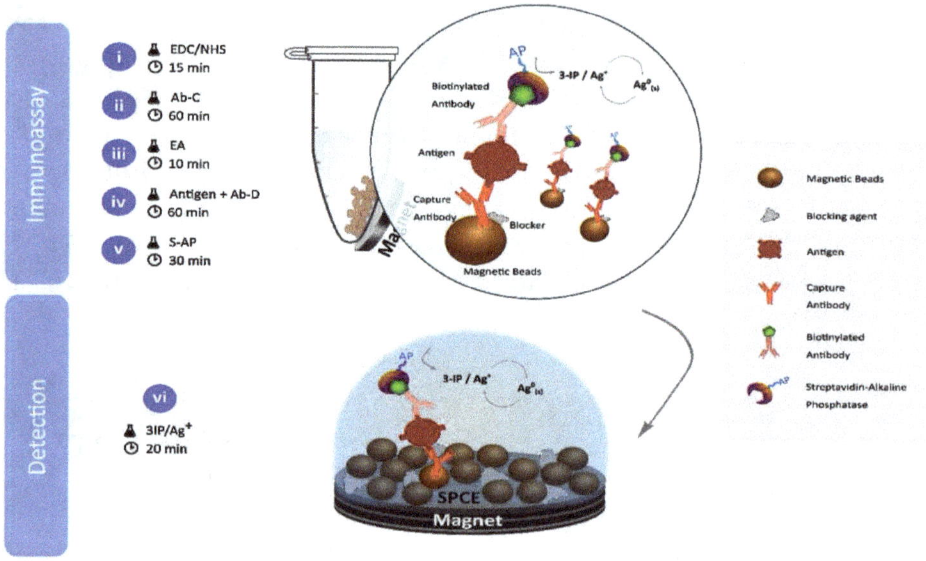

Figure 10. Graphical representation of operation of magnetic bead-based immunoassay.

The advanced approach was achieved employing the core/shell CdSe@ZnS QDs as an electroactive detection probe for HER2 biosensing, requiring a total time assay of 2 h [98]. The sandwich configuration was formed on the SPCE involving primary and secondary anti-HER2 antibodies. The biosensor required only 40 μL of a sample volume with an LOD down to 2.1 ng/mL. The biosensor was applied for the analysis of HER2 spiked into serum samples with a recovery index between 104% and 106% [98] (Approach 2).

In next paper, the authors combined magnetic beads and core/shell streptavidin-modified CdSe@ZnS QDs as an electroactive detection probe for the affinity-based detection of HER2 with LOD of 0.29 ng/mL (a linear range of 0.50–50 ng/mL) [99]. The device was applied for the detection of HER2 spiked into serum samples with a recovery index of 100%–108%, assay time of 90 min, and with a good agreement with the reference ELISA method, which took 285 min to complete [99] (Approach 2).

Hartati et al. used a bioconjugate prepared by the covalent immobilization of anti-HER2 antibodies onto cerium oxide NPs previously modified by 3-aminopropyl trimethoxysilane (APTES) and polyethylene glycol-α-maleimide-ω-NHS (PEG–NHS–maleimide) [103]. Then, such a bioconjugate was covalently attached to SPCE modified by AuNPs. The interaction of HER2 with the modified electrode was analyzed by CV with a decrease of the peak current in the presence of the analyte (a signal-off approach). The biosensor could detect HER2 with an LOD of 34.9 pg/mL. The biosensor was finally used for the analysis of HER2 spiked into serum samples with a recovery index close to 100% [103] (Approach 3).

4.5. Detection of Carcinoembryonic Antigen (CEA)

CEA (180–200 kDa) is a glycoprotein that participated in cell adhesion. Normally, it is expressed by normal fetal intestinal tissue, and after birth, its expression is inhibited. The serum level can be increased in non-malignant diseases such as inflammatory bowel disease and also in many types of human cancers, such as gastric cancer, breast cancer, ovarian cancer, lung cancer, pancreatic cancer, and colorectal cancer [104].

Wang et al. developed a label-free aptasensor based on an electrochemiluminescent (ECL) strategy with ZnS–CdS NP-decorated molybdenum disulfide (MoS_2, a 2D nanomaterial [105]) nanocomposite for CEA detection [106]. The GCE was firstly modified with layered MoS_2 as an electrode matrix, and then ZnS–CdS NPs were electrodeposited directly onto MoS_2/GCE. In the next step, chitosan and glutaraldehyde covered the electrode for the immobilization of an anti-CEA aptamer. The aptasensor was completed by a final incubation with BSA to suppress non-specific interactions. The ECL aptasensor showed a linear range from 0.05 to 20 ng/mL with an LOD of 0.031 ng/mL. CEA spiked into human serum was analyzed with a recovery index in the range from 80% to 111%. The method was also applied for the determination of CEA in 8 human serum samples with an excellent agreement with a reference analytical method, showing the clinical application of the approach [106] (Approach 1).

Paimard with co-workers developed an immunosensor for CEA detection based on the CPE surface covered by the core–shell nanofibers prepared by electrospinning [107]. A nanofiber was made of honey (a core) electrospun with polyvinylalcohol (a shell) formed by a coaxial approach. Electrospun nanofibers were decorated with AuNPs and MWCNTs. Subsequently, anti-CEA antibodies were immobilized on the electrode surface. The impedimetric immunosensor exhibited high sensitivity toward the CEA biomarker with LOD of 0.09 ng/mL and with a linear range up to 125 ng/mL. The biosensor was applied for the analysis of CEA in human serum samples. Significantly higher levels of CEA were found in the serum samples of cancer patients compared to control, which was also verified using ELISA [107] (Approach 1).

Wang with colleagues employed flower-like Ag/MoS_2/RGO nanocomposites deposited onto GCE for CEA label-free detection with LOD of 1.6 fg/mL through the electrocatalytic H_2O_2 reduction [108]. Firstly AgNPs and GO were synthesized by a seed-mediated Lee–Meisel method and by an improved Hummer's method, respectively. Next, MoS_2/RGO was synthesized by applying $Na_2MoO_4 \bullet 2H_2O$ and thiourea to obtain the final Ag/MoS_2/RGO nanocomposite. Anti-CEA antibodies were conjugated to the surface of AgNPs via amino groups for CEA determination in a wide concentration range from 0.01 pg/mL to 100 ng/mL. The analysis of CEA spiked into serum samples revealed a recovery index that was very close to 100% [108] (Approach 1). Another electrochemical platform for the detection of CEA using H_2O_2 reduction was developed by Su et al. [109]. Two-dimensional nanomaterial MoS_2 was modified by Prussian blue NPs, and such a hybrid nanomaterial was then deposited on GCE. The biosensor was finalized by the covalent immobilization of anti-CEA antibodies with subsequent surface blocking by BSA. CEA determination through the non-enzymatic detection of H_2O_2 offered LOD of 0.54 pg/mL (a linear range from 0.005 to 10 ng/mL). When the biosensor was applied for the detection of CEA spiked into human serum samples, a recovery index from 95% to 102% was obtained [109] (Approach 1).

Another sandwich-type electrochemical immunosensor for the determination of CEA was based on SPCE modified by AgNPs and RGO to which primary anti-CEA antibodies were immobilized [110]. After the electrode interface was incubated with an analyte, secondary anti-CEA antibodies labeled with HRP were added to complete a sandwich configuration, and a reduction of H_2O_2 was detected electrochemically. The modified SPCE-based biosensor detected CEA with LOD down to 0.035 μg/mL (a linear range of 0.05–0.50 μg/mL) [110] (Approach 1).

Rizwan et al. applied a layer-by-layer deposition of AuNPs, carbon nano-onions, SWCNTs, and chitosan layers onto GCE for the construction of a CEA immunosensor [111]. SWV was applied as an output signal in the presence of a soluble redox probe, and the device offered a linear range from 100 fg/mL to 400 ng/mL with LOD of 100 fg/mL for the detection of CEA. Only one serum sample spiked with three different CEA concentrations was applied for a clinical evaluation of the biosensor with recovery index in the range of 105%–110% [111] (Approach 1).

Wang and Hui [112] utilized the zwitterionic poly (carboxybetaine methacrylate) as a superhydrophilic matrix for the immobilization of anti-CEA antibodies and also as a layer resisting non-specific interactions. GCE was modified via electrodeposition by polyaniline nanowires, which were then activated to covalently graft zwitterionic monomers to the interfacial layer. In the subsequent step, a polymeric form of the zwitterions was prepared using UV irradiation. Finally, anti-CEA antibodies were immobilized via amine coupling. CEA concentration in the range from 1.0×10^{-14} g/mL to 1.0×10^{-10} g/mL with LOD of 3.05 fg/mL was determined by a DPV method. Four serum samples were analyzed by the biosensor, with the CEA values obtained being in excellent agreement with the reference ECL method, and when CEA was spiked in serum samples, a recovery index between 94% and 104% was obtained [112] (Approach 1).

Kumar et al. [113] functionalized ultrathin 2D nanomaterial Ti_3C_2 MXene nanosheets with aminosilane for the covalent immobilization of anti-CEA antibodies for ultrasensitive CEA detection with LOD down to 18 fg/mL (Figure 11). The label-free biosensor exhibited a linear detection range of 0.0001–2000 ng/mL using a soluble redox probe $[Ru(NH_3)_6]^{3+}$. The biosensor was applied for CEA detection when spiked into a human serum sample with a recovery index from 99% to 101% [113] (Approach 1).

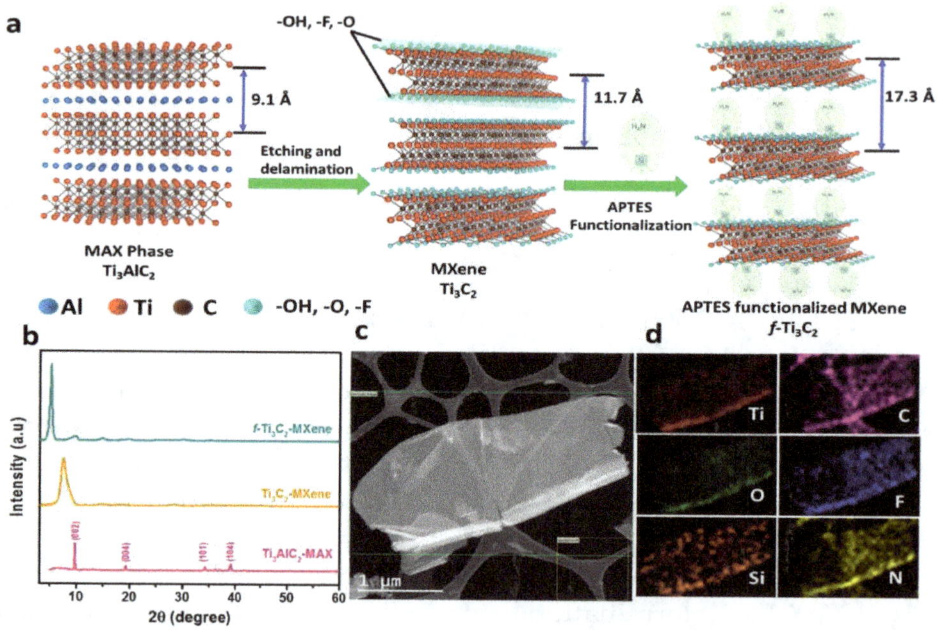

Figure 11. (**a**) Schematic illustration of MXene functionalization. Aluminum layered is etched from the Ti_3AlC_2-MAX phase, producing 2D nanosheets terminated with –OH, –O, and –F functional groups. Aminosilane (APTES) is then used to functionalize the MXene surface. (**b**) XRD pattern of the Ti_3AlC_2-MAX, MXene and functionalized MXene. (**c**,**d**) TEM image of a single MXene sheet and corresponding elemental map showing the uniform distribution of silicon (Si, brown), oxygen (O, green), and nitrogen (N, dark yellow), and revealing the homogenous functionalization of MXene with APTES.

Yang and co-workers utilized a label-free amplification strategy based on an Au-Ag/RGO nanohybrid prepared using dopamine as a reducing agent, which was deposited on GCE [114]. Such a modified electrode was then used for the immobilization of anti-CEA antibodies. CEA was detected by the decrease of an electrochemical signal due to the oxidation of AgNPs present on a signal probe upon incubation with an analyte with LOD of 0.286 pg/mL (a linear range from 0.001 ng/mL to 80 ng/mL). A serum sample spiked with 3 different CEA concentrations was successfully analyzed by the biosensor with a recovery index of 96%–107% with excellent agreement with an ELISA method [114] (Approach 1).

Gu et al. [115] integrated ferrocene (Fc) derivative and AuNPs into their biosensor for CEA detection in order to increase the conductivity of the sensing surfaces and increase ferrocene loading. Firstly, AuNPs were reduced from chloroauric acid with trisodium citrate as a reducing agent, and subsequently, polyclonal secondary anti-CEA antibodies were immobilized onto their surface via physisorption. Further chemisorption of the electroactive ferrocene molecules in a form of thiolated ferrocene chains was accomplished on AuNPs. Finally, PEG8000 was applied to stabilize AuNPs, and repeated centrifugation was applied to remove excess antibodies and Fc, and such a bioconjugate was applied as a signal probe. Pre-treated GEs were first modified with lipoic acid *N*-hydroxysuccinimide ester to attach primary antibodies, and the surface was blocked with ethanolamine. After CEA was affinity captured on the modified electrode, the sandwich configuration was completed by incubation with a signal probe. The developed biosensor exhibited LOD of approximately 0.01 ng/mL (a linear range up to 20 ng/mL), when detecting CEA using a SWV method with a good performance after storage for 3 weeks (91.8% of the original response) [115] (Approach 2).

Wei et al. developed an electrochemical ratiometric method for CEA detection [116]. The method was based on an AuNPs functionalized Cu_2S-CuS/graphene composite as a SPCE-modifying nanomaterial to which primary anti-CEA antibodies were immobilized. A signal probe was developed using CeO_2 NPs modified by deposited AuNPs to which secondary anti-CEA antibodies and toluidine blue (TB) as a redox mediator were covalently immobilized. The adsorption capacity toward toluidine blue was improved with carboxymethyl chitosan (CMC)-doped ionic liquids containing active groups such as –OH, –COOH, and $–NH_2$. The change of dual signals "$\Delta I = \Delta I_{TB} + |\Delta I_{Cu2S\text{-}CuS}|$" ($\Delta I_{TB}$ and $|\Delta I_{Cu2S\text{-}CuS}|$ present the change values of the oxidation peak currents of toluidine blue and Cu_2S-CuS, respectively) was applied as the response signal for the quantitative determination of CEA with LOD of 0.78 pg/mL (a linear range of 0.001–100 ng/mL) (Figure 12). The biosensor was applied for the analysis of CEA in one serum sample, and the CEA level found out by the biosensor device was in an excellent agreement with an ELISA method [116] (Approach 3).

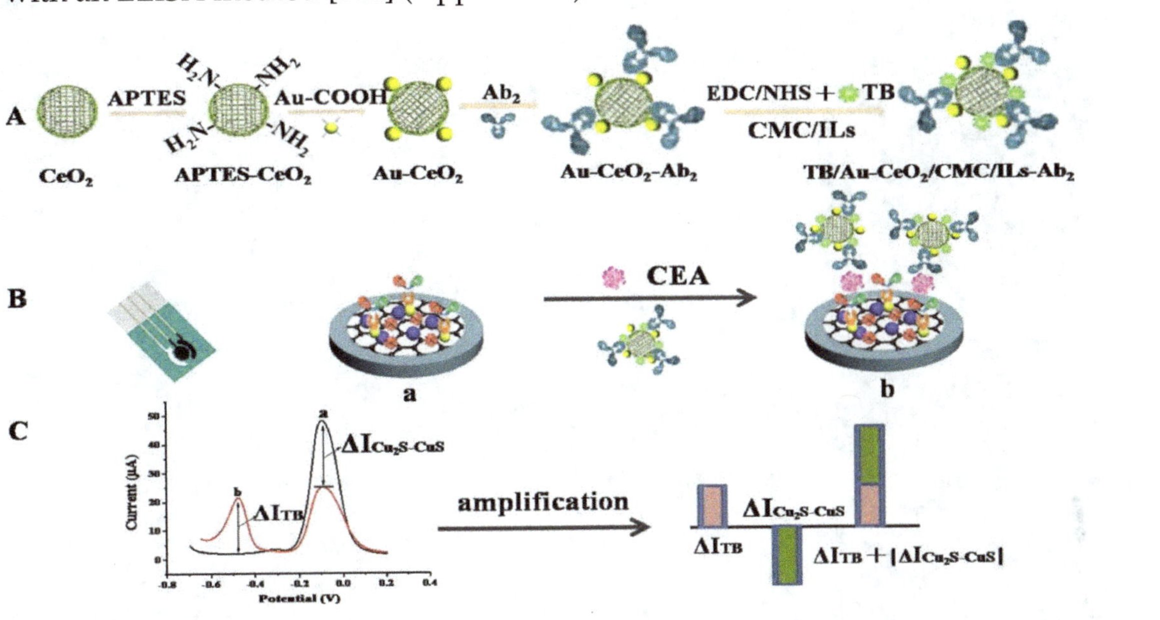

Figure 12. (**A**) Formation of a signal probe. (**B**) Schematic presentation of the immunosensor fabrication. (**C**) A dual-signaling amplification strategy.

Another type of a label-based sandwich-type electrochemical immunosensor for CEA determination was developed by Li et al. [117], who used amino functionalized magnetic graphene sheets loaded with Au@Ag core–shell NPs to adsorb Ni^{2+} and secondary anti-CEA antibodies as a signal probe to reduce H_2O_2. AuNPs electrodeposited from $HAuCl_4$ solution onto GCE improved the immobilization of primary anti-CEA antibodies and the device exhibited an LOD of 0.07 pg/mL (a linear range from 0.1 pg/mL to 100 ng/mL). The biosensor offered a recovery index close to 100% for the determination of CEA spiked into serum samples [117] (Approach 3).

A similar strategy based on the application of multiple types of nanoparticles for the detection of CEA was also applied by Wu et al. [118]. GCE was patterned by aminated-graphene sheets to which primary anti-CEA antibodies were covalently immobilized using glutaraldehyde. A signal probe was made of magnetic NPs covered by a shell made of a MnO_2 layer with a deposition of PtNPs to which secondary anti-CEA antibodies were immobilized. CEA was detected with an LOD of 0.16 pg/mL in a linear range from 0.5 pg/mL to 20 ng/mL. Serum samples spiked with different CEA concentration provided reliable results with a recovery index from 95% to 106%, and the assay was validated using an ELISA method [118] (Approach 3).

4.6. Dual-Target Analysis

The dual-target detection of miRNA-21 and MUC1 based on a dual catalytic hairpin assembly was performed by Li and co-workers [119]. GCE was modified by Au nanoflowers to which hybridization probe 1 was immobilized to recognize miRNA-21. After incubation with miRNA-21, the electrode was incubated with a hybridization probe 2 conjugated with QDs, resulting in an increase of ECL signal (Cycle I, Figure 13). When such an electrode was incubated with anti-MUC1 aptamer and MUC1, both molecules were attached to the modified electrode surface. Incubation with a hybridization probe 3 conjugated with AuNPs in the subsequent step replaced the anti-MUC1 aptamer from the electrode surface and due to a fluorescence resonance energy transfer between QDs and AuNPs, a decrease of ECL signal was observed (Cycle II, Figure 13). The biosensor detected miRNA-21 with LOD of 11 aM and MUC1 with LOD of 0.40 fg/mL. When both analytes were spiked into human serum samples, a recovery index between 98% and 103% was obtained [119] (Approach 3).

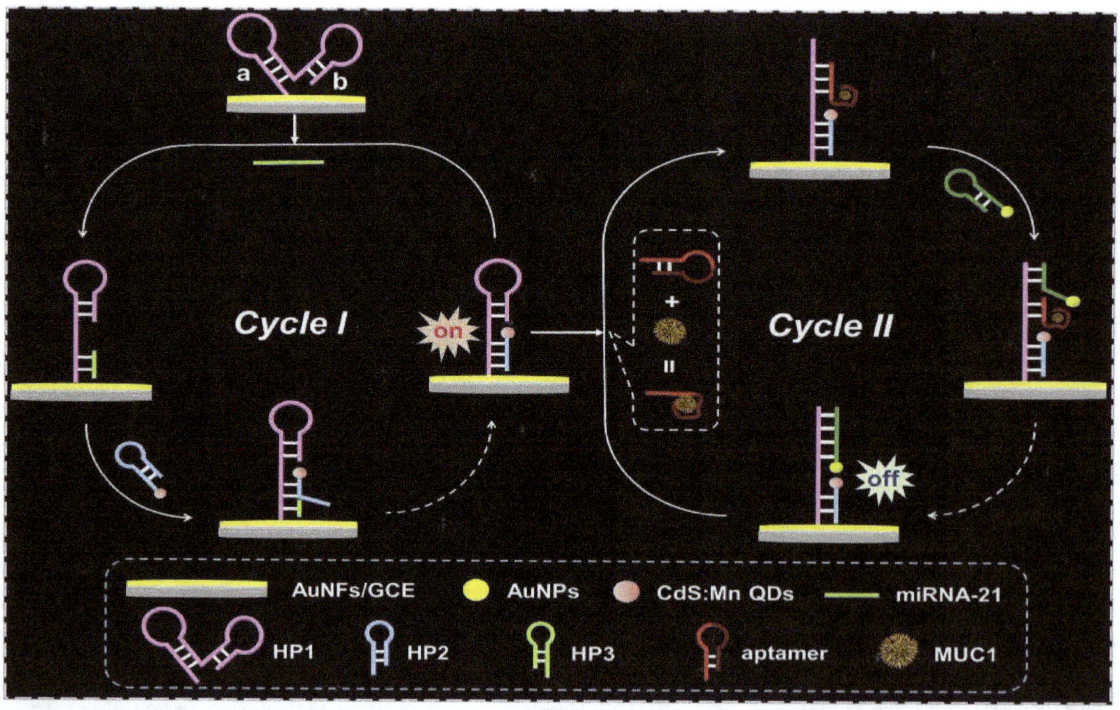

Figure 13. The principle of the fabricated biosensor for the sensitive detection of miRNA-21 and MUC1 based on dual catalytic hairpin assembly.

4.7. Detection of Other Potential BC Biomarkers

In the next part, we will focus on an electrochemical performance for the detection of less known biomarkers present in the serum of BC patients.

Cancer antigen 27.29 (CA27.29, 250–1000 kDa) is a soluble form of glycoprotein MUC1. It is expressed mainly in BC, but CA 27.29 levels can also be elevated by colon, stomach, kidney, lung, ovary, pancreas, and liver cancers as well as other non-cancerous conditions such as benign breast disease, kidney, and liver diseases [120]. Alarfaj et al. constructed a label-free electrochemical immunosensor based on an Au/MoS_2/RGO nanocomposite system [121]. First, a hybrid Au/MoS_2/RGO nanocomposite was deposited on the GCE surface. Then, anti-CA 27-29 antibodies were immobilized on the modified electrode surface for selective capture of the analyte via affinity interactions. A signal amplification strategy was achieved by a synergy of all nanomaterial components of the nanocomposite to reduce H_2O_2. The biosensor could detect analyte down to an LOD of 0.08 U/mL. The device was finally applied for analysis of the analyte in 25 human serum samples with an excellent agreement with an ELISA method, and when CA27.29 was spiked into serum samples, an excellent recovery index of 96%–100% was obtained [121] (Approach 1).

Urokinase-type plasminogen activator receptor (uPa) belongs to cell membrane receptors with their expression increased in a number of different types of human cancers, including BC [122]. An immunosensor based on fluorine-doped tin oxide was modified with graphene nanosheets to enhance the loading of covalently immobilized antibodies [122]. The immunosensor could detect the analyte down to 4.8 fM using DPV assays in the presence of a soluble redox probe. The device offered a good stability (75% of an initial activity observed after 4 weeks) with the ability to detect an analyte spiked into serum samples [122] (Approach 1).

Tissue plasminogen activator (tPa, 20–45 kDa) belongs to serine proteases (enzymes ensuring cleaving peptide bonds in proteins). As a result of this fact, the protein is essential in the human body in relation to angiogenesis in cancer cells [123]. The protein was detected with LOD of 0.026 ng/mL in a linear range from 0.1 to 1.0 ng/mL [124]. A label-free biosensor was fabricated by the functionalization of SWCNTs with antibodies immobilized, and such a bionanoconjugate was subsequently immobilized onto a GCE surface (Figure 14) [124] (Approach 1).

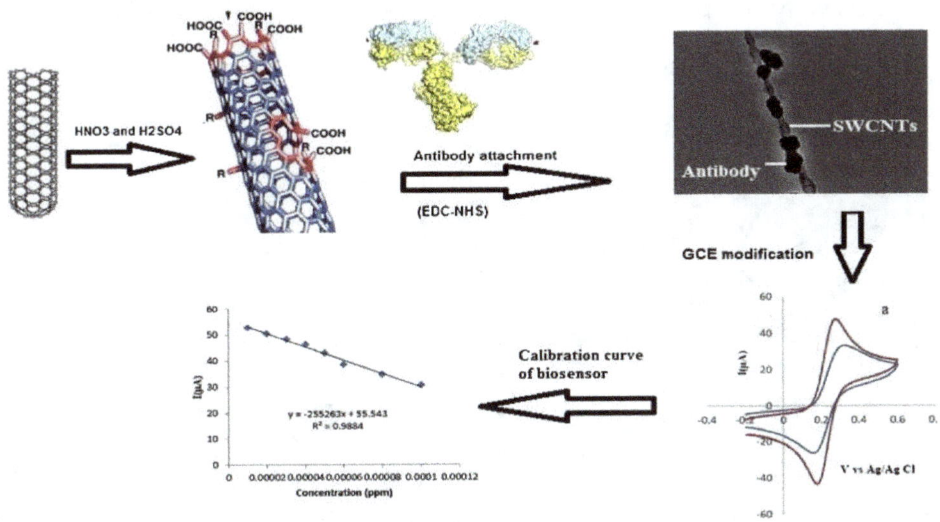

Figure 14. Fabrication of the biosensor for the determination of tissue plasminogen activator.

4.8. Detection of BC Cells

Circulatory tumor cells (CTC) are released from tumors and circulate in the bloodstream at a low concentration of up to 10 cells/mL, while the whole blood contains 10^9 erythrocytes and 10^6 leucocytes/mL [30]. This is why the detection of CTC is quite challenging.

The detection of CTCs, which are present in the blood at a very low level, is highly challenging and has not been done using affinity-based approaches. In the following text, we discuss some detection principles for the analysis of BC cells with some approaches potentially applicable for the analysis of CTCs. More details about the electrochemical detection of BC cells can be found elsewhere [125].

The Michigan Cancer Foundation-7 (MCF7) cell line is the most frequently studied BC cell line [126], since it is a suitable model for studying the development/progression of BC and anticancer drug therapies. The cells are non-invasive, expressing estrogen as well as progesterone receptors [127].

An interesting method for the electrochemical detection of CTCs within a microfluidic channel was proposed by Gurudatt et al. (Figure 15) [128]. Cells differing in their size, surface charge, and chemical state on the cell surface were effectively separated using such a device. In order to detect CTCs in an effective way, the surface of channels was chemically modified with an electrochemical polymerization of a monomer. In the subsequent step, a lipid layer by the deposition of phosphatidylserine was formed on the surface of the channels. In order to electrochemically detect cells, such cells were loaded with daunomycin prior to separation. Three different types of cancer cell lines were used for optimization of the assay, and optimized assay conditions allowed detecting single cells (approximately 7 cells/mL). Finally, the device was applied for the detection of CTCs from 37 cancer patients with (92.0 ± 0.5)% efficiency. The results showed differences in the retention time for different types of CTCs produced by different cancer types, suggesting differences in the size, surface charge, and chemical state on the cellular surface [128]. Another microfluidic electrochemical approach for the detection of CTCs was based on the measurement of changes in the impedance of the polydimethylsiloxane-based channel on a glass slide during the passage of CTCs [129]. A narrow constriction-based sensor was designed in a way allowing the passage of red and white blood cells without any restrictions, while much larger tumor cells needed to squeeze/deform in order to pass through the channel, causing changes in the impedance of the channel. As a result, only cancerous cells were able to generate an electrochemical signal in a label-free format, while smaller blood cells did not generate any measurable signal (Figure 16). The device was tested by an analysis of murine blood spiked with prostate or breast cancer cells with a throughput of 1 μL *per* min, but the throughput can be increased by analysis run in parallel. A signal processing of data generated was done automatically using MATLAB. The authors claim that false positive results can be obtained due to the presence of non-blood or non-cancer cells in blood such as epithelial cells, and this why the pre-enrichment of CTCs was suggested [129].

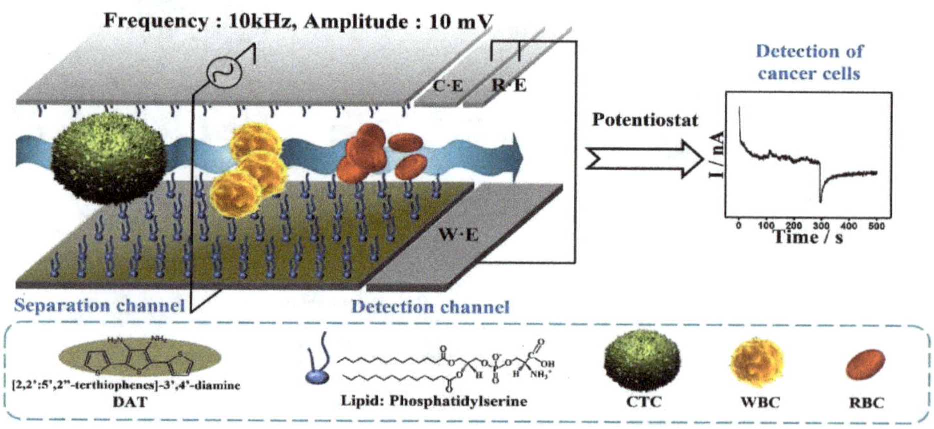

Figure 15. The schematic representation of the design and fabrication of the proposed microfluidic channel.

Anti-MUC1 aptamers, hybrid AuNPs, and carbon dots (Au@CDs) modifying GE were applied for the label-free ECL detection of circulating MCF-7 cells (MCF-7 CTCs) [130]. The biosensor detected MCF-7 CTCs down to 34 cells/mL with a linear range up to 10,000 cells/mL. MCF-7 cells spiked into serum samples were in addition clinically tested with an obtained recovery index of 93–117% [130] (Approach 1). Tian et al. [131] investigated MCF-7 CTCs by using a supporting RGO/AuNPs composite deposited on GCE with a catalytic CuO nanozyme used as a signal probe (Approach 3). MCF-7 CTCs membranes contain specific a MUC1 protein, which was recognized by the MUC-1 aptamer. The reached LOD was as low as 27 cells/mL (a linear range from 50 to 7×10^3 cells/mL). MCF-7 cells were further successfully studied and determined by applying aptamer-based electrochemical biosensors [132]. A DNA aptamer was immobilized onto AuNPs supported by α-cyclodextrin on GE (Approach 1). The aptasensor determined MCF-7 cells in the range of 328–593 cells/mL with LOD of 328 cells/mL, when cells were lysed and an intracellular level of platelet-derived growth factor was electrochemically determined [132]. Yang with colleagues [133] utilized GCE modified by several nanomaterials using a layer-by-layer deposition process incorporating 3D graphene, Au nanocages, and MWCNTs to which primary antibodies were immobilized (Approach 1). Once the biosensor was incubated with MCF-7 cells, a sandwich configuration was established by incubation with secondary antibodies linked to DNA. In the next step, complementary DNA was applied, and to double-stranded DNA, methylene blue as a redox mediator was intercalated and detected using SWV. The biosensor detected BC cells with LOD of 80 cells/mL (a linear range of 1.0×10^2–1.0×10^6 cells/mL) and exhibited satisfactory stability [133]. Wang et al. [134] fabricated a sensitive sandwich-based aptamer biosensor for the label-free electrochemical detection of cells (Approach 2). The sensor was based on GE modified with polyadenine (polydA)-aptamer recognizing MUC1 on the surface of cells. A signal probe was designed by the immobilization of an aptamer recognizing MUC1 protein on an AuNP/GO hybrid nanomaterial. MCF-7 cells were recognized by polydA-aptamer, and then, a sandwich configuration was completed by incubation with a signal probe. BC cells were detected via a DPV method with LOD of 8 cells/mL and a linear range from 10 to 10^5 cells/mL using a soluble redox probe with satisfactory selectivity [134]. An interesting approach in order to differentiate between different BC cell lines was based on the detection of H_2O_2 produced by the cells [135]. A sandwich consisting of synthesized Bi_2Se_3 NPs as 3D topological insulators between the gold electrode and another Au-deposited thin layer was designed by Mohammadniaei et al. as a nanostructured working electrode. In order to detect H_2O_2 in an ultrasensitive fashion, the immobilization of double-stranded DNA loaded with Ag^+ ions was established through the Au–thiol interaction of thiolated DNA (Figure 17) (Approach 1). The developed biosensor showed LOD of 10×10^{-9} M for H_2O_2 with a dynamic range from 0.10×10^{-6} M to 27.3×10^{-6} M and a short response time of 1.6 s. The biosensor could distinguish the MCF-7 cell line from the MDA-MB-231 cell line based on the H_2O_2 produced [135].

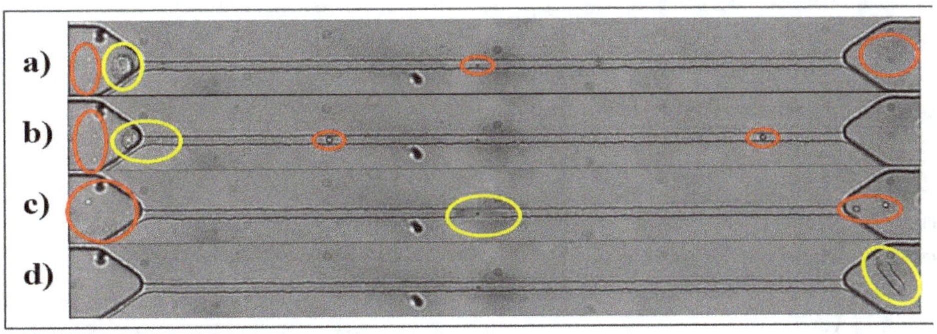

Figure 16. Transit of an MDA-MB-231 cell (circled in yellow) through the constriction region. (**a**) Cancer cell before deformation, (**b**) cell beginning to deform, (**c**) cell in constriction channel, and (**d**) cell after leaving the constriction channel. The surrounding white and red blood cells are indicated by the red circles.

In the next study, a H_2O_2 sensor employing a trimetallic AuPtPd nanocomposite and RGO nanosheets deposited on GCE was applied for the electrocatalytic detection of H_2O_2 reduction with LOD of 2 nM (a linear range from 0.005 μM to 6.5 mM) [136]. The biosensor was applied for the detection of H_2O_2 released by two BC cell lines (MDA-MB-231 and T47D) [137] (Approach 1).

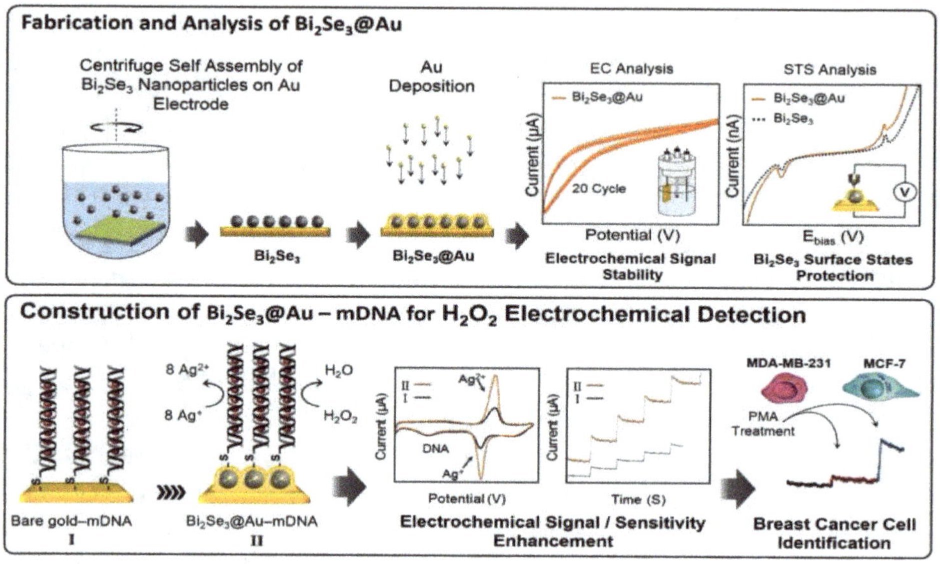

Figure 17. Fabrication process of a Bi_2Se_3@Au-DNA electrode, its electrical and electrochemical behavior, and the constitution for the electrochemical detection of H_2O_2.

Luo et al. applied hexagonal carbon nitride tubes as a photoactive material to determine the photocurrent in the presence of MCF-7 cells (Approach 1) [137]. The cells were detected down to 17 cells/mL (a linear range from 100 to 1×10^5 cells/mL). Glutaraldehyde was utilized as a cross-linker for the covalent immobilization of anti-MUC1 aptamers for the affinity capture of cells via surface-expressed MUC1. A clinical applicability of the biosensor was proved by the detection of cells spiked into blood samples at three different concentrations with a recovery index of 96%–104% [137].

Safavipour et al. developed an aptasensor using a hybrid nanomaterial composed of TiO_2 nanotubes attached to GO via UV irradiation [138]. GCE was modified by such a hybrid nanomaterial with the subsequent immobilization of anti-MUC1 aptamers for the affinity capture of MCF-7 cells via surface-expressed MUC1 proteins. An EIS-based device was able to ultrasensitively detect MCF-7 cells with LOD of 40 cells/mL within a linear concentration range from 10^3 to 10^7 cells/mL [138] (Approach 1).

GE modified by non-spherical AuNPs was made by electrodeposition in the presence of a shape-controlling agent for achieving an increased electrode active area [139]. A thiolated aptamer recognizing BC cells MDA-MB-231 was chemisorbed on the modified electrode surface, and the cells were electrochemically detected down to 2 cells/mL in an electrolyte using a soluble redox probe. The device was also applied for the analysis of cells spiked into blood serum samples with LOD of 5 cells/mL [139] (Approach 1).

Two immunomagnetic biosensors, which were described in Section 4.4. "Detection of HER2", were also applied for the detection of BC cells [97,99]. The first biosensor was applied for the determination of two BC cell lines: $HER2^+$ SK-BR-3 and $HER2^-$ MDA-MB-231 via surface-expressed HER2 proteins using Ag ions and 3-indoxyl phosphate for a signal generation [97] (Approach 2). The biosensor could detect cells in the linear range of 100–10,000 cells/mL with an LOD of 3 cells/mL [97]. Another immunomagnetic biosensor was applied for detection of the same BC cell lines as the first one [99] and an additional MCF-7 (a cell line with low HER2 expression) cell line via surface-expressed HER2 with a signal generated by a stripping voltammetry of Cd ions released from QDs (Approach 2). The selectivity toward SK-BR-3 cells was confirmed. A concentration-dependent signal that was 12.5× higher than the signal obtained for the HER2-negative cells (MDA-MB-231) and LOD of 2 cells/mL was obtained [99].

Cancer stem cells were discovered by Al-Hajj in 2003 [140]. Cancer stem cells were detected using a nanobiosensor with a thiolated aptamer against the CD44 surface protein immobilized on GE via chemisorption [141]. After stem-like cells were captured on the electrode surface, the electrode was modified by a self-assembled peptide-based multifunctional nanofiber containing CD44 binding protein and $-N_3$ groups, which were subsequently used for the clicking of AgNPs applied as a redox probe for an electrochemical signal generation. The LOD of the device was 6 cells/mL, and the device offered a wide linear range (from 10 cells/mL to 5×10^5 cells/mL). The selectivity of the device was successfully proved by the analysis of three different cancerous cell lines [141] (Approach 2).

4.9. Detection of Exosomes and Exosomal Content

Exosomes are characterized as endosome-derived vesicles involving the signal transduction within intercellular communication and in extracellular matrix remodeling. Exosomes are membrane-bound particles with a lipid bilayer structure carrying precious cargo: biomolecules that could be used as cancer biomarkers for more accurate cancer diagnostics in the future [51]. An increased number of exosomes circulating in body fluids was observed for cancer patients compared to healthy individuals, and a change in the exosome level can be applied as a diagnostic cancer biomarker on its own [51].

Kilic et al. fabricated a label-free electrochemical sensor to measure the increased release of nanoscale extracellular vesicles from the BC cell line, MCF-7, due to $CoCl_2$-induced hypoxia [142]. A pre-treated surface of AuSPE was modified with 11-mercaptoundenoic acid with the subsequent activation of –COOH groups for the attachment of neutravidin, which was applied for the immobilization of biotinylated anti-CD81 antibodies on the surface (Figure 18). Such a sensor was able to detect extracellular vesicles with LOD of 77 particles/mL or 379 particles/mL using EIS and DPV, respectively [142].

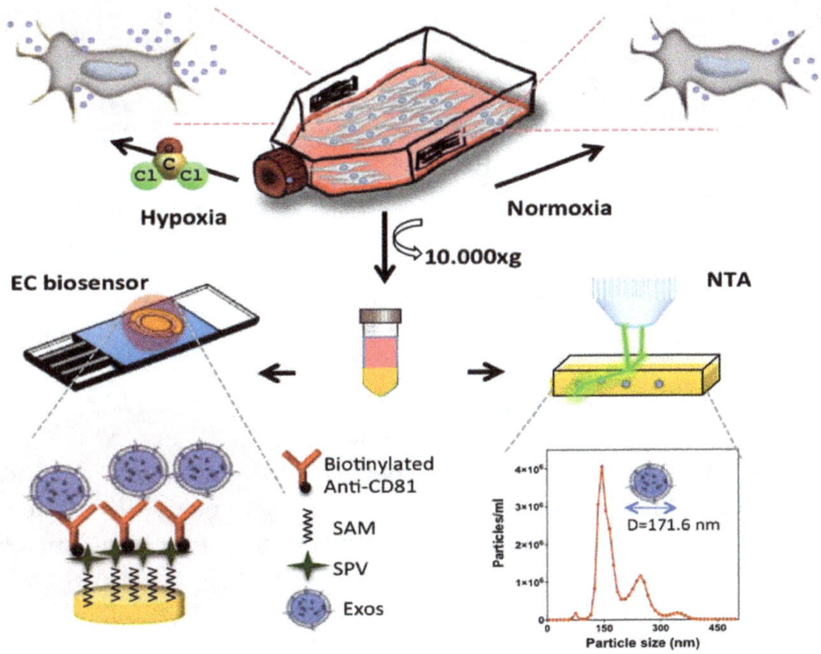

Figure 18. Experimental steps followed throughout the work. MCF-7 cells were exposed to either $CoCl_2$-induced hypoxic or normoxic conditions. The isolation of extracellular vesicles (EVs) was done via ultracentrifugation. The characterization and quantification of EVs were done via biosensors that are designed to capture exosomes on the electrode surface by antibodies raised against CD-81 protein expressed on the surface of exosomes. The gold electrode was patterned by thiolated SAM to which streptavidin was covalently immobilized, followed by the attachment of biotinylated anti-CD-81 antibodies.

Exosomes released from 4 BC cell lines were detected using a magneto-mediated electrochemical sensor [143]. Magnetic beads were modified with anti-CD63 aptamer for the capture of exosomes.

The selective detection of 4 proteins (MUC1, HER2, EpCAM, and CEA) on the exosomal surface was achieved by using silica NPs modified with respective aptamers. Silica NPs were also functionalized using mercapto–ferrocene derivative. The sandwich structure magnetic beads–exosomes–SiNPs was separated using a magnet, and the ferrocene derivatives were released from the sandwich using dithiothreitol. Ferrocene derivatives released from the sandwich were electrochemically detected on SPCE modified by a GO layer. Using this approach, 4 different biomarkers on 4 different cell lines were sensitively detected (Figure 19) (Approach 2). The sensor was clinically tested by the analysis of expression profile of 4 proteins on exosomes isolated from one BC patient and one healthy individual, confirming statistically higher levels of all 4 exosomal proteins when using BC serum compared to the serum of a healthy individual [143].

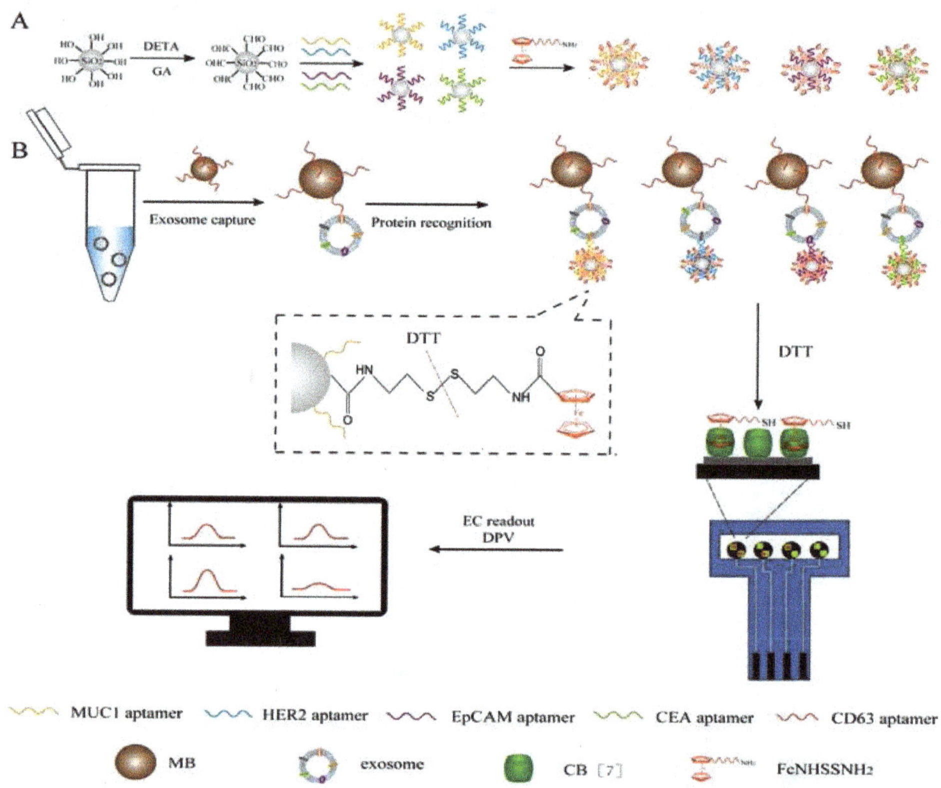

Figure 19. (**A**) Preparation of SiO2 NPs Probes; (**B**) Differential pulse voltammetry (DPV) responses of the magneto-mediated electrochemical sensor for MUC1, HER2, EpCAM, and carcinoembryonic antigen (CEA) markers. Magneto-mediated electrochemical sensor for exosomal proteins analysis based on host–guest recognition. Differential pulse voltammetry (DPV) responses of the magneto-mediated electrochemical sensor for MUC1, HER2, EpCAM, and carcinoembryonic antigen (CEA) markers for the MCF7, SKBR-3, MDA-MB-231, and BT474 cells-derived exosomes at a concentration of 1.2×10^6 particles/μL

Moura et al. prepared an electrochemical immunosensor for the detection of exosomes derived from three cell lines (MCF7, MDA-MB-231, and SKBR3) [144]. Exosomes were captured to MPs, which were modified with antibodies against general tetraspanins CD9, CD63, and CD81, as well as against specific receptors of cancer (CD24, CD44, CD54, CD326, and CD340) (Figure 20). Exosomes were immobilized on magnetic particles (MPs) in a direct and in an indirect format. The direct format was based on incubation of the exosomes–MP with the antiCD63-HRP antibodies with a final electrochemical signal readout. The indirect format was based on incubation of the exosomes–MPs with antiCDX mouse monoclonal antibodies (CDX being either CD9, CD24, CD44, CD54, CD63, CD81, CD326, or CD340 biomarkers) and the indirect labeling with antimouse–HRP antibodies. Hydroquinone was used as a mediator. The study also found out that there are differences in the size and amount of exosomes depending on the exosome origin. Moreover, the level and size distribution of exosomes purified from healthy individuals was strikingly different from the exosomes purified from BC patients. The approach offered LOD as low as 81 exosomes/μL. The method could be applied to distinguish exosomes from healthy donors and those isolated from BC patients [144] (Approach 2).

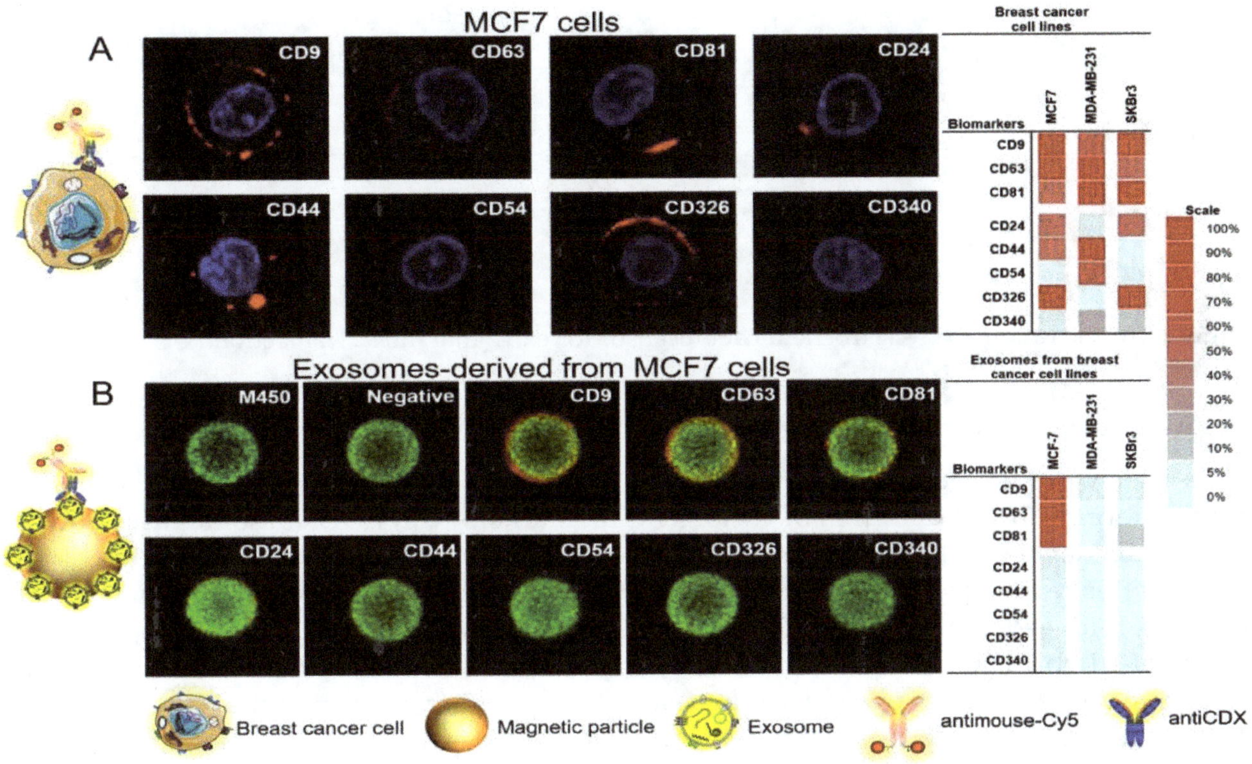

Figure 20. Confocal microscopy study for (**A**) MCF7 breast cancer cell lines and (**B**) their corresponding exosomes covalently immobilized on MPs (exosomes–MPs), followed by indirect labeling with mouse antiCDX antibodies (being CDX either CD9, CD24, CD44, CD54, CD63, CD81, CD326, and CD340 biomarkers) and antimouse-Cy5. The concentration of exosomes was set as 4×10^9 *per* assay. The scale indicates the percentage of positive entities (cells and exosomes-coated MPs in panels A and B, respectively).

Luo et al. developed a ratiometric electrochemical DNA biosensor employing an immobilized locked nucleic acid (LNA)-modified in a form of a "Y" shape-like structure for the detection of miR-21 present in exosomes released by MCF-7 cell lines [145] (Approach 1). GCE was modified by a polylysine film to which a DNA probe 1 labeled with methylene blue was covalently attached followed by hybridization with a DNA probe 2 labeled with ferrocene. The DNA probe 2 was attached to the electrode in a way such that the ferrocene redox moiety was in proximity to the electrode surface, while methylene blue redox moiety was exposed to the solution phase (Figure 21). Upon binding of the analyte miRNA-21, a DNA probe 2 labeled with ferrocene was released from the electrode surface, leaving behind only a DNA probe 1 with a surface-confined methylene blue redox moiety. Thus, upon analyte binding, an increase ("signal-on" response) in the DPV signal for methylene blue was observed with a decrease ("signal-off" response) of the DPV peak attributed to ferrocene. Both single signal responses (i.e., "signal-on" response and "signal-off" response) exhibited significant signal variation, while a ratiometric signal was highly stable. When the biosensor response was expressed in a form of a ratiometric signal, the device offered LOD of 2.3 fM with a linear range from 10 to 70 fM. The biosensor exhibited high specificity with a negligible response obtained for single- and double-mismatched RNA sequences. The device showed high assay accuracy for the analysis of miRNA-21 released from exosomes produced by a MCF-7 cell line, which was confirmed by a reference analytical method [145].

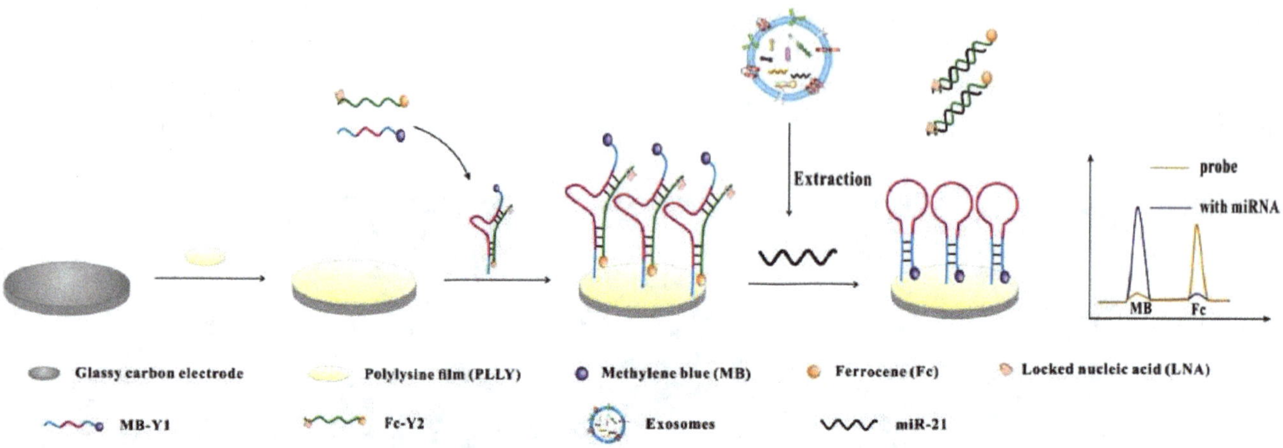

Figure 21. The ratiometric electrochemical biosensor for exosomal miR-21 detection.

5. Conclusions and Perspectives

This review provides evidence that electrochemical detection principles can offer ultrasensitive detection platforms for the detection of various BC biomarkers with LODs in some cases down to the single molecule level thanks to the use of a wide range of nanoparticles (Table 3). Such biosensors discussed in this review were mainly based on modification of the electrodes by nanomaterials (i.e., Approach 1), followed by the design of signal probes based on nanomaterials (i.e., Approach 2) with the design of a hybrid approach using nanomaterials for the modification of electrodes and for the design of signal probes (i.e., Approach 3). In a significant number of studies, the clinical performance of the nanobiosensors was validated by using human serum samples. Unfortunately, only a minor fraction of papers was focused on the detection of true concentration of BC biomarkers in human serum, but rather analyte spiking into serum samples was applied to validate the clinical usefulness of the nanobiosensors developed. Furthermore, only a limited number of papers dealt with the validation of nanobiosensing by a standard reference method i.e., ELISA. Such comparison is really needed to verify the reliability of nanobiosensors for the analysis of cancer biomarkers in complex samples such as serum samples from BC patients.

In order to really verify the clinical usefulness of the nanobiosensing approach, a larger number of human serum samples divided into two cohorts—BC patients and healthy (non-cancerous) individuals—need to be analyzed for the level of BC biomarkers in order to see if a particular biomarker is present in serum samples of BC patients at a statistically higher level compared to serum samples of healthy individuals. At the same time, such a comparison needs to be evaluated in the form of an ROC (Receiver Operating Curve) with an AUC (Area Under Curve) determined, and only such information can be then applied for the direct comparison of a clinical performance of nanobiosensing with standard immunoassays. The other aspect worth investigating in the future is a multiplexed format of analysis, when several samples are run in a parallel or when several biomarkers are detected in a single sample in parallel. So far, there is only one study describing the simultaneous analysis of miRNA-21 and MUC1, and only one study that determined the level of 4 different proteins on an exosomal surface. Although the electrochemical sensing approach is an ideal tool for integration into lab-on-a-chip platforms, we have not identified any single study analyzing BC biosensors in such an advanced assay platform using electrochemical sensing.

It is also of the utmost importance to deal with the non-specific binding of proteins from complex samples especially in cases when an electrochemical signal readout is not done in a sandwich configuration and rather detects changes in the interfacial properties of the interfacial layer after incubation with a sample i.e., impedimetric signal reading.

Table 2. Key characteristics of electrochemical nanobiosensors for the detection of BC biomarkers.

Target Biomarker (Biomolecule)	Bare Electrode	Electrode Modification	Detection	LR	LOD	Refs.
BRCA 1	MBCPE	Fe_3O_4@Ag, DNA probe	EIS	100 aM–10 nM	30 aM	[63]
	GCE	RGO, MWCNTs, PANHS	CV, EIS	100 aM–10 nM	37 aM	[64]
PIK3CA gene	CPE	ssDNA/PIn6COOH/ MoS_2	CV, EIS	100 aM–10 pM	15 aM	[72]
	GCE	GO, GNR	EIS	15 fM–148 pM	4.5 fM	[77]
	GCE	ZrO_2-RGO	EIS	10 fM–100 pM	4.3 fM	[78]
MUC MUC	SPCE	CNTs	CV, EIS	0.1–2 U/mL	0.02 U/mL	[83]
	GCE	ferrocene-loaded polymeric micelle	CV	1–1000 cells/mL	10 cells/mL	[85]
	GCE	cDNA-Fc/MXene/Apt/Au	EIS, SWV	1.0 pM–10 mM	0.33 pM	[86]
CA15-3	GE	streptavidin-coated magnetic beads	CV, EIS	ND	15×10^{-12} U/mL	[87]
	GE	GO/Py-COOH, MWCNTs	DPV	0.1–20 U/mL	0.01 U/mL	[90]
HER2	ITO	APTES/MoO_3@RGO	CV, DPV, EIS	0.001–500 ng/mL	0.001 ng/mL (~5.41 fM)	[92]
	GCE	AuNP-ERGO-SWCNTs	EIS	0.1 pg/mL–1 ng/mL	50 fg/mL (~0.27 fM)	[93]
	SPGE	MIP	CV	10–70 ng/mL	1.6 ng/L (~8.65 fM)	[95]
	GE	GNR@Pd SSs—Apt—HRP	EIS	10–200 ng/mL	0.15 ng/mL (~0.81 pM)	[101]
	SPCE	MBs and CdSe@ZnS QDs	DPASV	0.50–50 ng/mL	0.29 ng/mL (~1.57 pM)	[99]
CEA	GCE	aptamer/GLD/CS/ZnS-CdS/MoS_2	CV	0.05–20 ng/mL	0.031 ng/mL (~0.16 pM)	[106]
	CPE	GNPs and MWCNTs.	CV, EIS	0.4–125 ng/mL	0.09 ng/mL (~0.45 pM)	[107]
	GCE	Au-AgNPs/RGO	CV	0.001–80 ng/mL	0.29 pg/mL (~1.45 fM)	[114]
miRNA-21 and MUC1	GCE	Au nanoflowers	ECL	20 aM–50 pM (miRNA-21) 1 fg mL^{-1}–10 ng mL^{-1} (MUC1)	11 aM (miRNA-21) 0.4 fg/mL (~7.27 aM) (MUC1)	[119]
CA 27-29	GCE	Au/MoS_2/RGO	CV	0.1–100 U/mL	0.08 U/mL	[121]
uPA	FTO	GNS	DPV, CV	1 fM–1 μM	4.8 fM	[122]

Table 3. Key characteristics of electrochemical nanobiosensors for the detection of BC biomarkers.

Target Biomarker (Biomolecule)	Bare Electrode	Electrode Modification	Detection	LR	LOD	Refs.
tPA	GCE	SWCNTs	CV, EIS	0.1–1.0 ng/mL	0.026 ng/mL (~0.37 pM)	[124]
MCF-7/CTC		RGO/AuNPs/CuO	CV, CA	50–7000 cells/mL	27 cells/mL	[131]
MCF-7	GCE	Au NCs/amino-functionalized MWCNT-NH_2	CV, EIS	100–1.0 × 10^6 cells/mL	80 cells/mL	[133]
	GE	Bi_2Se_3@Au-mDNA	CV, EIS	100 nM–27 µM	10 nM	[135]
	GCE	Hexagonal carbon nitride tubes	Photo-current	100–1 × 10^5 cells/mL	17 cells/mL	[137]
	GCE	TiO_2 nanotubes with graphene	EIS	1000–1 × 10^7 cells/mL	40 cells/mL	[138]
MDA-MB-231	GE	Non-spherical AuNPs	DPV	10–1 × 10^6 cells/mL	2 cells/mL	[139]
Cancer stem cells	GE	AgNPs	DPV	10–5 × 10^5 cells/mL	6 cells/mL	[141]
Exosomes Exosomal miRNA-21	Au SPE	11-MUA	EIS, DPV	10^2–10^9 particles/mL	77 particles/mL	[142]
	SPCE	MB SiO_2 NPs	DPC, EIS	1.2 × 10^3–1.2 × 10^7 particles/µL	1.0 × 10^7 particles/µL	[143]
	m-GEC magnetic	MPs	Ampero-metry	0–1 × 10^6 particles/µL	10^5 particles/µL	[144]
	GCE	Polylysine	DPV	10–70 fM	2.3 fM	[145]

Abbreviations

Apt	aptamer
APTES	3-aminopropyltriethoxysilane
Ar-CH_2-COOH	p-aminophenylacetic acid
AuNCs	gold nanocages
AuNPs	gold nanoparticles
Au-SPE	gold screen-printed electrode
BRCA1	BReast CAncer Type 1 gene
CA15-3	cancer antigen 15-3
CA 27-29	cancer antigen 27-29
CA	chronoamperometry
CEA	carcinoembryonic antigen
CdSe@ZnS QDs	core/shell quantum dots
CNTs	carbon nanotubes
CPE	carbon paste electrode
CV	cyclic voltammetry
CysA	cysteamine
CTES	carboxyethylsilanetriol
DPV	differential pulse voltammetry
DPASV	differential pulse anodic stripping voltammetry
EIS	electrochemical impedance spectroscopy
ERGO	electrochemically reduced graphene oxide
Fc	ferrocene
FTO	fluorine doped tin oxide
GE	gold electrode
GCE	glassy carbon electrode
GLD	glutaraldehyde
GNR	gold nanorods
GNS	graphene nanosheets
GO	graphene oxide
3-GOPE	3-glycidoxypropyl triethoxysilane
GSPE	Graphite-based screen-printed electrode
GQDs	graphene quantum dots
HER2	human epidermal growth factor receptor 2
HRP	horseradish peroxidase
ITO	indium tin oxide
mDNA	mediated double-stranded DNA
m-GEC	magnetic electrode—magneto-actuated graphite epoxy composite
MBs	magnetic beads
MAM	mammaglobin
MBCPE	magnetic bar carbon paste electrode
MPs	magnetic particles
11-MUA	11-mercaptoundenoic acid
MIP	molecularly imprinted polymer
Mt-HSA NCs	clay–protein based composite nanoparticles
MWCNTs	multi-walled carbon nanotubes
OM	one order of magnitude
OPN	osteopontin
PANHS	1-pyrenebutyric acid-*N*-hydroxysuccinimide ester

Pd SSs	Pd superstructures
PEG	polyethylene glycol
PGE	pencil graphite electrode
PIK3CA gene	phosphatidylinositol-4,5-bisphosphate 3-kinase catalytic subunit alpha gene
Ppy	polypyrrole polymer
Py-COOH	1-pyrenecarboxylic acid
RGO	reduced graphene oxide
SAM	self-assembled monolayer
SPCE	screen-printed carbon electrode
SPGE	screen-printed gold electrode
ssDNA	single-stranded deoxyribonucleic acid
SOX2	sex-determining region Y-box 2
SWCNTs	single-walled carbon nanotubes
SWV	square wave voltammetry
tPA	tissue plasminogen activator
uPA	urokinase plasminogen activator

References

1. Siegel, R.L.; Miller, K.D.; Jemal, A. Cancer statistics, 2019. *CA Cancer J. Clin.* **2019**, *69*, 7–34. [CrossRef] [PubMed]
2. Rahman, S.A.; Al-Marzouki, A.; Otim, M.; Khalil Khayat, N.E.H.; Yousuf, R.; Rahman, P. Awareness about Breast Cancer and Breast Self-Examination among Female Students at the University of Sharjah: A Cross-Sectional Study. *Asian Pac. J. Cancer Prev.* **2019**, *20*, 1901–1908. [CrossRef] [PubMed]
3. Dos Anjos Pultz, B.; da Luz, F.A.; de Faria, P.R.; Oliveira, A.P.; de Araujo, R.A.; Silva, M.J. Far beyond the usual biomarkers in breast cancer: A review. *J. Cancer* **2014**, *5*, 559–571. [CrossRef] [PubMed]
4. Khorrami, S.; Tavakoli, M.; Safari, E. Clinical Value of Serum S100A8/A9 and CA15-3 in the Diagnosis of Breast Cancer. *Iran. J. Pathol.* **2019**, *14*, 104–112. [CrossRef]
5. Begum, M.; Karim, S.; Malik, A.; Khurshid, R.; Asif, M.; Salim, A.; Nagra, S.A.; Zaheer, A.; Iqbal, Z.; Abuzenadah, A.M.; et al. CA 15–3 (Mucin-1) and physiological characteristics of breast cancer from Lahore, Pakistan. *Asian Pac. J. Cancer Prev.* **2012**, *13*, 5257–5261. [CrossRef]
6. Scott, D.A.; Drake, R.R. Glycosylation and its implications in breast cancer. *Expert Rev. Proteom.* **2019**, *16*, 665–680. [CrossRef]
7. Núñez, C. Blood-based protein biomarkers in breast cancer. *Clin. Chim. Acta* **2019**, *490*, 113–127. [CrossRef]
8. Torre, L.A.; Trabert, B.; DeSantis, C.E.; Miller, K.D.; Samimi, G.; Runowicz, C.D.; Gaudet, M.M.; Jemal, A.; Siegel, R.L. Ovarian Cancer statistics, 2018. *CA Cancer J. Clin.* **2018**, *68*, 284–296. [CrossRef]
9. Becker, S. A historic and scientific review of breast cancer: The next global healthcare challenge. *Int. J. Gynaecol. Obstet.* **2015**, *131* (Suppl. 1), S36–S39. [CrossRef]
10. Schopper, D.; de Wolf, C. How effective are breast cancer screening programmes by mammography? Review of the current evidence. *Eur. J. Cancer* **2009**, *45*, 1916–1923. [CrossRef]
11. Gebrehiwot, A.G.; Melka, D.S.; Kassaye, Y.M.; Gemechu, T.; Lako, W.; Hinou, H.; Nishimura, S.-I. Exploring serum and immunoglobulin G N-glycome as diagnostic biomarkers for early detection of breast cancer in Ethiopian women. *BMC Cancer* **2019**, *19*, 588. [CrossRef] [PubMed]
12. Sadighbayan, D.; Sadighbayan, K.; Khosroushahi, A.Y.; Hasanzadeh, M. Recent advances on the DNA-based electrochemical biosensing of cancer biomarkers: Analytical approach. *Trends Anal. Chem.* **2019**, *119*, 115609. [CrossRef]
13. Sadighbayan, D.; Sadighbayan, K.; Tohid-kia, M.R.; Khosroushahi, A.Y.; Hasanzadeh, M. Development of electrochemical biosensors for tumor marker determination towards cancer diagnosis: Recent progress. *Trends Anal. Chem.* **2019**, *118*, 73–88. [CrossRef]
14. Sharifi, M.; Avadi, M.R.; Attar, F.; Dashtestani, F.; Ghorchian, H.; Rezayat, S.M.; Saboury, A.A.; Falahati, M. Cancer diagnosis using nanomaterials based electrochemical nanobiosensors. *Biosens. Bioelectron.* **2019**, *126*, 773–784. [CrossRef] [PubMed]

15. Freitas, M.; Nouws, H.P.A.; Delerue-Matos, C. Electrochemical Biosensing in Cancer Diagnostics and Follow-up. *Electroanalysis* **2018**, *30*, 1584–1603. [CrossRef]
16. Sharifi, M.; Hasan, A.; Attar, F.; Taghizadeh, A.; Falahati, M. Development of point-of-care nanobiosensors for breast cancers diagnosis. *Talanta* **2020**, *217*, 121091. [CrossRef]
17. Campuzano, S.; Pedrero, M.; Pingarron, J.M. Non-invasive breast cancer diagnosis through electrochemical biosensing at different molecular levels. *Sensors* **2017**, *17*, 1993. [CrossRef]
18. Hasanzadeh, M.; Shadjou, N.; de la Guardia, M. Early stage screening of breast cancer using electrochemical biomarker detection. *Trends Anal. Chem.* **2017**, *91*, 67–76. [CrossRef]
19. Barber, M.D.; Thomas, J.S.J.; Dixon, J.M. *Breast Cancer: An Atlas of Investigation and Management*; Clinical Pub.: Oxford, UK, 2008; pp. 1–5.
20. Mills, D.; Gomberawalla, A.; Gordon, E.J.; Tondre, J.; Nejad, M.; Nguyen, T.; Pogoda, J.M.; Rao, J.; Chatterton, R.; Henning, S.; et al. Examination of Duct Physiology in the Human Mammary Gland. *PLoS ONE* **2016**, *11*, e0150653. [CrossRef]
21. Love, S.; Barsky, S. Anatomy of the nipple and breast ducts revisited. *Cancer* **2004**, *101*, 1947–1957. [CrossRef]
22. Bombonati, A.; Sgroi, D.C. The molecular pathology of breast cancer progression. *J. Pathol.* **2011**, *223*, 307–317. [CrossRef] [PubMed]
23. Rakha, E.A.; Putti, T.C.; Abd El-Rehim, D.M.; Paish, C.; Green, A.R.; Powe, D.G.; Lee, A.H.; Robertson, J.F.; Ellis, I.O. Morphological and immunophenotypic analysis of breast carcinomas with basal and myoepithelial differentiation. *J. Pathol.* **2006**, *208*, 495–506. [CrossRef] [PubMed]
24. Barroso-Sousa, R.; Metzger-Filho, O. Differences between invasive lobular and invasive ductal carcinoma of the breast: Results and therapeutic implications. *Ther. Adv. Med. Oncol.* **2016**, *8*, 261–266. [CrossRef] [PubMed]
25. Li, Q.; Li, G.; Zhou, Y.; Zhang, X.; Sun, M.; Jiang, H.; Yu, G. Comprehensive N-Glycome Profiling of Cells and Tissues for Breast Cancer Diagnosis. *J. Proteome Res.* **2019**, *18*, 2559–2570. [CrossRef]
26. Harbeck, N.; Penault-Llorca, F.; Cortes, J.; Gnant, M.; Houssami, N.; Poortmans, P.; Ruddy, K.; Tsang, J.; Cardoso, F. Breast cancer. *Nat. Rev. Dis. Primers* **2019**, *5*, 66. [CrossRef]
27. Ludwig, J.A.; Weinstein, J.N. Biomarkers in cancer staging, prognosis and treatment selection. *Nat. Rev. Cancer* **2005**, *5*, 845–856. [CrossRef]
28. Tzitzikos, G.; Saridi, M.; Filippopoulou, T.; Makri, A.; Goulioti, A.; Stavropoulos, T.; Stamatiou, K. Measurement of tumor markers in chronic hemodialysis patients. *Saudi J. Kidney Dis. Transplant.* **2010**, *21*, 50–53.
29. Estakhri, R.; Ghahramanzade, A.; Vahedi, A.; Nourazarian, A. Serum levels of CA15-3, AFP, CA19-9 and CEA tumor markers in cancer care and treatment of patients with impaired renal function on hemodialysis. *Asian Pac. J. Cancer Prev.* **2013**, *14*, 1597–1599. [CrossRef]
30. Mittal, S.; Kaur, H.; Gautam, N.; Mantha, A.K. Biosensors for breast cancer diagnosis: A review of bioreceptors, biotransducers and signal amplification strategies. *Biosens. Bioelectron.* **2017**, *88*, 217–231. [CrossRef]
31. Tkac, J.; Gajdosova, V.; Hroncekova, S.; Bertok, T.; Hires, M.; Jane, E.; Lorencova, L.; Kasak, P. Prostate-specific antigen glycoprofiling as diagnostic and prognostic biomarker of prostate cancer. *Interface Focus* **2019**, *9*, 20180077. [CrossRef]
32. Au, G.H.; Mejias, L.; Swami, V.K.; Brooks, A.D.; Shih, W.Y.; Shih, W.H. Quantitative assessment of Tn antigen in breast tissue micro-arrays using CdSe aqueous quantum dots. *Biomaterials* **2014**, *35*, 2971–2980. [CrossRef] [PubMed]
33. Christiansen, M.N.; Chik, J.; Lee, L.; Anugraham, M.; Abrahams, J.L.; Packer, N.H. Cell surface protein glycosylation in cancer. *Proteomics* **2014**, *14*, 525–546. [CrossRef] [PubMed]
34. Tousi, F.; Bones, J.; Hancock, W.S.; Hincapie, M. Differential Chemical Derivatization Integrated with Chromatographic Separation for Analysis of Isomeric Sialylated N-Glycans: A Nano-Hydrophilic Interaction Liquid Chromatography-MS Platform. *Anal. Chem.* **2013**, *85*, 8421–8428. [CrossRef] [PubMed]
35. Ju, L.L.; Wang, Y.P.; Xie, Q.; Xu, X.K.; Li, Y.; Chen, Z.J.; Li, Y.S. Elevated level of serum glycoprotein bifucosylation and prognostic value in Chinese breast cancer. *Glycobiology* **2016**, *26*, 460–471. [CrossRef] [PubMed]
36. Ideo, H.; Hinoda, Y.; Sakai, K.; Hoshi, I.; Yamamoto, S.; Oka, M.; Maeda, K.; Maeda, N.; Hazama, S.; Amano, J. Expression of mucin 1 possessing a 3′-sulfated core1 in recurrent and metastatic breast cancer. *Int. J. Cancer* **2015**, *137*, 1652–1660. [CrossRef] [PubMed]

37. Imamura, M.; Morimoto, T.; Nomura, T.; Michishita, S.; Nishimukai, A.; Higuchi, T.; Fujimoto, Y.; Miyagawa, Y.; Kira, A.; Murase, K.; et al. Independent prognostic impact of preoperative serum carcinoembryonic antigen and cancer antigen 15–3 levels for early breast cancer subtypes. *World J. Oncol.* **2018**, *16*, 26. [CrossRef]
38. Park, B.-J.; Cha, M.-K.; Kim, I.-H. Thioredoxin 1 as a serum marker for breast cancer and its use in combination with CEA or CA15-3 for improving the sensitivity of breast cancer diagnoses. *BMC Res. Notes* **2014**, *7*. [CrossRef]
39. Bernstein, J.L.; Godbold, J.H.; Raptis, G.; Watson, M.A.; Levinson, B.; Aaronson, S.A.; Fleming, T.P. Identification of mammaglobin as a novel serum marker for breast cancer. *Clin. Cancer Res.* **2005**, *11*, 6528–6535. [CrossRef]
40. Yan, X.; Lin, Y.; Liu, S.; Aziz, F.; Yan, Q. Fucosyltransferase IV (FUT4) as an effective biomarker for the diagnosis of breast cancer. *Biomed. Pharmacother.* **2015**, *70*, 299–304. [CrossRef]
41. Koo, J.H. (Ed.) An Overview of Nanomaterials. In *Fundamentals, Properties, and Applications of Polymer Nanocomposites*; Cambridge University Press: Cambridge, UK, 2016; pp. 22–108.
42. Pacheco-Torgal, F.; Jalali, S. Nanotechnology: Advantages and drawbacks in the field of construction and building materials. *Constr. Build. Mater.* **2011**, *25*, 582–590. [CrossRef]
43. Gajdosova, V.; Lorencova, L.; Prochazka, M.; Omastova, M.; Micusik, M.; Prochazkova, S.; Kveton, F.; Jerigova, M.; Velic, D.; Kasak, P.; et al. Remarkable differences in the voltammetric response towards hydrogen peroxide, oxygen and Ru(NH(3))(6)(3+) of electrode interfaces modified with HF or LiF-HCl etched Ti(3)C(2)T(x) MXene. *Mikrochim. Acta* **2019**, *187*, 52. [CrossRef] [PubMed]
44. Hughes, G.; Westmacott, K.; Honeychurch, K.C.; Crew, A.; Pemberton, R.M.; Hart, J.P. Recent Advances in the Fabrication and Application of Screen-Printed Electrochemical (Bio)Sensors Based on Carbon Materials for Biomedical, Agri-Food and Environmental Analyses. *Biosensors* **2016**, *6*, 50. [CrossRef]
45. Taleat, Z.; Khoshroo, A. Screen-printed electrodes for biosensing: A review (2008–2013). *Microchim. Acta* **2014**, *181*, 865–891. [CrossRef]
46. Arduini, F.; Micheli, L.; Moscone, D.; Palleschi, G.; Piermarini, S.; Ricci, F.; Volpe, G. Electrochemical biosensors based on nanomodified screen-printed electrodes: Recent applications in clinical analysis. *TrAC Trends Anal. Chem.* **2016**, *79*, 114–126. [CrossRef]
47. Renedo, O.D.; Alonso-Lomillo, M.A.; Martínez, M.J.A. Recent developments in the field of screen-printed electrodes and their related applications. *Talanta* **2007**, *73*, 202–219. [CrossRef] [PubMed]
48. Grieshaber, D.; MacKenzie, R.; Vörös, J.; Reimhult, E. Electrochemical Biosensors-Sensor Principles and Architectures. *Sensors* **2008**, *8*, 1400–1458. [CrossRef]
49. Tang, Y.; Ouyang, M. Tailoring properties and functionalities of metal nanoparticles through crystallinity engineering. *Nat. Mater.* **2007**, *6*, 754–759. [CrossRef]
50. Bertok, T.; Lorencova, L.; Chocholova, E.; Jane, E.; Vikartovska, A.; Kasak, P.; Tkac, J. Electrochemical Impedance Spectroscopy Based Biosensors: Mechanistic Principles, Analytical Examples and Challenges towards Commercialization for Assays of Protein Cancer Biomarkers. *ChemElectroChem* **2019**, *6*, 989–1003. [CrossRef]
51. Lorencova, L.; Bertok, T.; Bertokova, A.; Gajdosova, V.; Hroncekova, S.; Vikartovska, A.; Kasak, P.; Tkac, J. Exosomes as a Source of Cancer Biomarkers: Advances in Electrochemical Biosensing of Exosomes. *ChemElectroChem* **2020**, *7*, 1956–1973. [CrossRef]
52. Reddy, K.K.; Bandal, H.; Satyanarayana, M.; Goud, K.Y.; Gobi, K.V.; Jayaramudu, T.; Amalraj, J.; Kim, H. Recent Trends in Electrochemical Sensors for Vital Biomedical Markers Using Hybrid Nanostructured Materials. *Adv. Sci.* **2020**. [CrossRef]
53. Lorencova, L.; Gajdosova, V.; Hroncekova, S.; Bertok, T.; Blahutova, J.; Vikartovska, A.; Parrakova, L.; Gemeiner, P.; Kasak, P.; Tkac, J. 2D MXenes as Perspective Immobilization Platforms for Design of Electrochemical Nanobiosensors. *Electroanalysis* **2019**, *31*, 1833–1844. [CrossRef]
54. Maia, F.R.; Reis, R.L.; Oliveira, J.M.; Maia, F.R.; Reis, R.L.; Oliveira, J.M.; Maia, F.R.; Reis, R.L.; Oliveira, J.M. Nanoparticles and Microfluidic Devices in Cancer Research. *Adv. Exp. Med. Biol.* **2020**, *1230*, 161–171. [PubMed]
55. Meng, L.; Turner, A.P.F.; Mak, W.C. Soft and flexible material-based affinity sensors. *Biotechnol. Adv.* **2020**, *39*, 107398. [CrossRef]

56. Siemer, S.; Wunsch, D.; Khamis, A.; Lu, Q.; Hagemann, J.; Stauber, R.H.; Gribko, A.; Scherberich, A.; Filippi, M.; Krafft, M.P.; et al. Nano Meets Micro-Translational Nanotechnology in Medicine: Nano-Based Applications for Early Tumor Detection and Therapy. *Nanomaterials* **2020**, *10*, 383. [CrossRef]
57. Sierra, J.; Rodriguez-Trujillo, R.; Mir, M.; Samitier, J.; Sierra, J.; Marrugo-Ramirez, J.; Rodriguez-Trujillo, R.; Mir, M.; Samitier, J.; Mir, M.; et al. Sensor-Integrated Microfluidic Approaches for Liquid Biopsies Applications in Early Detection of Cancer. *Sensors* **2020**, *20*, 1317. [CrossRef]
58. Agnolon, V.; Contato, A.; Meneghello, A.; Tagliabue, E.; Toffoli, G.; Gion, M.; Polo, F.; Fabricio, A.S.C. ELISA assay employing epitope-specific monoclonal antibodies to quantify circulating HER2 with potential application in monitoring cancer patients undergoing therapy with trastuzumab. *Sci. Rep.* **2020**, *10*, 3016. [CrossRef] [PubMed]
59. Yousef, G.; Polymeris, M.-E.; Grass, L.; Soosaipillai, A.; Chan, P.-C.; Scorilas, A.; Borgoño, C.; Harbeck, N.; Schmalfeldt, B.; Dorn, J.; et al. Human Kallikrein 5 A Potential Novel Serum Biomarker for Breast and Ovarian Cancer. *Cancer Res.* **2003**, *63*, 3958–3965.
60. Kumar, J.K.; Aronsson, A.C.; Pilko, G.; Zupan, M.; Kumer, K.; Fabjan, T.; Osredkar, J.; Eriksson, S. A clinical evaluation of the TK 210 ELISA in sera from breast cancer patients demonstrates high sensitivity and specificity in all stages of disease. *Tumour Biol. J. Int. Soc. Oncodev. Biol. Med.* **2016**, *37*, 11937–11945. [CrossRef]
61. Li, D.; Harlan-Williams, L.M.; Kumaraswamy, E.; Jensen, R.A. BRCA1-No Matter How You Splice It. *Cancer Res.* **2019**, *79*, 2091–2098. [CrossRef]
62. Benvidi, A.; Dehghani Firouzabadi, A.; Dehghan Tezerjani, M.; Moshtaghiun, S.M.; Mazloum-Ardakani, M.; Ansarin, A. A highly sensitive and selective electrochemical DNA biosensor to diagnose breast cancer. *J. Electroanal. Chem.* **2015**, *750*, 57–64. [CrossRef]
63. Benvidi, A.; Jahanbani, S. Self-assembled monolayer of SH-DNA strand on a magnetic bar carbon paste electrode modified with Fe3O4@Ag nanoparticles for detection of breast cancer mutation. *J. Electroanal. Chem.* **2016**, *768*, 47–54. [CrossRef]
64. Benvidi, A.; Tezerjani, M.D.; Jahanbani, S.; Mazloum Ardakani, M.; Moshtaghioun, S.M. Comparison of impedimetric detection of DNA hybridization on the various biosensors based on modified glassy carbon electrodes with PANHS and nanomaterials of RGO and MWCNTs. *Talanta* **2016**, *147*, 621–627. [CrossRef] [PubMed]
65. Benvidi, A.; Abbasi, Z.; Tezerjani, M.; Banaei, M.; Zare, H.; Molahosseini, H.; Jahanbani, S. A Highly Selective DNA Sensor Based on Graphene Oxide-Silk Fibroin Composite and AuNPs as a Probe Oligonucleotide Immobilization Platform. *Acta Chim. Slov.* **2018**, *65*, 278–288. [CrossRef] [PubMed]
66. Chen, L.; Liu, X.; Chen, C. Impedimetric biosensor modified with hydrophilic material of tannic acid/polyethylene glycol and dopamine-assisted deposition for detection of breast cancer-related BRCA1 gene. *J. Electroanal. Chem.* **2017**, *791*, 204–210. [CrossRef]
67. Ehzari, H.; Safari, M.; Shahlaei, M. A simple and label-free genosensor for BRCA1 related sequence based on electrospinned ribbon conductive nanofibers. *Microchem. J.* **2018**, *143*, 118–126. [CrossRef]
68. Kazerooni, H.; Nassernejad, B. A novel biosensor nanomaterial for the ultraselective and ultrasensitive electrochemical diagnosis of the breast cancer-related BRCA1 gene. *Anal. Methods* **2016**, *8*, 3069–3074. [CrossRef]
69. Benvidi, A.; Firouzabadi, A.D.; Moshtaghiun, S.M.; Mazloum-Ardakani, M.; Tezerjani, M.D. Ultrasensitive DNA sensor based on gold nanoparticles/reduced graphene oxide/glassy carbon electrode. *Anal. Biochem.* **2015**, *484*, 24–30. [CrossRef]
70. Shahrokhian, S.; Salimian, R. Ultrasensitive detection of cancer biomarkers using conducting polymer/electrochemically reduced graphene oxide-based biosensor: Application toward BRCA1 sensing. *Sens. Actuators B Chem.* **2018**, *266*, 160–169. [CrossRef]
71. Saeed, A.A.; Sánchez, J.L.A.; O'Sullivan, C.K.; Abbas, M.N. DNA biosensors based on gold nanoparticles-modified graphene oxide for the detection of breast cancer biomarkers for early diagnosis. *Bioelectrochemistry* **2017**, *118*, 91–99. [CrossRef]
72. Yang, J.; Yin, X.; Zhang, W. Electrochemical determination of PIK3CA gene associated with breast cancer based on molybdenum disulfide nanosheet-supported poly(indole-6-carboxylic acid). *Anal. Methods* **2019**, *11*, 157–162. [CrossRef]

73. Babaei, K.; Shams, S.; Keymoradzadeh, A.; Vahidi, S.; Hamami, P.; Khaksar, R.; Norollahi, S.E.; Samadani, A.A. An insight of microRNAs performance in carcinogenesis and tumorigenesis; an overview of cancer therapy. *Life Sci.* **2020**, *240*, 117077. [CrossRef]
74. Kashyap, D.; Kaur, H. Cell-free miRNAs as non-invasive biomarkers in breast cancer: Significance in early diagnosis and metastasis prediction. *Life Sci.* **2020**, *246*, 117417. [CrossRef] [PubMed]
75. Valihrach, L.; Androvic, P.; Kubista, M. Circulating miRNA analysis for cancer diagnostics and therapy. *Mol. Asp. Med.* **2020**, *72*, 100825. [CrossRef] [PubMed]
76. Cardoso, A.R.; Moreira, F.T.C.; Fernandes, R.; Sales, M.G.F. Novel and simple electrochemical biosensor monitoring attomolar levels of miRNA-155 in breast cancer. *Biosens. Bioelectron.* **2016**, *80*, 621–630. [CrossRef] [PubMed]
77. Ebrahimi, A.; Nikokar, I.; Zokaei, M.; Bozorgzadeh, E. Design, development and evaluation of microRNA-199a-5p detecting electrochemical nanobiosensor with diagnostic application in Triple Negative Breast Cancer. *Talanta* **2018**, *189*, 592–598. [CrossRef] [PubMed]
78. Zhang, K.; Zhang, N.; Zhang, L.; Wang, H.; Shi, H.; Liu, Q. Label-free impedimetric sensing platform for microRNA-21 based on ZrO 2 -reduced graphene oxide nanohybrids coupled with catalytic hairpin assembly amplification. *RSC Adv.* **2018**, *8*, 16146–16151. [CrossRef]
79. Rafiee-Pour, H.A.; Behpour, M.; Keshavarz, M. A novel label-free electrochemical miRNA biosensor using methylene blue as redox indicator: Application to breast cancer biomarker miRNA-21. *Biosens. Bioelectron.* **2016**, *77*, 202–207. [CrossRef]
80. Kilic, T.; Erdem, A.; Erac, Y.; Seydibeyoglu, M.O.; Okur, S.; Ozsoz, M. Electrochemical Detection of a Cancer Biomarker mir-21 in Cell Lysates Using Graphene Modified Sensors. *Electroanalysis* **2015**, *27*, 317–326. [CrossRef]
81. Zouari, M.; Campuzano, S.; Pingarrón, J.M.; Raouafi, N. Femtomolar direct voltammetric determination of circulating miRNAs in sera of cancer patients using an enzymeless biosensor. *Anal. Chim. Acta* **2020**, *1104*, 188–198. [CrossRef]
82. Nath, S.; Mukherjee, P. MUC1: A multifaceted oncoprotein with a key role in cancer progression. *Trends Mol. Med.* **2014**, *20*, 332–342. [CrossRef]
83. Nawaz, M.A.H.; Rauf, S.; Catanante, G.; Nawaz, M.H.; Nunes, G.; Marty, J.L.; Hayat, A. One Step Assembly of Thin Films of Carbon Nanotubes on Screen Printed Interface for Electrochemical Aptasensing of Breast Cancer Biomarker. *Sensors* **2016**, *16*, 1651. [CrossRef] [PubMed]
84. Paimard, G.; Shahlaei, M.; Moradipour, P.; Karamali, V.; Arkan, E. Impedimetric aptamer based determination of the tumor marker MUC1 by using electrospun core-shell nanofibers. *Microchim. Acta* **2019**, *187*. [CrossRef] [PubMed]
85. Mouffouk, F.; Aouabdi, S.; Al-Hetlani, E.; Serrai, H.; Alrefae, T.; Leo Chen, L. New generation of electrochemical immunoassay based on polymeric nanoparticles for early detection of breast cancer. *Int. J. Nanomed.* **2017**, *12*, 3037–3047. [CrossRef] [PubMed]
86. Wang, H.; Sun, J.; Lu, L.; Yang, X.; Xia, J.; Zhang, F.; Wang, Z. Competitive electrochemical aptasensor based on a cDNA-ferrocene/MXene probe for detection of breast cancer marker Mucin1. *Anal. Chim. Acta* **2020**, *1094*, 18–25. [CrossRef]
87. Akbari Nakhjavani, S.; Khalilzadeh, B.; Samadi Pakchin, P.; Saber, R.; Ghahremani, M.H.; Omidi, Y. A highly sensitive and reliable detection of CA15-3 in patient plasma with electrochemical biosensor labeled with magnetic beads. *Biosens. Bioelectron.* **2018**, *122*, 8–15. [CrossRef] [PubMed]
88. Santos, A.R.T.; Moreira, F.T.C.; Helguero, L.A.; Sales, M.G.F. Antibody Biomimetic Material Made of Pyrrole for CA 15–3 and Its Application as Sensing Material in Ion-Selective Electrodes for Potentiometric Detection. *Biosensors* **2018**, *8*, 8. [CrossRef]
89. Amani, J.; Khoshroo, A.; Rahimi-Nasrabadi, M. Electrochemical immunosensor for the breast cancer marker CA 15–3 based on the catalytic activity of a CuS/reduced graphene oxide nanocomposite towards the electrooxidation of catechol. *Microchim. Acta* **2018**, *185*. [CrossRef]
90. Akter, R.; Jeong, B.; Choi, J.S.; Rahman, M.A. Ultrasensitive Nanoimmunosensor by coupling non-covalent functionalized graphene oxide platform and numerous ferritin labels on carbon nanotubes. *Biosens. Bioelectron.* **2016**, *80*, 123–130. [CrossRef]

91. Goutsouliak, K.; Veeraraghavan, J.; Sethunath, V.; De Angelis, C.; Osborne, C.K.; Rimawi, M.F.; Schiff, R. Towards personalized treatment for early stage HER2-positive breast cancer. *Nat. Rev. Clin. Oncol.* **2020**, *17*, 233–250. [CrossRef]
92. Augustine, S.; Kumar, P.; Malhotra, B.D. Amine-Functionalized MoO3@RGO Nanohybrid-Based Biosensor for Breast Cancer Detection. *ACS Appl. Bio Mater.* **2019**, *2*, 5366–5378. [CrossRef]
93. Rostamabadi, P.; Heydari-Bafrooei, E. Impedimetric aptasensing of the breast cancer biomarker HER2 using a glassy carbon electrode modified with gold nanoparticles in a composite consisting of electrochemically reduced graphene oxide and single-walled carbon nanotubes. *Microchim. Acta* **2019**, *186*. [CrossRef] [PubMed]
94. Arkan, E.; Saber, R.; Karimi, Z.; Shamsipur, M. A novel antibody-antigen based impedimetric immunosensor for low level detection of HER2 in serum samples of breast cancer patients via modification of a gold nanoparticles decorated multiwall carbon nanotube-ionic liquid electrode. *Anal. Chim. Acta* **2015**, *874*, 66–74. [CrossRef] [PubMed]
95. Pacheco, J.G.; Rebelo, P.; Freitas, M.; Nouws, H.P.A.; Delerue-Matos, C. Breast cancer biomarker (HER2-ECD) detection using a molecularly imprinted electrochemical sensor. *Sens. Actuators B Chem.* **2018**, *273*, 1008–1014. [CrossRef]
96. Freitas, M.; Nouws, H.P.A.; Delerue-Matos, C. Electrochemical Sensing Platforms for HER2-ECD Breast Cancer Biomarker Detection. *Electroanalysis* **2019**, *31*, 121–128. [CrossRef]
97. Freitas, M.; Nouws, H.P.A.; Keating, E.; Delerue-Matos, C. High-performance electrochemical immunomagnetic assay for breast cancer analysis. *Sens. Actuators B Chem.* **2020**, *308*, 127667. [CrossRef]
98. Freitas, M.; Neves, M.; Nouws, H.; Delerue-Matos, C. Quantum dots as nanolabels for breast cancer biomarker HER2-ECD analysis in human serum. *Talanta* **2019**, *208*, 120430. [CrossRef]
99. Freitas, M.; Nouws, H.P.A.; Keating, E.; Fernandes, V.C.; Delerue-Matos, C. Immunomagnetic bead-based bioassay for the voltammetric analysis of the breast cancer biomarker HER2-ECD and tumour cells using quantum dots as detection labels. *Microchim. Acta* **2020**, *187*. [CrossRef]
100. Malecka, K.; Pankratov, D.; Ferapontova, E.E. Femtomolar electroanalysis of a breast cancer biomarker HER-2/neu protein in human serum by the cellulase-linked sandwich assay on magnetic beads. *Anal. Chim. Acta* **2019**, *1077*, 140–149. [CrossRef]
101. Chen, D.; Wang, D.; Hu, X.; Long, G.; Zhang, Y.; Zhou, L. A DNA nanostructured biosensor for electrochemical analysis of HER2 using bioconjugate of GNR@Pd SSs—Apt—HRP. *Sens. Actuators B Chem.* **2019**, *296*, 126650. [CrossRef]
102. Lah, Z.M.A.N.H.; Ahmad, S.A.A.; Zaini, M.S.; Kamarudin, M.A. An Electrochemical Sandwich Immunosensor for the Detection of HER2 using Antibody-Conjugated PbS Quantum Dot as a label. *J. Pharm. Biomed. Anal.* **2019**, *174*, 608–617. [CrossRef]
103. Hartati, Y.W.; Letelay, L.K.; Gaffar, S.; Wyantuti, S.; Bahti, H.H. Cerium oxide-monoclonal antibody bioconjugate for electrochemical immunosensing of HER2 as a breast cancer biomarker. *Sens. BioSens. Res.* **2020**, *27*, 100316. [CrossRef]
104. Xiang, W.; Lv, Q.; Shi, H.; Xie, B.; Gao, L. Aptamer-based biosensor for detecting carcinoembryonic antigen. *Talanta* **2020**, *214*, 120716. [CrossRef] [PubMed]
105. Dalila, R.N.; Arshad, M.K.M.; Gopinath, S.C.B.; Norhaimi, W.M.W.; Fathil, M.F.M. Current and future envision on developing biosensors aided by 2D molybdenum disulfide (MoS2) productions. *Biosens. Bioelectron.* **2019**, *132*, 248–264. [CrossRef] [PubMed]
106. Wang, Y.-L.; Cao, J.-T.; Chen, Y.-H.; Liu, Y.-M. A label-free electrochemiluminescence aptasensor for carcinoembryonic antigen detection based on electrodeposited ZnS–CdS on MoS2 decorated electrode. *Anal. Methods* **2016**, *8*, 5242–5247. [CrossRef]
107. Paimard, G.; Shahlaei, M.; Moradipour, P.; Akbari, H.; Jafari, M.; Arkan, E. An Impedimetric Immunosensor modified with electrospun core-shell nanofibers for determination of the carcinoma embryonic antigen. *Sens. Actuators B Chem.* **2020**, *311*, 127928. [CrossRef]
108. Wang, Y.; Wang, Y.; Wu, D.; Ma, H.; Zhang, Y.; Fan, D.; Pang, X.; Du, B.; Wei, Q. Label-free electrochemical immunosensor based on flower-like Ag/MoS2/rGO nanocomposites for ultrasensitive detection of carcinoembryonic antigen. *Sens. Actuators B Chem.* **2018**, *255*, 125–132. [CrossRef]

109. Su, S.; Han, X.; Lu, Z.; Liu, W.; Zhu, D.; Chao, J.; Fan, C.; Wang, L.; Song, S.; Weng, L.; et al. Facile Synthesis of a MoS2–Prussian Blue Nanocube Nanohybrid-Based Electrochemical Sensing Platform for Hydrogen Peroxide and Carcinoembryonic Antigen Detection. *ACS Appl. Mater. Interfaces* **2017**, *9*, 12773–12781. [CrossRef]
110. Lee, S.X.; Lim, H.N.; Ibrahim, I.; Jamil, A.; Pandikumar, A.; Huang, N.M. Horseradish peroxidase-labeled silver/reduced graphene oxide thin film-modified screen-printed electrode for detection of carcinoembryonic antigen. *Biosens. Bioelectron.* **2017**, *89*, 673–680. [CrossRef]
111. Rizwan, M.; Elma, S.; Lim, S.A.; Ahmed, M.U. AuNPs/CNOs/SWCNTs/chitosan-nanocomposite modified electrochemical sensor for the label-free detection of carcinoembryonic antigen. *Biosens. Bioelectron.* **2018**, *107*, 211–217. [CrossRef]
112. Wang, J.; Hui, N. Zwitterionic poly(carboxybetaine) functionalized conducting polymer polyaniline nanowires for the electrochemical detection of carcinoembryonic antigen in undiluted blood serum. *Bioelectrochemistry* **2019**, *125*, 90–96. [CrossRef]
113. Kumar, S.; Lei, Y.; Alshareef, N.H.; Quevedo-Lopez, M.A.; Salama, K.N. Biofunctionalized two-dimensional Ti3C2 MXenes for ultrasensitive detection of cancer biomarker. *Biosens. Bioelectron.* **2018**, *121*, 243–249. [CrossRef] [PubMed]
114. Yang, Y.; Jiang, M.; Cao, K.; Wu, M.; Zhao, C.; Li, H.; Hong, C. An electrochemical immunosensor for CEA detection based on Au-Ag/rGO@ PDA nanocomposites as integrated double signal amplification strategy. *Microchem. J.* **2019**, *151*, 104223. [CrossRef]
115. Gu, X.; She, Z.; Ma, T.; Tian, S.; Kraatz, H.-B. Electrochemical detection of carcinoembryonic antigen. *Biosens. Bioelectron.* **2018**, *102*, 610–616. [CrossRef] [PubMed]
116. Wei, Y.; Ma, H.; Ren, X.; Ding, C.; Wang, H.; Sun, X.; Du, B.; Zhang, Y.; Wei, Q. A dual-signaling electrochemical ratiometric method for sensitive detection of carcinoembryonic antigen based on Au-Cu2S-CuS/graphene and Au-CeO2 supported toluidine blue complex. *Sens. Actuators B Chem.* **2018**, *256*, 504–511. [CrossRef]
117. Li, Y.; Zhang, Y.; Li, F.; Li, M.; Chen, L.; Dong, Y.; Wei, Q. Sandwich-type amperometric immunosensor using functionalized magnetic graphene loaded gold and silver core-shell nanocomposites for the detection of Carcinoembryonic antigen. *J. Electroanal. Chem.* **2017**, *795*, 1–9. [CrossRef]
118. Wu, D.; Ma, H.; Zhang, Y.; Jia, H.; Yan, T.; Wei, Q. Corallite-like Magnetic Fe3O4@MnO2@Pt Nanocomposites as Multiple Signal Amplifiers for the Detection of Carcinoembryonic Antigen. *ACS Appl. Mater. Interfaces* **2015**, *7*, 18786–18793. [CrossRef]
119. Li, J.; Liu, J.; Bi, Y.; Sun, M.; Bai, J.; Zhou, M. Ultrasensitive electrochemiluminescence biosensing platform for miRNA-21 and MUC1 detection based on dual catalytic hairpin assembly. *Anal. Chim. Acta* **2020**, *1105*, 87–94. [CrossRef]
120. Jeong, S.; Park, M.-J.; Song, W.; Kim, H.-S. Current immunoassay methods and their applications to clinically used biomarkers of breast cancer. *Clin. Biochem.* **2020**, *78*, 43–57. [CrossRef]
121. Alarfaj, N.A.; El-Tohamy, M.F.; Oraby, H. New label-free ultrasensitive electrochemical immunosensor-based Au/MoS2/rGO nanocomposites for CA 27–29 breast cancer antigen detection. *New J. Chem.* **2018**, *42*, 11046–11053. [CrossRef]
122. Roberts, A.; Tripathi, P.P.; Gandhi, S. Graphene nanosheets as an electric mediator for ultrafast sensing of urokinase plasminogen activator receptor-A biomarker of cancer. *Biosens. Bioelectron.* **2019**, *141*, 111398. [CrossRef]
123. Jilani, T.N.; Siddiqui, A.H. Tissue Plasminogen Activator. In *StatPearls*; StatPearls Publishing Copyright ©: Treasure Island, FL, USA, 2020; pp. 159–170.
124. Saify Nabiabad, H.; Piri, K.; Kafrashi, F.; Afkhami, A.; Madrakian, T. Fabrication of an immunosensor for early and ultrasensitive determination of human tissue plasminogen activator (tPA) in myocardial infraction and breast cancer patients. *Anal. Bioanal. Chem.* **2018**, *410*, 3683–3691. [CrossRef] [PubMed]
125. Vajhadin, F.; Ahadian, S.; Travas-Sejdic, J.; Lee, J.; Mazloum-Ardakani, M.; Salvador, J.; Aninwene, G.E., II; Bandaru, P.; Sun, W.; Khademhossieni, A. Electrochemical cytosensors for detection of breast cancer cells. *Biosens. Bioelectron.* **2019**, *151*, 111984. [CrossRef]
126. Lee, A.V.; Oesterreich, S.; Davidson, N.E. MCF-7 Cells—Changing the Course of Breast Cancer Research and Care for 45 Years. *J. Natl. Cancer Inst.* **2015**, *107*. [CrossRef] [PubMed]
127. Comşa, Ş.; Cîmpean, A.M.; Raica, M. The Story of MCF-7 Breast Cancer Cell Line: 40 years of Experience in Research. *Anticancer Res.* **2015**, *35*, 3147–3154. [PubMed]

128. Gurudatt, N.G.; Chung, S.; Kim, J.-M.; Kim, M.-H.; Jung, D.-K.; Han, J.-Y.; Shim, Y.-B. Separation detection of different circulating tumor cells in the blood using an electrochemical microfluidic channel modified with a lipid-bonded conducting polymer. *Biosens. Bioelectron.* **2019**, *146*, 111746. [CrossRef] [PubMed]
129. Ghassemi, P.; Ren, X.; Foster, B.M.; Kerr, B.A.; Agah, M. Post-enrichment circulating tumor cell detection and enumeration via deformability impedance cytometry. *Biosens. Bioelectron.* **2020**, *150*, 111868. [CrossRef] [PubMed]
130. Liu, P.; Wang, L.; Zhao, K.; Liu, Z.; Cao, H.; Ye, S.; Liang, G. High luminous efficiency Au@CDs for sensitive and label-free electrochemiluminescent detection of circulating tumor cells in serum. *Sens. Actuators B Chem.* **2020**, *316*, 128131. [CrossRef]
131. Tian, L.; Qi, J.; Qian, K.; Oderinde, O.; Liu, Q.; Yao, C.; Song, W.; Wang, Y. Copper (II) oxide nanozyme based electrochemical cytosensor for high sensitive detection of circulating tumor cells in breast cancer. *J. Electroanal. Chem.* **2018**, *812*, 1–9. [CrossRef]
132. Hasanzadeh, M.; Razmi, N.; Mokhtarzadeh, A.; Shadjou, N.; Mahboob, S. Aptamer based assay of plated-derived grow factor in unprocessed human plasma sample and MCF-7 breast cancer cell lysates using gold nanoparticle supported alpha-cyclodextrin. *Int. J. Biol. Macromol.* **2018**, *108*, 69–80. [CrossRef]
133. Yang, Y.; Fu, Y.; Su, H.; Mao, L.; Chen, M. Sensitive detection of MCF-7 human breast cancer cells by using a novel DNA-labeled sandwich electrochemical biosensor. *Biosens. Bioelectron.* **2018**, *122*, 175–182. [CrossRef]
134. Wang, K.; He, M.-Q.; Zhai, F.-H.; He, R.-H.; Yu, Y.-L. A novel electrochemical biosensor based on polyadenine modified aptamer for label-free and ultrasensitive detection of human breast cancer cells. *Talanta* **2017**, *166*, 87–92. [CrossRef] [PubMed]
135. Mohammadniaei, M.; Yoon, J.; Lee, T.; Bharate, B.G.; Jo, J.; Lee, D.; Choi, J.-W. Electrochemical Biosensor Composed of Silver Ion-Mediated dsDNA on Au-Encapsulated Bi2Se3 Nanoparticles for the Detection of H2O2 Released from Breast Cancer Cells. *Small* **2018**, *14*, 1703970. [CrossRef] [PubMed]
136. Dong, W.; Ren, Y.; Bai, Z.; Yang, Y.; Wang, Z.; Zhang, C.; Chen, Q. Trimetallic AuPtPd nanocomposites platform on graphene: Applied to electrochemical detection and breast cancer diagnosis. *Talanta* **2018**, *189*, 79–85. [CrossRef] [PubMed]
137. Luo, J.; Liang, D.; Li, X.; Deng, L.; Wang, Z.; Yang, M. Aptamer-based photoelectrochemical assay for the determination of MCF-7. *Microchim. Acta* **2020**, *187*. [CrossRef] [PubMed]
138. Safavipour, M.; Kharaziha, M.; Amjadi, E.; Karimzadeh, F.; Allafchian, A. TiO2 nanotubes/reduced GO nanoparticles for sensitive detection of breast cancer cells and photothermal performance. *Talanta* **2020**, *208*, 120369. [CrossRef]
139. Akhtartavan, S.; Karimi, M.; Sattarahmady, N.; Heli, H. An electrochemical signal-on apta-cyto-sensor for quantitation of circulating human MDA-MB-231 breast cancer cells by transduction of electro-deposited non-spherical nanoparticles of gold. *J. Pharm. Biomed. Anal.* **2020**, *178*, 112948. [CrossRef] [PubMed]
140. Al-Hajj, M.; Wicha, M.S.; Benito-Hernandez, A.; Morrison, S.J.; Clarke, M.F. Prospective identification of tumorigenic breast cancer cells. *Proc. Natl. Acad. Sci. USA* **2003**, *100*, 3983–3988. [CrossRef]
141. Tang, Y.; Dai, Y.; Huang, X.; Li, L.; Han, B.; Cao, Y.; Zhao, J. Self-assembling peptide-based multifunctional nanofibers for electrochemical identification of breast cancer stem-like cells. *Anal. Chem.* **2019**, *91*, 7531–7537. [CrossRef]
142. Kilic, T.; Valinhas, A.T.D.S.; Wall, I.; Renaud, P.; Carrara, S. Label-free detection of hypoxia-induced extracellular vesicle secretion from MCF-7 cells. *Sci. Rep.* **2018**, *8*, 9402. [CrossRef] [PubMed]
143. An, Y.; Li, R.; Zhang, F.; He, P. Magneto-Mediated Electrochemical Sensor for Simultaneous Analysis of Breast Cancer Exosomal Proteins. *Anal. Chem.* **2020**, *92*, 5404–5410. [CrossRef] [PubMed]
144. Moura, S.L.; Martín, C.G.; Martí, M.; Pividori, M.I. Electrochemical immunosensing of nanovesicles as biomarkers for breast cancer. *Biosens. Bioelectron.* **2020**, *150*, 111882. [CrossRef] [PubMed]
145. Luo, L.; Wang, L.; Zeng, L.; Wang, Y.; Weng, Y.; Liao, Y.; Chen, T.; Xia, Y.; Zhang, J.; Chen, J. A ratiometric electrochemical DNA biosensor for detection of exosomal MicroRNA. *Talanta* **2020**, *207*, 120298. [CrossRef] [PubMed]

Permissions

All chapters in this book were first published by MDPI; hereby published with permission under the Creative Commons Attribution License or equivalent. Every chapter published in this book has been scrutinized by our experts. Their significance has been extensively debated. The topics covered herein carry significant findings which will fuel the growth of the discipline. They may even be implemented as practical applications or may be referred to as a beginning point for another development.

The contributors of this book come from diverse backgrounds, making this book a truly international effort. This book will bring forth new frontiers with its revolutionizing research information and detailed analysis of the nascent developments around the world.

We would like to thank all the contributing authors for lending their expertise to make the book truly unique. They have played a crucial role in the development of this book. Without their invaluable contributions this book wouldn't have been possible. They have made vital efforts to compile up to date information on the varied aspects of this subject to make this book a valuable addition to the collection of many professionals and students.

This book was conceptualized with the vision of imparting up-to-date information and advanced data in this field. To ensure the same, a matchless editorial board was set up. Every individual on the board went through rigorous rounds of assessment to prove their worth. After which they invested a large part of their time researching and compiling the most relevant data for our readers.

The editorial board has been involved in producing this book since its inception. They have spent rigorous hours researching and exploring the diverse topics which have resulted in the successful publishing of this book. They have passed on their knowledge of decades through this book. To expedite this challenging task, the publisher supported the team at every step. A small team of assistant editors was also appointed to further simplify the editing procedure and attain best results for the readers.

Apart from the editorial board, the designing team has also invested a significant amount of their time in understanding the subject and creating the most relevant covers. They scrutinized every image to scout for the most suitable representation of the subject and create an appropriate cover for the book.

The publishing team has been an ardent support to the editorial, designing and production team. Their endless efforts to recruit the best for this project, has resulted in the accomplishment of this book. They are a veteran in the field of academics and their pool of knowledge is as vast as their experience in printing. Their expertise and guidance has proved useful at every step. Their uncompromising quality standards have made this book an exceptional effort. Their encouragement from time to time has been an inspiration for everyone.

The publisher and the editorial board hope that this book will prove to be a valuable piece of knowledge for researchers, students, practitioners and scholars across the globe.

List of Contributors

Shipra Suman, Fawnizu Azmadi Hussin and Aamir Saeed Malik
Center for Intelligent Signal & Imaging Research, Universiti Teknologi PETRONAS, Seri Iskandar 32610, Malaysia

Shiaw Hooi Ho, Ida Hilmi, Alex Hwong-Ruey Leow and Khean-Lee Goh
Department of Medicine, University of Malaya Medical Center, Kuala Lumpur 50603, Malaysia

Penghui Fan, Yilin Song, Shengwei Xu, Yuchuan Dai, Yiding Wang, Botao Lu, Jingyu Xie, Hao Wang and Xinxia Cai
Aerospace Information Research Institute, Chinese Academy of Sciences, Beijing 100190, China
University of the Chinese Academy of Sciences, Beijing 100049, China

Lucia Sarcina
Dipartimento di Chimica, Università degli Studi di Bari Aldo Moro, 70125 Bari, Italy

Luisa Torsi
Dipartimento di Chimica, Università degli Studi di Bari Aldo Moro, 70125 Bari, Italy
CSGI (Centre for Colloid and Surface Science), Department of Chemistry, 70125 Bari, Italy
The Faculty of Science and Engineering, Åbo Akademi University, FI-20500 Turku, Finland

Rosaria Anna Picca and Kyriaki Manoli
Dipartimento di Chimica, Università degli Studi di Bari Aldo Moro, 70125 Bari, Italy
2SGI (Centre for Colloid and Surface Science), Department of Chemistry, 70125 Bari, Italy

Eleonora Macchia
The Faculty of Science and Engineering, Åbo Akademi University, FI-20500 Turku, Finland

Marco Bassoli, Valentina Bianchi and Ilaria De Munari
Department of Engineering and Architecture, University of Parma, Parco Area delle Scienze, 181/A, 43124 Parma, Italy

Babagana Modu, Yang Lan and Savas Konur
School of Electrical Engineering and Computer Science, University of Bradford, Bradford BD7 1DP, UK

Nereida Polovina
Manchester Metropolitan University Business School, Manchester Metropolitan University, Manchester M15 6BH, UK

A. Taufiq Asyhari
Centre for Electronic Warfare, Information and Cyber, Cranfield University, Shrivenham SN6 8LA, UK

Yonghong Peng
Faculty of Computer Science, University of Sunderland, St Peters Campus, Sunderland SR6 0DD, UK

Junsang Yuh
R&D Center, Begas, Seoul 06179, Korea
School of Industrial Management Engineering, Korea University, Seoul 02841, Korea

Seokhyun Chung and Taesu Cheong
School of Industrial Management Engineering, Korea University, Seoul 02841, Korea

Chiara Calamanti, Sara Moccia, Lucia Migliorelli, Marina Paolanti and Emanuele Frontoni
Department of Information Engineering, Universitá Politecnica delle Marche, 60121 Ancona, Italy

Emanuele Torti, Giordana Florimbi, Francesca Castelli and Francesco Leporati
Department of Electrical, Computer and Biomedical Engineering, University of Pavia, I-27100 Pavia, Italy

Samuel Ortega, Himar Fabelo, Gustavo Marrero Callicó and Margarita Marrero-Martin
Institute for Applied Microelectronics (IUMA), University of Las Palmas de Gran Canaria (ULPGC), 35017 Las Palmas de Gran Canaria, Spain

Jinhee Lee, Ellie D. Wilson and Koji Sode
Joint Department of Biomedical Engineering, The University of North Carolina at Chapel Hill and North Carolina State University, Chapel Hill, NC 27599, USA

Atsuro Tatsumi, Kaori Tsukakoshi, Koichi Abe and Kazunori Ikebukuro
Department of Biotechnology and Life Science, Graduate School of Engineering, Tokyo University of Agriculture and Technology, 2-24-16 Naka-cho, Koganei, Tokyo 184-8588, Japan

Valentina Bianchi, Andrea Boni and Ilaria De Munari
Department of Engineering and Architecture, University of Parma, 43124 Parma, Italy

Monica Mattarozzi, Marco Giannetto and Maria Careri
Department of Chemistry, Life Sciences and Environmental Sustainability, University of Parma, 43124 Parma, Italy

Zahid Mahmood, Huansheng Ning and Xuanxia Yao
School of Computer and Communication Engineering University of Science and Technology, Beijing (USTB), Beijing 10008, China

Ata Ullah
Department of Computer Science, National University of Modern Languages, Islamabad 44000, Pakistan

Yuan-Kai Wang
Graduate Institute of Applied Science and Engineering, Fu Jen Catholic University, New Taipei 24205, Taiwan Electrical Engineering, Fu Jen Catholic University, New Taipei 24205, Taiwan

Hung-Yu Chen and Jian-Ru Chen
Graduate Institute of Applied Science and Engineering, Fu Jen Catholic University, New Taipei 24205, Taiwan

Stefano Ricci and Valentino Meacci
Information Engineering Department (DINFO), University of Florence, Florence 50139, Italy

Xianghan Zheng and Lingting Wu
College of Mathematics and Computer Science, Fuzhou University, Fuzhou 350116, China
Fujian Key Laboratory of Network Computing and Intelligent Information Processing, Fuzhou 350116, China

Shaozhen Ye
College of Mathematics and Computer Science, Fuzhou University, Fuzhou 350116, China

Riqing Chen
College of Computer and Information, Fujian Agriculture and Forestry University, Fuzhou 350002, China

Veronika Gajdosova, Lenka Lorencova and Jan Tkac
Institute of Chemistry, Slovak Academy of Sciences, Dubravska cesta 9, 845 38 Bratislava, Slovakia

Peter Kasak
Center for Advanced Materials, Qatar University, Doha 2713, Qatar

Index

www.ingramcontent.com/pod-product-compliance
Lightning Source LLC
LaVergne TN
LVHW081014210926
848485LV00004B/862